Introduction *to* Surgery

Introduction *to* Surgery

THIRD EDITION

DAVID H. LEVIEN, M.D., F.A.C.S.
Director, Department of Surgery
Episcopal Hospital
Clinical Professor of Surgery
Jefferson Medical College and Thomas Jefferson University
Philadelphia, Pennsylvania

W.B. SAUNDERS COMPANY
A Division of Harcourt Brace & Company
Philadelphia London Toronto Montreal Sydney Tokyo

W.B. SAUNDERS COMPANY
A Division of Harcourt Brace & Company

The Curtis Center
Independence Square West
Philadelphia, Pennsylvania 19106

Library of Congress Cataloging-in-Publication Data

Levien, David H.

Introduction to surgery / David H. Levien.—3rd ed.

p.   cm.

Includes index.

ISBN 0–7216–7652–9

1. Surgery. [DNLM: 1. Surgery.   WO 100L664i 1999]

RD31.L49 1999   617—dc21

DNLM/DLC   98–36803

INTRODUCTION TO SURGERY   ISBN 0–7216–7652–9

Printed in the United States of America.

Last digit is the print number: 9   8   7   6   5   4   3   2   1

Foreword to the Third Edition

The most important task of medical educators is to teach and prepare the next generation of physicians to become practitioners in the field of medicine and teachers of future generations of medical students, residents, and the lay public. Each specialty of medicine must provide medical students with a sufficient background of didactic information and clinical experience that the student can then use in making career decisions as well as in caring for future patients. The purpose of the surgical clerkships is not to train medical students to become surgeons, but rather to provide a broad base of information and experience in the pathophysiology of diseases treated by surgeons that can be broadly applied by the student.

One challenge facing authors of surgical textbooks is to provide sufficient information that the student can then apply to common clinical situations encountered in the surgical rotations. In the preceding editions of *Introduction to Surgery*, Dr. David Levien has given students and junior-level general surgical residents an ideal combination of knowledge and case-oriented and problem-oriented case presentations. This unique format has provided an excellent, well-written text that focuses on the basic principles and management of patients with common surgical problems. This approach has proven popular with students as well as with first- and second-year surgical residents. The third edition of *Introduction to Surgery* retains this unique format and has been updated to reflect the rapid changes occurring in surgery, especially the advances that have been made in the care of patients with biliary and breast disease. Dr. Levien places emphasis on how the student can use this book as a baseline. The text's well-written format allows it to be read quickly at the beginning of the surgical rotations, and the text can then be used as a reference throughout the surgical rotation. The illustrations are also very clearly presented and aid the students in interpreting the data and cases provided.

The third edition of *Introduction to Surgery* continues to be exactly as promised in the title. Consistent with the first two editions, it is written for use by students and beginning residents. This edition reflects the long history and interest that Dr. Levien has had in the education of students and residents. I strongly urge you to read this edition of *Introduction to Surgery* as it will provide a strong foundation for someone starting the clinical rotation in surgery.

STUART MYERS, M.D., FACS
Professor and Chairman
Department of Surgery
Temple University School of Medicine
Philadelphia, Pennsylvania

Foreword to the Second Edition

Where does one start? How do you introduce bright and inquisitive students and trainees to a discipline that they have not been previously exposed to? How do you provide information and the building blocks for learning that are so essential for all physicians, regardless of their career goals, in an area that is as large and encompassing as general surgery? These are the questions that we all ask ourselves as we attempt to develop and structure a curriculum and meaningful educational experience for our teaching programs. In this, the second edition of "Introduction to Surgery," Dr. David Levien has met these challenges and has provided an outstanding, straightforward, and well-written text that focuses on the basic principles and management of patients with surgical problems.

In recent years, there has been an increasing emphasis not on what we teach but rather how we teach it, and the most effective way of communicating information. The concept of a clinically oriented book that is also problem- and case-oriented is refreshing and represents a novel but contemporary approach to surgical education. The book starts out by describing how one takes a history and physical examination; it progresses through the assessment of specific clinical problems and concludes with wonderfully apt descriptions of the various stages and steps that individuals would follow in order to complete their surgical education and training. The book is easy to read and the text is greatly enhanced by the illustrations. Unlike many texts, this book is not cluttered with data and numbers. Dr. Levien has given his readers only what they need to know.

Many books claim to be things that they are not. *Introduction to Surgery* is exactly what its title indicates. This book is intended for students and junior housestaff who are beginning their surgical experience. It is the perfect way to begin one's education and journey into the discipline that we call surgery. I invite you to read through this book and learn about a fascinating area in the biological sciences, as told by a master educator.

JOEL J. ROSLYN, M.D.
Alma Dea Morani Professor and Chairman
Department of Surgery
The Medical College of Pennsylvania
Philadelphia, Pennsylvania

Foreword to the First Edition

Other titles come to mind for this concise and lucid introduction to surgery—"How to Get an A in Surgery" or "How to Survive the Pyramid System." Having been a teacher of medical students and surgical residents for the past 27 years, and as Chairman of the Department in which Dr. Levien is one of our best surgical education coordinators, I can state that reading this book is the perfect way to begin a surgical clerkship or internship. It is not the sort of textbook that should be studied; rather, it should be read from cover to cover, preferably at one sitting, so that the entire broad surgical experience can be anticipated and appreciated.

The purpose of a surgical clerkship is not to prepare medical students to become surgeons, because few of them have that intention. The surgical clerkship should be considered a clinical laboratory in which physiology-in-action and pathology-in-situ can be demonstrated to the student in a manner that remains vividly in the memory for many years. The format of Dr. Levien's book with pertinent examples of clinical problems and concise case discussions is the perfect way to prepare a student for the demanding tasks of surgery. The many practical details regarding the writing of orders and the efficient diagnostic work-up reflect the current state of the art in surgery. The illustrations correlate well with the textual material and are so succinct and clear that they can be used by themselves as a quick review of the field.

In reading this book, it is easy to see why Dr. Levien's students and residents do so well. The clear explanations of pertinent detail and the rational presentation of time-honored principles as well as the new and the modern provide a good foundation for what should be a rewarding and exciting experience for someone starting a clinical rotation in surgery.

LOUIS R. M. DEL GUERCIO, M.D.
Professor and Chairman
Department of Surgery
New York Medical College
Valhalla, New York

Preface

I have written this book in order to provide an introduction to surgery. It is my hope that it will be read easily and quickly and will provide a modicum of enjoyment to the reader. It is intended to provide a framework upon which medical students or beginning residents can build and to provide them with a sense of confidence when they step onto the surgical wards. It should provide a common ground with which they can converse with their mentors and should generally increase the enjoyment of the surgical rotation. The case histories, which are composites, should very quickly provide the student with a sense of familiarity with the cases to be encountered on a busy surgical service.

DAVID H. LEVIEN, M.D.

Acknowledgments

I would like to thank Drs. H. Brownell Wheeler, William J. McCann, Louis R. M. Del Guercio, Joel Roslyn, Francis Rosato, and Stuart Myers for their leadership in surgical education. Drs. Ajit Sachdeva and Philip Wolfson deserve great praise for their leadership role in ensuring that medical student education in surgery receives proper emphasis.

I would like to thank my wife, Merril, and my children, Michael, Billy, and Rachel, for allowing me the time to write this book.

It is fitting to acknowledge the surgical residents at Episcopal Hospital and the many medical students who provide constant stimulation and for whom this book is written.

I would like to thank the staff at the W.B. Saunders Company for their assistance, including Lisette Bralow, Editor-in-Chief, Medical Books, and Natalie Ware, Production Manager. As always, I have greatly enjoyed working with the highly accomplished staff at the W.B. Saunders Company.

I would also like to thank Toni Riley, Elaine Kradzinski, and Mary Lee Dougherty for their hard work.

DAVID H. LEVIEN, M.D.

Contents

Abbreviations

ABG	arterial blood gases
ARDS	adult respiratory distress syndrome
bid	bis in die (twice a day)
BP	blood pressure
BUN	blood urea nitrogen
CBC	complete blood count
cc	cubic centimeter
CCU	coronary care unit
cm	centimeter
CMF	cyclophosphamide, methotrexate, 5-fluorouracil
CPAP	continuous positive airway pressure
CT	computed tomography
CVA	cerebrovascular accident
CVP	central venous pressure
D/C	discontinue
DDAVP	desmopressin
DIC	diffuse intravascular coagulation
dL	deciliter
D5W	5% dextrose in water
D5-½NS	5% dextrose in one half normal saline
D5NS	5% dextrose in normal saline
D50W	50% dextrose in water
DSA	digital subtraction angiography
DTR	deep tendon reflex
DVT	deep vein thrombosis
Dx	diagnosis
EBL	estimated blood loss
ECG	electrocardiogram
EMT	emergency medical technician
ER	estrogen receptor
ERCP	endoscopic retrograde pancreatocholangiography
FIo_2	fractional inspired oxygen
FIP	forced inspiratory pressure
GI	gastrointestinal
g	gram
Hct	hematocrit

Hg	mercury
HR	heart rate
ICU	intensive care unit
IM	intramuscular
IMV	intermittent mandatory ventilation
IPG	impedance plethysmography
IV	intravenous
IVP	intravenous pyelography
JVD	jugular venous distention
kg	kilogram
L	liter
LDH	lactate dehydrogenase
MAST	military antishock trousers
μg	microgram
mEq	milliequivalent
mg	milligram
mL	milliliter
mm	millimeter
MRI	magnetic resonance imaging
NG	nasogastric
NPO	nothing by mouth
NS	normal saline
PaO_2	partial pressure of oxygen in arterial blood
$PaCO_2$	partial pressure of carbon dioxide in arterial blood
PEEP	positive end-expiratory pressure
PND	paroxysmal nocturnal dyspnea
PO	per os (by mouth)
PRN	as needed
PT	prothrombin time
PTC	percutaneous transhepatic cholangiography
PTT	partial thromboplastin time
PVC	premature ventricular contractions
q	quaque (every)
qhs	every evening
qid	quarter in die (4 times a day)
q2h	every 2 hours
RBC	red blood cells
RUQ	right upper quadrant
SGPT	serum glutamate pyruvate transaminase
SOAP	*s*ubjective and *o*bjective data, *a*ssessment, and *p*lan (components of a progress note)
TIA	transient ischemic attack
TPN	total parenteral nutrition
US	ultrasonography
WBC	white blood cells
WNL	within normal limits

1

Introduction

This book is written to introduce students and first-year residents to general surgery. It is easily read over the course of a few days and should allow the reader to get a "running start" on surgical rotations. This book makes no attempt to be encyclopedic, but, the reader who finishes it will have a foundation for starting surgical training and will better understand the action that will quickly follow.

Surgery and medicine are two inextricably interwoven disciplines; a good surgeon must be thoroughly familiar with medicine. Any given disease may best be treated with medical intervention during one stage and with surgery at another. In most instances, practitioners of medicine and surgery attempt to restore the patient to homeostasis by creating a "second lesion" to counterbalance the first. An operation often affects an alteration in the patient's physiologic state by altering structure.

It is my conviction that assimilation of the information contained in this book will enable readers to establish a relationship with their mentors on a foundation of shared principles. The development of a surgeon is a much more protracted process: It probably lasts a lifetime. In this work, I aspire to foster a good beginning.

2

The History and Physical Examination

The history and physical examination are among the most basic aspects of medicine, and even in this era of advanced technology they are the cornerstones of diagnosis. The lingo of computer scientists has found its way into medicine, and one hears talk of acquiring a "data base" from which to make a diagnosis. This, in fact, is exactly what one must do. Careful acquisition of this information allows for accurate assessment and a rational plan of management.

The medical history consists of several elements: a *chief complaint, history of present illness, medical history, review of systems, family history,* and *social history.* It has been tradition in many institutions that, while medical students are assigned to medical clerkship, they faithfully obtain from each patient an encyclopedic history and dutifully record it on a form. However, during this assignment to the surgical service, they often cut many corners, so as to spend more time in the operating room or to participate in ward procedures. In point of fact, with a little practice, a complete and relevant history can be obtained quite quickly, and it allows surgical clerks to be productive without sacrificing accuracy or completeness.

A confident demeanor on the part of surgical clerks or junior house officers helps to facilitate the interview. Students need not feel superfluous, since their presence on the surgical service contributes a great deal. First, the inquiring nature of students, by necessity, keeps the intellectual atmosphere at a high pitch on the involved service. Second, it is not uncommon for students to discover, during the interview or examination, a historical fact or a physical finding that has been overlooked by senior clinicians. Third, the attendings and senior residents did not attain their abilities *de novo:* they developed them as students and junior house staff. Fourth, students owe it to their future patients to be intimately involved with all activities of patient care, within the limits set by the faculty. Most patients understand this and accept it.

A significant percentage of diagnoses can be made on the basis of history alone; this speaks to the importance of this phase of the diagnostic workup. Many patients have some insight into the pathogenesis of their problem, and allowing them to talk for a few minutes, offering them little in the way of direction, can be productive and can provide psychological catharsis. They may supply much useful information in this fashion, but, even if they do not, their need to tell their story will have been fulfilled, and, thus relieved, they may better respond to the questions the examiner believes are relevant.

COMPONENTS OF THE HISTORY

The *chief complaint* (CC) is the symptom that prompts the patient to seek medical attention. When adding this to the form it is usually couched in the patient's own words, as in the statement, "This 51-year-old man is being admitted with the chief complaint of vomiting blood." On many efficient surgical services, however, often the diagnosis has been established in the surgeon's office or in the clinic. In this situation a chief complaint might read, "This 49-year-old man with a known right inguinal hernia is to undergo elective right inguinal herniorrhaphy as an outpatient next week." It could have been stated that he presented with a chief complaint of a bulge in his right groin, but this seems needlessly cryptic. Although in many instance, it is better to use the patient's own words, there are times when it is preferable merely to describe the purpose of admission.

The *history of present illness* (HPI) should begin at the earliest event that pertains to the disease entity for which the patient is being admitted. To formulate the HPI intelligently, one often must make a judgment on the disease entity responsible for the present admission, so that one can decide which events are relevant. Types of events that must be catalogued include previous treatment (as an outpatient or in hospital) and onset of various symptoms. The patient and the family can often provide information about these factors, but the medical record (the "old chart") should be consulted if possible. In modern institutions it is often easier to order computed tomography (CT) or angiography than to obtain an old chart that well could contain valuable information about previous diagnostic endeavors.

The chief complaint and history of present illness of a patient with upper gastrointestinal bleeding might read something like this:

CASE 2–1

Example of a Chief Complaint and History of Present Illness in a Patient with Upper Gastrointestinal Bleeding

CC: J.M. is a 54-year-old man admitted with a 4-day history of black, tarry stools.

HPI: Nine years before admission, the patient underwent upper GI series because of severe epigastric pain. He was told at that time that he had a duodenal ulcer and was treated with a bland diet and

H2 blockers, with resolution of his symptoms. Other than occasional dyspepsia, he had no further episodes until 1 week before admission, when he began to develop epigastric pain radiating to the back and associated with nausea. In spite of self-administered H2 blockers, the pain became constant. He consulted his family physician, who made arrangements for elective endoscopy. Four days before the scheduled procedure his stools began to turn black and he developed dizziness when he stood up, prompting urgent admission.

The *past medical history* (PMH) follows the history of present illness, and is a necessary part of the subjective data base. The interviewer often relies heavily on information obtained from the patient and family, but this part should include information supplied by the referring physician and, if possible, by the old chart. These facts about associated illnesses are required to ensure good preoperative, intraoperative, and postoperative care to the surgical patient.

The past medical history can be broken down into more specific categories, such as medical illnesses, and can include data on medications and special diets, operations, hospitalizations, and allergies. Special emphasis should be placed on factors that might have some influence on the care to be given in the perioperative period. It is important to include significant *negatives* (e.g., "history negative for heart disease"), as this is the only way that someone reading the form containing the history and data from the physical can be sure that the examiner has asked all the correct questions. I would suggest that questions about bleeding tendencies be asked in the past medical history section rather than in the review of systems, since a bleeding diathesis could significantly affect safe conduct of an operation.

What follows is an example of a chief complaint, history of present illness, and past medical history for a 35-year-old woman admitted for elective cholecystectomy.

CASE 2–2

Example of a Chief Complaint, History of Present Illness, and Past Medical History in a Patient Admitted for Elective Cholecystectomy

CC: J.T. is a 35-year-old woman admitted with a chief complaint of right upper-quadrant abdominal pain.

HPI: During the 3 years before admission the patient has experienced episodes of colicky right upper-quadrant abdominal pain, precipitated by fatty foods, radiating to the right subscapular region and associated with nausea and vomiting. During the 2 months before admission the episodes became more frequent, prompting her to seek medical attention. An ultrasound of the gallbladder ordered by her family physician demonstrated cholelithiasis. An upper GI series was unremarkable. There has been no history of jaundice, dark urine, or clay-colored stools. She is now admitted for elective laparoscopic cholecystectomy this morning.

PMH: There is no history of heart disease, diabetes mellitus, or hypertension. The patient has been taking prednisone, 20 mg daily, for a collagen vascular disease. Her only previous surgery was a bilateral inguinal herniorrhaphy during infancy. There are no known allergies and no bleeding tendencies. She underwent tooth extraction a year before admission, without undue bleeding.

This example demonstrates some principles of history taking. There are several adjectives that should be elicited about pain if the examiner is to acquire the most information available, and they can be remembered by the following aid to learning: **PPQRST A.**

P*recipitating* and p*alliating* factors can give the clinician clues to the cause of the pain. Pain precipitated by hunger or spicy foods may tip off to peptic ulcer disease, especially if food or antacids provide palliation.

The q*uality* of the pain may aid in the diagnosis. The pain of intestinal obstruction is often described as crampy; the pain of a peptic ulcer as gnawing.

R*adiation* of the pain can also provide useful information. The pain of cholecystitis often radiates to the right subscapular region, and pain of urolithiasis (stones in the urinary system) can radiate to the testicles.

S*everity* of the pain is also informative, as is t*iming*. For example, a perforated ulcer often presents as severe pain of sudden onset, whereas pain from other causes may be gradual in onset.

A*ssociated symptoms* may also give clues to the diagnosis. For instance, in a patient with left lower quadrant abdominal pain, increasing constipation over the last 6 months might indicate carcinoma of the sigmoid colon. In the sample case report given, the absence of the associated symptoms of jaundice, dark urine, and clay-colored stools argues against common bile duct obstruction.

Important negatives are noted in the past medical history, and the knowledge that there is no history of heart disease or diabetes helps in patient management in the perioperative period. It is extremely important to know that the patient has been taking steroids within the last year, because the surgeon then realizes that he or she must administer steroids during the perioperative period, to prevent addisonian crisis.

The clinical clerk often forgets the difference between the *past medical history* and the *review of systems.* The former is a chronicle of the patient's medical problems, as diagnosed by the patient's physician, whereas, the latter is a systematic determination of symptoms that might help uncover previously unsuspected disease in a given body system. A patient with no history of diagnosed atherosclerotic cardiovascular disease may tell the admitting house officer that he does develop substernal pain radiating to the left arm when he walks uphill on a cold day.

Although he may have never told his family physician of this, it nevertheless suggests to the admitting house officer that the patient might have ischemic heart disease and that further preoperative evaluation is indicated.

This is an example of a disease entity involving a physiologic system (cardiovascular) that is discovered only on careful review of systems, even though it was not previously suspected and, thus, not to be found in the past medical history. Similarly, orthopnea, dyspnea on exertion, paroxysmal nocturnal dyspnea, and syncope may suggest left ventricular failure. Chronic productive cough may indicate chronic lung disease or carcinoma of the lung. Preoperative pulmonary function–and room air blood gas testing—should be considered; these findings can facilitate postoperative management, as can chest radiographs.

Polydipsia, polyphagia, and polyuria suggest diabetes mellitus, and the astute house officer may be responsible for the diagnosis of this entity when it was not previously suspected. Certainly, changes in bowel habits, such as increasing constipation, constipation alternating with diarrhea, or a history of blood per rectum, arouse suspicion of carcinoma of the colon, and when this is an early incidental finding in a patient admitted for another cause, the clinician has certainly done the patient a service. Men should be asked about frequency, hesitancy, and nocturia, as benign prostatic hypertrophy can be responsible for postoperative urine retention.

Symptoms referable to the central nervous system should be elicited preoperatively, as they can affect the patient's perioperative care and may require intervention in their own right. Examples of such symptoms include seizures, syncope, and any suggestive of transient ischemic attacks (e.g., hemiparesis, aphasia, loss of vision in one eye [amaurosis fugax] lasting less than 24 hours).

Family history may elucidate the health of the patient in question. Many disorders are familial, even if they are not transmitted in direct mendelian fashion. Many such disorders have marked surgical significance, either because they are amenable to surgical intervention or because they influence the course of operations performed for other reasons.

Familial adenomatous polyposis is a lesion that carpets the entire colon with adenomatous polyps, each with a small—but real—malignant potential. Thus, familial adenomatous polyposis requires either subtotal colectomy and ileorectal anastomosis plus very frequent proctoscopic screening of the rectal remnant for cancer, restorative proctocolectomy (ileal pouch–anal anastomosis), or total proctocolectomy and permanent ileostomy, to avoid otherwise inevitable carcinoma of the colon. Although inflammatory bowel disease (Crohn's disease or ulcerative colitis) can affect an isolated individual, there is certainly a familial relationship. Likewise, carcinoma of the breast is many times more likely to occur in a woman whose mother, sisters, or maternal aunts have had breast cancer.

Multiple endocrine neoplasias (MEN) types I and II are fascinating and tend to run in families. Type I consists of the "Ps" (*p*ituitary tumor, *p*ancreatic involvement with a gastrinoma causing Zollinger-Ellison syndrome, and hyper*p*arathyroidism); whereas, type II consists of pheochromocytoma, medullary carcinoma of the thyroid, and hyperparathyroidism. Since medullary carcinoma of the thyroid secretes the tumor marker calcitonin, relatives of patients with MEN II can be screened by calcitonin assay.

Social history, especially that relating to cigarette smoking, alcohol intake, and drug abuse, is exceedingly meaningful because of the vast array of disorders that are referable to these habits. Because a stigma is attached to each, the physician should have established a solid relationship before questioning the patient about smoking or drinking. (This relationship can often be established in a few minutes with a little skill and the right instincts.) The patient must be convinced that the physician is not being judgmental, only concerned; then the patient is likely to answer honestly.

As the history is elicited—by students or physicians—answers to earlier questions allow them to formulate a tentative list of diagnoses from which they can "zero in" on areas to be emphasized during the remainder of the history, physical, and diagnostic testing.

PHYSICAL EXAMINATION

Physical examination remains very important, even in this technologic age. The information gained might obviate more costly and invasive studies. Physical examination might yield findings that are not apparent even with the most sophisticated imaging studies. For instance, a small number of breast cancers are palpable but not visible on mammography. In addition, the "laying on of hands" can help demonstrate to the patient that this is a caring physician.

The conducting of the physical examination is described in many fine books on physical diagnosis. It should be approached as an art, and surgeons can take pride in their ability to discover subtle physical findings. Many classic physical signs are described in the appropriate chapters of this book. The surgical clerk or house officer who encounters these signs in patients should introduce his compatriots to the patient, so that each can learn from this case. Certainly this can be done without sacrificing the dignity of the patient.

Rectal and pelvic examinations are part of any complete history and physical examination. Because of the emotional significance attached to these anatomic areas, students and junior house officers in some centers forego these parts of the examination. When this happens, the patient loses out, because an important part of the physical examination is omitted, and doctors-in-training—perhaps through false modesty—shortchange future patients, who are counting on their experience. The clinician must respect the patient's wishes in this matter, however, and must respect the custom of the institution.

Medical educators no longer place much emphasis on eponyms (a person's name associated, in this case, with a physical finding), but they are fun to learn and they remind clerks to look for certain pertinent physical findings that might be significant. *Battle's sign* is ecchymosis (blue discoloration from blood in the tissues) behind the ear, signifying the presence of a basilar skull fracture. This should be sought in trauma patients. *Cullen's sign,* ecchymosis of the skin around the umbilicus, indicates blood in the peritoneal cavity. *Grey Turner's sign* is ecchymoses at the costovertebral angles secondary bleeding into the retroperitoneum, such as one might see in hemorrhagic pancreatitis, renal contusion, or leaking from an abdominal aortic aneurysm that is temporarily under tamponade. *Homans' sign* is pain in the calf on dorsiflexion of the foot. Although previously it was believed to suggest deep vein thrombosis, it is exceedingly unreliable, since inflammation of any cause in this area provokes this sign. *Kehr's sign* is pain in the left shoulder caused by diaphragmatic irritation from a ruptured spleen. *Rovsing's sign* is pain over *McBurney's point* (in the right lower abdominal quadrant) elicited by palpation of the left lower quadrant, and is believed to suggest acute appendicitis. *Trousseau's sign,* tetany of the hand elicited when the brachial artery is occluded for 3 minutes with a blood pressure cuff, indicates hypocalcemia, which might occur following excision of a parathyroid adenoma.

On the basis of a good history and physical examination, many diseases can be diagnosed without extensive laboratory testing. Even if tests are necessary, the history and physical examination findings usually indicate which tests will be most helpful.

3

Progress Notes: Preoperative, Operative, Postoperative, Daily, and Procedure Notes

Progress notes are written to facilitate continuity of care. Simply stated, they allow another doctor who reads the chart to comprehend quickly what has occurred to date. Accurate note writing is important to good patient care.

Although the medical record has acquired great legal significance in our litigious society, that is a peripheral issue. Progress notes are meant to:

Help physicians organize their thoughts and prepare a plan of action
Orient:
    Consultants who are called upon to give an opinion
    House officers who will assume management of the patient's case at the beginning of a new rotation
    Surgeons or physicians who will care for the patient during a future admission

It has long been recognized that through language people not only communicate but also organize their understanding of the world. Similarly, a physician comprehends a patient's problems and formulates a plan through information recorded in the progress notes. On some services, the problem-oriented record has been adopted. This format, sometimes nicknamed the SOAP format, consists of enumerating the patient's problems and describing a *subjective* and an *objective* data base. Subjective information is that gleaned from the history, including chief complaint, history of present illness, past medical history, family history, social history, and review of systems. Objective data include findings (signs) elicited on physical examination. Laboratory tests and radiologic evaluation are other examples of objective data. The physician then makes an assessment and formulates a plan for each of the patient's problems.

An example of how one might use the problem-oriented record in a 54-year-old man with upper GI bleeding, chronic obstructive lung disease, cirrhosis of the liver, and atherosclerotic heart disease might read like this:

Problem 1: Upper GI Bleeding
Subjective: Coffee-ground emesis, melena, and orthostatic symptoms.
Objective: Blood pressure drops to 80 systolic when head of bed elevated, hemoglobin is 6 g. Endoscopy shows active bleeding from large esophageal varices.
Assessment: Bleeding esophageal varices due to portal hypertension. Hypovolemia.
Plan: Resuscitation with packed red blood cells and fresh-frozen plasma. Endoscopy with possible sclerotherapy or rubber band ligation of varices. Administration of intravenous pitressin or somatostatin. Insertion of a Sengstaken-Blakemore tube if these measures fail to stop bleeding. Other measures to consider include transjugular intrahepatic portasystemic shunt (TIPS), operative portasystemic shunt, and liver transplantation.

Problem 2: Chronic Obstructive Pulmonary Disease
Subjective: Chronic productive cough and dyspnea; 40–pack-year history of cigarette smoking.
Objective: Distant breath sounds. Chest hyperresonant to percussion. Increased AP diameter of the chest. CO_2 retention on arterial blood gases.
Assessment: Severe chronic obstructive pulmonary disease.
Plan: Low-flow oxygen via nasal cannula. Careful monitoring of respiratory rate and blood gases. Intubation may be required. Careful attention to pulmonary toilet.

Problem 3: Liver enlargement
Subjective: Patient gives a history of ingestion of a fifth of bourbon daily.
Objective: The liver is palpable five finger-breadths below the right costal margin. SGPT, alkaline phosphatase, LDH, and total bilirubin are elevated, as is the blood ammonia level. Present are spider angiomas, palmar erythema, caput medusae, gynecomastia, and testicular atrophy.
Assessment: Cirrhosis of the liver.
Plan: Cathartics and enemas to clear the colon of blood. Neomycin or lactulose to prevent hepatic encephalopathy. More branched-chain and less aromatic amino acids in diet.

Problem 4: Chest pain
Subjective: Substernal pain radiating down the left arm, associated with dyspnea and diaphoresis, lasting 3 minutes and relieved by nitroglycerine.
Objective: ST-T wave changes on ECG.
Assessment: Angina pectoris due to atherosclerotic cardiovascular disease and exacerbated by hypovolemia.
Plan: Serial ECGs and cardiac enzymes. Consider insertion of Swan-Ganz catheter and arterial line if patient's condition becomes hemodynamically unstable. Cardiology consultation.

Signed _____

Patients admitted to a surgical service often have a single problem that is to be dealt with on the admission in question. It may be needlessly cumbersome to employ the problem-oriented method just outlined for a healthy, young person who presents for cholecystectomy. In fact, it may be only the extraordinary patient admitted to the surgical service who requires this method. However, as will be shown in Chapter 17, patients in the intensive care unit certainly benefit from such a record. In fact, each daily progress note can take the form of a matrix in which, for each physiologic system, subjective and objective data are catalogued, along with an assessment and plan for maintenance of each system.

Many different types of notes are required to chronicle the patient's admission from beginning to end. The *admitting note* is traditionally written by a more senior house officer and by the attending surgeon. It is more concise than the history and physical, and it is meant to summarize the patient's status and to outline a plan for further diagnosis and treatment. The *chief complaint* and *history of present illness* may be combined in a single paragraph. The *past medical history* as it relates to the present management of the patient's case is described, and only pertinent physical findings are mentioned. *Important lab work is* summarized, and a *brief assessment* and *plan* are outlined. An example of such an admitting note is:

M.H. is a 41-year-old premenopausal woman admitted with carcinoma of the left breast documented by needle biopsy obtained in the office. Both the patient's mother and sister have undergone mastectomy for breast carcinoma. The patient was 31 years of age at the time of her first pregnancy, and she had taken oral contraceptives for 10 years.

PMH: Hypertension controlled by diet; otherwise unremarkable.

On physical examination, there is a 3-cm mobile, hard, nontender mass in the upper outer quadrant of the left breast with a small, hard, left axillary lymph node palpable. No nodes are palpable in the supraclavicular areas, and the liver is not clinically enlarged.

Chest x-ray, bone and liver scans, and alkaline phosphatase are within normal limits.

It is my impression that the patient has stage II carcinoma of the left breast. Alternative treatments have been explained to her. She refuses radiation therapy and wishes to undergo left modified radical mastectomy. Estrogen and progesterone receptors will be obtained, and administration of adjuvant chemotherapy will be considered.

If the patient is in the hospital, a *preoperative note* should be written the evening before surgery by the house officer who will be involved with the operative procedure. It should state the diagnosis, associated illnesses, and contemplated procedure in a sentence. It should summarize the laboratory work with reference to the tests required for safe conduct of anesthesia and surgery. If appropriate it should document that blood is available in the blood bank and that the consent form has been signed. A typical preoperative note might look something like this:

F.R. is a 64-year-old nondiabetic man admitted with ischemic rest pain and impending gangrene of the right leg. Angiography showed a right iliac artery stenosis and occlusion of the right superficial femoral artery at its takeoff. He underwent a transluminal angioplasty for the former today and is scheduled for a right femoral popliteal bypass for the latter tomorrow.

CBC: Hct 39.1, WBC 8500

SMA6: Na 143, k 4.2, Cl 105, CO_2 25, glucose 110, BUN 14, creatinine 1.0

Urinalysis: WNL [within normal limits]

Prothrombin and partial thromboplastin times: Normal

Chest x-ray: No acute disease

ECG: Occasional atrial premature contractions; otherwise WNL (within normal limits)

Persantin-thallium stress test: No ischemic areas amenable to revascularization

Two units of packed red blood cells are available in blood bank.

Consent: Signed

Preoperative orders written

Patient ready for OR tomorrow

To minimize waste and decrease costs, many institutions try to mandate only those preoperative tests that genuinely contribute to the patient's care. For example, some institutions require preoperative chest x-ray and urinalysis only if there is a specific indication.

Increasingly, even patients scheduled to undergo major surgery are being admitted on the morning of surgery, and the history is taken and physical examination performed in the office or clinic well in advance of the scheduled procedure. Relevant laboratory work, x-rays, and consultations are also obtained on an outpatient basis before surgery. When significant time has elapsed between (1) history taking and physical examination and (2) the patient's arrival for the scheduled ambulatory or same-day surgery, it is sometimes a requirement that a note be written to indicate that the patient's status has not changed from the time the H&P was written.

At the conclusion of the operation, a *brief operative note* is written. Because either the attending surgeon or the resident will dictate a comprehensive operative note, the brief operative note need include only the essentials of the operation, so that the patient's hospital course can be readily ascertained by anyone assuming responsibility for this patient's care. Such a note includes the preoperative and postoperative diagnoses, procedure, names of surgeon and assistants, type of anesthesia, estimated blood loss, amount of fluid replacement and blood transfusions (if any), types of drains, specimens obtained, complications, and the patient's condition. A typical brief operative note might read like this:

Preoperative diagnosis: Right inguinal hernia

Postoperative diagnosis: Same

Procedure: Right inguinal herniorrhaphy

Surgeon: Dr. B. Jones

Assistant: Dr. J. Smith

Anesthesia: Local with Marcaine by surgeon

Estimated blood loss [EBL]: Minimal

Drains: None

Specimen: Indirect sac to pathology

Complications: None

Condition: Patient tolerated procedure well and was taken to recovery room in satisfactory condition

On the evening after surgery, the patient should be seen by either the house officer who scrubbed on the case or the house officer covering the service, or by both. The *postoperative note* should read like a check-list of those things that require attention on the first postoperative night. Obviously the vital signs and respiratory status need to be checked. The dressing should be examined. Since it is not uncommon for patients to develop urinary retention postoperatively, it is important to make sure the patient has voided within approximately 8 hours after surgery or at least before distention of the bladder creates discomfort. If the patient's state of hydration is questionable, a Foley catheter should be placed to monitor hourly urine output, and the urine output should be documented in the postoperative note. It may be appropriate to check laboratory studies, depending on the magnitude of the procedure and the nature of any associated conditions that might exist. An example of a postoperative note on a patient with chronic obstructive lung disease who underwent low anterior resection earlier in the day is as follows:

Vital signs stable
Lungs clear to auscultation, no respiratory distress. Respiratory rate 18. Arterial blood gases satisfactory.
Dressing dry and intact
Urine output 50–60 cc per hour
Hemoglobin 14 g

Following surgery, *progress notes* must be written on a daily basis that summarize the care given to the patient. If the problem-oriented record is used, each problem should be addressed, subjective and objective data bases should be updated, and an impression should be recorded for each problem, along with a plan for further diagnosis and treatment of each. In point of fact, this is not always desirable, and it is common for a daily progress note to be limited to the most pertinent information. A progress note for a 55-year-old woman 4 days after resection of the sigmoid colon with end-to-end anastomosis during a quiescent phase for the second attack of sigmoid diverticulitis might read something like this:

POD #4 vital signs stable. Afebrile
Lungs clear to auscultation
Abdomen soft, nontender, nondistended
Incision clean and healing well
Jackson-Pratt drain removed yesterday
Tolerating regular diet, moving bowels
Ambulatory. Voiding well with good urine output after Foley catheter removed. No calf tenderness
For discharge tomorrow

In addition to routine daily progress notes, a note should be written whenever a procedure is performed or the patient is seen because of a change in status. An example of such a note is this:

Brought to intensive care unit because of pleuritic chest pain and dyspnea 6 days after a left above-knee amputation. Blood pressure 80 systolic on arrival. Because of suspected pulmonary embolus, patient underwent anticoagulation with heparin, 10,000 units IV push, and was given continuous infusion of heparin 1000 units per hour, on which his partial thromboplastin time was 56. A Swan-Ganz catheter was inserted, and his pulmonary artery pressure was high, and pulmonary capillary wedge pressure and cardiac output were low. He was volume expanded with normal saline. Cardiac output increased from 3.2 to 4.6 L per minute, with an increase in urine output and improvement in blood pressure to 120 systolic. Perfusion scan revealed multiple filling defects involving the left lung. These defects were absent on ventilation scan, confirming pulmonary embolus as the source of the patient's signs and symptoms.

As one can readily see, this note makes the situation immediately clear to any doctor just coming on the scene, helping to ensure continuity of care. This, in fact, is the purpose of note writing, and good notes can make a substantial contribution to quality of care.

4

The Science of Order Writing

The writing of orders is the means by which the physician directs the management of the hospitalized patient's care. On the surgical service, orders can be grouped into (1) admission orders, (2) preoperative orders, (3) postoperative orders, and (4) daily orders. Although the nursing staff are responsible for executing the doctor's orders, it is a good idea to discuss the orders with the nurse to make sure that they are understood and duly registered. One must often double-check, to make sure that the orders are carried out properly.

It is important that the doctor have a system of order writing, to minimize the possibility that important instructions are left out. One good system is outlined here. Some memorization is required, but the effort pays off.

The body of any comprehensive system of orders should be organized into *nursing orders, medication orders* (standing and PRN [as needed]), and orders for *laboratory tests.* Examples of nursing orders are instructions for the nurse to measure intake and output, to have the patient ambulate with assistance, to weigh the patient daily, to connect the nasogastric sump tube to low continuous suction, and to irrigate it every 2 hours with 50 ml of normal saline (NS). An example of standing medication orders would be to infuse D5–1/3NS + 20 mEq of KCl per liter at 100 ml per hour, or to administer cefazolin, 1 g IV q8h. An example of a PRN medication order would be demerol, 75 mg IM q3h PRN pain. Notice that PRN alone is not enough: the order must indicate PRN *for* something—be it pain, lack of sleep, or blood pressure over a certain level.

ADMISSION ORDERS

Admission orders are organized as follows:

1. Admit to Dr. _____
2. Diagnosis (Dx)
3. Condition
4. Allergies
5. Associated conditions
6. Vital signs

7. Diet
8. Ambulation
9. Nursing orders
10. Medication orders
11. Lab orders

Notice that Orders 2 through 5 are not really *orders* at all; they summarize information about the patient—information that is available in detail in the admitting history and physical examination. The purpose of these "orders" is twofold. First, they inform the nurse about the patient, even if the nurse does not read the admission history and physical. Second, they remind others of things to be aware of when writing other orders. As a very obvious example, you are unlikely to order penicillin if you have just written that the patient is allergic to penicillin. If you have just written that the patient is diabetic, you are likely to remember to order appropriate blood sugar determinations and insulin or an oral hypoglycemic, if indicated.

Order 6, vital signs, usually includes blood pressure, respirations, pulse, and temperature. What is *ordered* here is the frequency with which they should be monitored, and the frequency should be appropriate for the degree of stability that the patient's condition indicates. Under *nursing orders,* the physician may indicate the upper and lower limits of acceptable vital signs by stating that the physician should be called when values deviate from the acceptable range.

Below are the admitting orders for a hypothetical male patient who had been taking steroids for Crohn's disease and who developed an enterocutaneous fistula while at home, 3 months after ileocolic resection for intestinal obstruction:

1. Admit to Dr. Smith
2. Dx: Crohn's disease with enterocutaneous fistula
3. Condition: Satisfactory
4. Allergies: *Penicillin*
5. Associated conditions: Steroid dependence, asthma
6. Vital signs: q4h
7. NPO
8. May be out of bed with assistance
9. Strict [measuring of] intake and output
10. Weigh daily
11. Finger-stick blood sugars q6h × 72h
12. Ileostomy bag to enterocutaneous fistula—record effluent volume q shift
13. Protect skin around fistula with aluminum paste
14. Call MD for T 101.5 or greater; p 110 or greater; systolic BP <100; diastolic BP <60; or urine output <240 ml per shift
15. Please have subclavian catheter tray on floor in AM
16. D5 Ringer's lactate solution at 125 ml per hour for the next 8 hours; then check with MD
17. Hydrocortisone, 100 mg IV q8h

18. Dalmane 30 mg PO qhs PRN sleep (may take with 30 ml of water)
19. CBC, electrolytes, BUN, blood sugar, creatinine today
20. Repeat serum potassium, liver function tests, calcium, magnesium, TIBC, B_{12}, folate, protime, partial thromboplastin time in AM
21. PA and lateral chest x-ray and flat and upright abdominal x-rays today

Orders 1 and 2 are self-explanatory. Order 3 alerts the staff to the condition of the patient and provides a gross baseline. Order 4 alerts doctors and nurses to the fact that the patient is allergic to penicillin. This order should always be underlined if the patient is allergic to a medication. An alternative entry, if appropriate, would be "None known." In addition, allergies are usually noted on the front of the patient's chart. A true allergic reaction must be distinguished from an untoward reaction such as nausea from codeine, since the two have different significances.

Order 5 is very significant. It is vitally important for the doctor to know that the patient has been on steroids, because failure to order and administer them could precipitate addisonian crisis. Here, 300 mg of hydrocortisone daily is begun, since this is what a patient with normal adrenal glands is able to secrete under the influence of maximal stress. It is assumed, for safety's sake, that this patient, who has been admitted with an enterocutaneous fistula, may have a septic component to his illness, and thus is under maximal stress. The steroids are both to prevent addisonian crisis and to treat the Crohn's disease. It is possible that the steroids can be tapered significantly over the ensuing few days. Notice again that "orders" 2 through 5 are not *orders* in the true sense of the word but do serve useful functions.

Order 17, the steroid order, is written with the mental stimulus of order 5.

Orders 6 to 8 fall under the categories of *vital signs, diet,* and *ambulation.* In this example the admitting resident believes that once every 4 hours would be a safe and appropriate interval for the nurse to take the vital signs, which include temperature.

Order 7 is the diet order and indicates that this patient is to be kept NPO (given nothing by mouth). This is done in this case in the hope of decreasing or totally stopping fistula output. Order 8 deals with ambulation. In this case there is no reason to keep the patient at bed rest, and ambulation is desirable to prevent such complications as atelectasis and deep vein thrombosis. It is requested that assistance be given, at least at first, since the patient may be weak and unsteady because of the underlying disease process, and the patient must be prevented from falling and possibly sustaining injury. Ambulation is required to prevent or reverse deconditioning and to help achieve a state of anabolism, when total parenteral nutrition is begun.

Orders 9 through 14 represent *nursing orders,* orders that the nursing staff are to carry out. Orders 9 and 10 promote proper fluid management; this will become especially important when total parenteral nutrition is initiated. Order 11 is written because it is anticipated that intravenous hyperalimentation will be started the next day, and the large glucose load that the patient given total parenteral nutrition (TPN) receives may cause hyperglycemia and glycosuria—and even hyperglycemic, hyperosmolar, nonketotic coma. In this patient, hydrocortisone would be expected to exacerbate glucose intolerance. Frequent checks of finger-stick blood sugar values may alert the physician early to this development. Order 12 is significant to the fluid management of the patient, since fistula loss must be replaced if the patient is not to become hypovolemic. Gastrointestinal losses are usually isotonic.

Order 14 tells the nurse about which parameters the physician wishes to be notified. The specific ones listed are predicated on the patient's baseline values and are not meant to apply to every patient. In addition, the nurse should be encouraged to call the physician for any change in the patient's status that seems worrisome.

Order 16 relates to the patient's fluid management. To determine the patient's requirements, one must take into consideration his maintenance requirements, the original deficit, and any ongoing losses as from this patient's enterocutaneous fistula. Ringer's lactated solution was chosen here because the patient has obviously lost salt and bicarbonate from the small bowel.

The lab work, which includes radiographic studies, is meant to provide a baseline. Some of the tests ordered are required to guide proper institution of parenteral nutrition.

PREOPERATIVE ORDERS

Preoperative orders are written the night before surgery and are meant to set the stage for the operation the next day. A typical set of preoperative orders might read as follows:

1. NPO after midnight
2. Shave and prep, nipple to midthigh in early AM
3. Void on call to operating room
4. Premeds per anesthesia
5. Consent form for fundoplication by Dr. Jones
6. Apply external pneumatic compression boots

The patient is given nothing to eat after midnight, so that the stomach will be empty at the time of induction of anesthesia, thus preventing vomiting and aspiration of gastric contents.

The practice of shaving and prepping the night before surgery has—rightly—come under criticism, since it seems to increase the incidence of wound infection in clean surgical procedures. Presumably, this occurs because the little nicks made by shaving become infected with skin flora such as staphylococci, and these bacteria proliferate overnight, contributing to infection. Possible solutions to this problem are (1) to shave and prep the patient the morning of surgery, (2) to use a depilatory cream instead of a razor, and (3) to forego shaving altogether.

The patient urinates on call to the operating room to avoid a full bladder postoperatively, as this could lead to urinary retention. Order 4 reminds the nurse to make sure that the anesthesiologist has ordered premedication, such as a sedative, if the anesthesiologist deems it appropriate for that patient. Practice varies among institutions in terms of who obtains the consent and whether it is *ordered* at all or just *obtained.*

POSTOPERATIVE ORDERS

Postoperative orders again include four orders that are not true "orders" but that serve to orient physician and nurses, and that are superimposed on the core of *vital signs, diet, ambulation, nursing orders, medication orders,* and *laboratory orders.* Postoperative orders for a patient who has just undergone right colon resection might read as follows:

1. Procedure: Right hemicolectomy
2. Condition: Satisfactory
3. Allergies: None known
4. Associated conditions: COPD
5. Routine recovery room vital signs, VS q4h on floor
6. NPO
7. Out of bed with assistance tonight, ambulate with assistance at least qid in AM
8. Call MD for no void by 6:00 PM
9. Encourage turn, cough, and deep breathe, and incentive spirometer q2h while awake
10. Strict [measuring of] intake and output
11. Weigh daily
12. D/C NG tube in recovery room
13. D5–1/4 NS plus 20 mEq of KCl per liter at 100 ml per hour
14. Cefazolin 1 g at 2 PM, then D/C
15. Demerol 75 mg IM q3h PRN pain
16. CBC, serum potassium in AM

"Orders" 1 through 4, again, serve to orient the physician and nursing staff; 5 through 7 fall under the categories of *vital signs, diet,* and *ambulation.* Orders 8 through 12 are *nursing orders,* and 13 through 15 are *medication orders* (both standing and PRN). Order 16 is laboratory orders.

It is noted in Order 4 that the patient has chronic obstructive pulmonary disease, and this sets the stage for orders 7 and 9, which are calculated to prevent atelectasis and to mobilize pulmonary secretions. The patient is given nothing to eat or drink (NPO), because after colon resection, adequate peristalsis would not have returned by the first postoperative night. After a laparotomy without peritonitis, peristalsis of the small bowel returns immediately, that of the stomach in 24 to 36 hours, and that of the colon in 48 to 72 hours. However inexplicably, in some patients peristalsis takes much longer to return. Order 8 deals with the fact that a patient may have difficulty voiding on the first postoperative night, because the anticholinergic agents given by the anesthesiologist decrease the bladder's ability to contract, postoperative pain makes it harder for the patient to strain, and preexisting benign prostatic hypertrophy in older men may have made voiding marginal in the first place.

Asking the nurse to measure intake and output helps the doctor to monitor the patient's fluid status, as does daily taking of weights, since fluid retention is manifested by increasing weight. The fluid order (No. 13) is not arbitrary but is based on the fact that humans require as maintenance fluid 100 ml/kg body weight for the first 10 kg, 50 ml/kg for the next 10 kg, and 20 ml/kg thereafter. A 70-kg person, thus requires 1000 ml plus 500 ml plus 1000 ml, which equals 2500 ml of maintenance fluid in 24 hours. As can readily be seen, 100 ml of fluid per hour approximates this amount over 24 hours. A normal healthy person requires 30 mEq/L of sodium and 20 mEq/L of potassium of maintenance fluid. Since normal saline has approximately 150 mEq/L of sodium, one-quarter normal saline approximates closely enough the 30 mEq/L required for fluid maintenance. Many surgeons are now omitting the nasogastric tube after routine colon surgery. If a patient undergoing gastrointestinal surgery does have a large postoperative nasogastric output, it can be replaced, cubic centimeter for cubic centimeter, with normal or half-normal saline, which approximates the electrolyte content of nasogastric juice.

Order 15 deals with the fact that parenteral prophylactic antibiotics have been shown to reduce the incidence of septic complications such as wound infection after colon surgery. One dose should be given preoperatively, one dose intraoperatively, and one dose postoperatively. No benefit—and some harm—can come from giving more than three doses of prophylactic antibiotics. The harms include predisposing to resistant organisms in a given patient and in the environment in general, exposing the patient to increased risk of side effects such as allergic reaction or nephrotoxicity, and increased cost. Sometimes when a foreign body is inserted operatively (e.g., vascular prosthesis) the benefits of prolonged prophylaxis can outweigh the risks). This is the exception. In addition to order 17, one could argue that an arterial blood gas reading should be obtained in the early postoperative period and the findings compared with the preoperative blood gas values, to make sure that the patient is ventilating and oxygenating adequately.

Daily Orders

The *routine orders* appropriate for this patient on the first or second postoperative day might include renewal of the intravenous orders. Clear fluids could be started by mouth, if there were no abdominal distention and if there were evidence to suggest that peristalsis had returned, such as the presence of bowel sounds or flatus.

5

Wound Management

Healed wounds and healed anastomoses are primary goals of the surgeon. To be sure, surgical trauma is directed toward correcting a preexisting lesion, to achieve homeostasis; but the incision must heal and the anastomosis must not leak if the surgical intervention is to be effective. Surgical science provides insight into how the surgeon can maximize the likelihood of a successful outcome.

Much of what is known about surgical technique has been learned during wartime, and it was Ambrose Paré who discovered that amputations healed better when hemostasis was achieved by ligating bleeding vessels rather than merely by applying boiling oil to the amputation stump. This advance in surgical science was not only a blessing to the wounded of the day but an important example of how gentle technique promotes healing.

CASE 5–1

Primary Closure

A 53-year-old man was seen in the emergency department after being slashed in the right cheek with a straight razor. There was no history of trauma to the chest, abdomen, or head, and past medical history was unremarkable.

The site was prepped with povidone-iodine, and local anesthesia was achieved by injection of 1% Xylocaine. The wound was irrigated with saline. Devitalized tissue was minimal. Hemostasis was achieved by suture ligature of bleeding vessels using No. 5–0 polyglycolic acid sutures, and the skin was closed with No. 6–0 nylon on a fine needle. A sterile dressing was applied. The patient was given an intramuscular injection of tetanus toxoid, because it had been more than 10 years since a previous immunization. Careful wound precautions were given, and the patient was told to make an appointment to be seen in the office for suture removal in 5 days' time.

DISCUSSION OF CASE 5–1

History. A laceration by a razor suggests a clean injury with a minimum of devitalized tissue. Moreover, one would not expect much dirt or other foreign bodies in the wound. This is akin to a surgical incision with a scalpel, although sterility is more likely in the latter instance. Thus, extensive débridement, with the attendant further tissue loss, can be avoided. There was no history of diabetes or malnutrition to suggest that wound healing would be impaired. The face is highly vascular; therefore, facial injuries have a high probability of healing primarily. Since the patient had had no tetanus toxoid immunization within the last 10 years, a booster was given. In a tetanus-prone wound, active immunization with hyperimmune globulin is a prudent measure. Since there was no history of injury to other parts of the body, meticulous attention to the facial wound could be given, especially if physical examination had confirmed that the patient's condition was stable.

Physical Examination. Physical examination must be directed toward confirming the absence of distant injuries, identifying devitalized tissue that must be débrided and any foreign body that must be removed if infection is to be avoided, and making sure that adjacent structures are not involved. A facial laceration that crosses a line between the ear and the angle of the mouth may involve the parotid duct; this must be recognized if a parotid fistula is to be avoided.

Laboratory Examination and Diagnostic Imaging. Diagnostic studies would not be indicated in this instance unless trauma to remote body parts was believed to be present or an associated illness were suspected.

Treatment: Primary Closure. Primary closure is performed when there has been minimal tissue loss. This is sometimes called *healing by primary intention,* and it occurs when a clean laceration is sutured (Fig. 5–1). As in all wounds, *coagulation* occurs first and achieves hemostasis. Platelets aggregate and thrombus forms. *Inflammation* is the next crucial step. As the permeability of the local vasculature increases, polymorphonuclear leukocytes and macrophages migrate into the local milieu to phagocytose devitalized tissue, foreign bodies, and any bacteria that may be present.

Fibroblasts are then stimulated to provide the next step in wound healing, *collagen synthesis.* Transforming growth factor-beta and platelet-derived growth factor are cytokines found in platelets and other cells that accelerate the wound-healing process. Collagen is secreted from the fibroblasts, and cross-linking, involving hydroxylation of proline and lysine to hydroxyproline and hydroxylysine, occurs. Extracellular matrix is deposited. Ingrowth of capillaries—

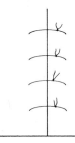

Figure 5–1. Primary closure of an incised wound. There is minimal loss of tissue; thus, epithelialization and contraction play minor roles. Coagulation, inflammation, angiogenesis, collagen formation, and remodeling all contribute to wound healing.

angiogenesis—provides oxygen and nutrition to the nascent connective tissue. In wounds that can be closed by primary intention there is minimal loss of tissue. *Epithelialization* plays a relatively minor role, as there is only a small gap to traverse. Similarly, *contraction,* which can be so important in wounds closed by secondary intention, is not required for primary closure.

CASE 5–2

Secondary Closure

A 23-year-old man underwent repair of a liver laceration and resection of a devitalized segment of small bowel after a motorcycle accident. On the posterior thorax were multiple full-thickness skin defects, ranging from 0.5 to 0.8 cm in diameter, caused by abrasion with gravel as the patient slid along the ground after being thrown from his motorcycle. Following closure of the laparotomy incision, while still under anesthesia the patient was turned prone and the abrasions and skin defects were cleansed and débrided of foreign bodies such as dirt, gravel, and shreds of clothing, and of devitalized tissue. A nonadherent dressing and antibiotic ointment were applied. While the patient was in the hospital, the dressings were changed three times daily, and after discharge this was continued by a visiting nurse and the patient's wife. On a follow-up visit to the surgeon's office 6 weeks later, the defects were found to be completely healed.

DISCUSSION OF CASE 5–2

When there is full-thickness skin, loss healing can occur by *secondary intention.* The same processes of *coagulation, inflammation, angiogenesis, collagen formation,* and *deposition of extracellular matrix* must occur, just as they do with primary closure. In healing by secondary intention, however, the processes of *wound contraction* and *epithelialization* play important roles. The former process is mediated by myofibroblasts that cause the wound edges to contract, moving toward the center of the wound, in effect shrinking it. The latter phenomenon occurs as epithelial cells migrate from the edge of the wound across the defect until it is healed. When the defect is completely covered, contact inhibition occurs and the epithelial cells stop multiplying.

Wound remodeling occurs in most wounds over the course of many months as well-organized collagen replaces the less well-organized collagen, giving the wound greater tensile strength. It is reasonable to allow small wounds to heal by secondary intention, especially in a patient such as the one described, whose major organ trauma must take priority, whose defects are small, and for whom gross contamination makes primary closure likely to fail because of infection. However, healing by secondary intention causes contractures and this must be avoided if the wound crosses a joint, as such contractures would limit motion across that joint. A defect near the eyelids should not be allowed to heal by secondary intention, as the resultant contracture could produce ectropion. Closing the defect with a split-thickness skin graft would cause less contracture, and closing it with a full-thickness graft or flap would cause even less.

Another reason not to allow large defects to close secondarily is that "scar carcinomas," also called *Marjolin's ulcers* have been known to develop many years later in burns or areas of chronic osteomyelitis or in scars from large defects that were allowed to heal by secondary intention. These lesions are squamous cell carcinomas.

CASE 5–3
Delayed Primary Closure

A 35-year-old man underwent appendectomy through McBurney's incision for gangrenous appendicitis. Because a large amount of pus lay free in the peritoneal cavity the surgeon closed the fascia with monofilament nylon sutures. The skin was left open and packed loosely with gauze. Nylon skin sutures were placed, but not tied. On the 5th postoperative day delayed primary closure was accomplished by tying the skin sutures. The patient was discharged to home on the 7th postoperative day.

DISCUSSION OF CASE 5–3

When there is established infection at the time of laparotomy, the case is said to be *dirty*. If a tubular structure harboring bacteria, such as the colon or the trachea, is traversed but there is no undue spillage, the case is said to be *clean-contaminated*. If there is spillage of the contents of the tubular organ, the wound is said to be *contaminated*. If no tubular structure is traversed and there is no preexisting infection or break in operative technique, the case is said to be *clean*. A breast biopsy is a clean case; a left hemicolectomy is a clean-contaminated case unless gross spillage has occurred. In Case 5–3, pus was encountered when the peritoneum was entered; thus, the case was dirty.

In a dirty case such as Case 5–3, the chances of developing a wound infection are extraordinarily high when the wound is closed primarily. If an infection should occur, the surgeon would be forced to open the incision to drain the pus. Moreover, he would be exposing the patient to the risks of sepsis, necrotizing fasciitis, and wound dehiscence. To avoid this, the wound could be left open to heal by secondary intention. This is likely to avert infection, but complete healing would be delayed until the process of wound contraction and epithelialization could occur. In fact, abdominal wounds closed by secondary intention usually heal well, ultimately.

In Case 5–3, an intermediate method—delayed primary closure— was chosen (Fig. 5–2). For the first 5 days the wound was packed

Figure 5–2. Delayed primary closure of a heavily contaminated wound. Sutures may be placed at the time of surgery and the wound left open and packed. Approximately 5 days later, when a large number of inflammatory cells are present, the sutures can be tied in the hope of avoiding infection. If this is successful, the time required for healing should be not different from that required for healing of a wound closed primarily.

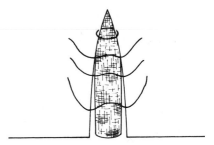

open, allowing polymorphonuclear leukocytes and macrophages to accumulate. Thus, when the sutures were tied on the fifth postoperative day, the wound was relatively resistant to infection. Instead of placing the skin sutures at the time of surgery, the wound could be closed with sterile paper strips (Steri-Strips) on postoperative day 5.

Infection is the enemy of wound healing. It perpetuates the inflammatory phase and delays collagen synthesis. It may increase collagenase activity. To avoid infection, it is necessary to understand its pathogenesis. The probability of developing infection is directly proportional to the *number* and *virulence* of organisms present and inversely proportional to *host resistance*. Host resistance can be divided into local and systemic factors.

The number of organisms can be minimized during laparotomy by aseptic techniques such as prepping the skin with povidone-iodine, using sterile gloves, and avoiding spillage of gastrointestinal contents when hollow organs are opened. The number of organisms in traumatic wounds can be decreased by irrigation under pressure and by débridement of tissue impregnated with contaminated material. It is generally said that a density of 10^5 organisms per gram of tissue is required to set up an invasive infection.

The surgeon has some control over the virulence of organisms that are likely to cause infection. A shorter preoperative hospital stay protects from nosocomial (hospital) organisms, which tend to be selected for antibiotic resistance because of the quantity of antibiotics utilized in the hospital environment. Along the same line, the surgeon can avoid indiscriminate use of antibiotics in an effort to avoid selecting out resistant strains.

Host resistance is influenced by both systemic and local factors. Malnutrition, diabetes, steroid therapy, chemotherapy, heavy tumor burden, and congenital abnormalities of the immune system such as chronic granulomatous disease are systemic factors that decrease host resistance and predispose to wound infection. Local factors that decrease the number of organisms required to set up an invasive infection include ischemia, foreign bodies, and hematomas.

Good surgical technique includes minimizing the amount of devitalized tissue, as such tissue cannot fight infection. The surgeon accomplishes this by refraining from ligating large areas of tissue and by avoiding parallel incisions, which cut off the blood supply to the tissue between them. The amount of suture material left in wounds is minimized, as these act as foreign bodies and reduce the number of organisms required to establish infection.

Monofilament nylon and polypropylene are nonabsorbable and nonreactive and have several advantages over absorbable suture material such as catgut and polyglycolic acid. For the first few weeks the wound relies on the suture for its strength. Thus, it makes more sense to use a nonabsorbable suture that retains its strength over this period when strength is required, as for closure of the fascia. Moreover, the fact that they are monofilament rather than braided is helpful as there are no interstices in which bacteria can lodge. (Monofiliment sutures are more difficult to tie than braided ones.) Absorbable suture can be helpful when suture removal is inconvenient and when the native tissues are expected to regain acceptable strength quickly.

Silk was originally believed to be nonabsorbable, but we know now that it does lose its strength over time. In addition, it sets up a marked inflammatory response that delays wound healing and can be responsible for chronically draining suture sinuses. Wounds closed with silk sutures have been known to "spit silk" months—even years—after closure.

The abdominal cavity can be entered by many types of incisions, and each has its advocates (Fig. 5–3). None is ideal for every situation, and the choice of incision must be individualized. A *midline incision* is rapidly made, and since it is through the linea alba (a relatively avascular structure), blood loss is minimized. Moreover, it can be extended upward as far as the xiphoid process and downward as far as the symphysis pubis, so that almost any abdominal operation can be performed through it. Accordingly, it is especially suitable for exploratory laparotomy and for trauma.

A *subcostal incision (Kocher's incision)* provides excellent exposure of the gallbladder fossa and is entirely suitable for cholecystectomy. Right and left *paramedian incisions* are preferred by some surgeons for right and left colectomy, respectively. *McBurney's incision* is a muscle-splitting incision; the muscles tend to come together naturally postoperatively, so this incision has a low incidence of

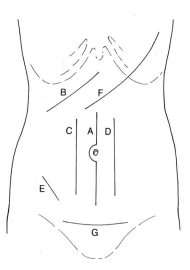

Figure 5–3. Abdominal incisions. (A) Midline; (B) subcostal (Kocher's incision); (C) right paramedian; (D) left paramedian; (E) McBurney; (F) thoracoabdominal; (G) Pfannenstiel's.

dehiscence and incisional hernia and is ideal for appendectomy. Exposure through it can be limited, however. If it is suspected that a lesion other than appendicitis may be responsible for the patient's findings, it may be prudent to use a right paramedian or a midline incision, should more extensive surgery be required.

A *thoracoabdominal incision* may be used for esophagogastrectomy for carcinoma of the cardia of the stomach. *Pfannenstiel's incision* is a transverse incision utilized in gynecologic procedures. It provides good exposure to the uterus and fallopian tubes, and, because it is in the skin crease above the pubis, it usually yields a good cosmetic result.

Understanding the physiology of wound healing and the pathophysiology of infection is central to a good surgical outcome. Wound healing must be achieved if surgical intervention is to be successful.

Recommended Reading

1. Adzick NS: Wound healing: Biological and clinical features. In Sabiston DC (ed): *Textbook of Surgery: The Biological Basis of Modern Surgical Practice,* ed 15. Philadelphia: W.B. Saunders, 1997, pp 207–220.
2. Lawrence WT: Wound healing biology and its application to wound management. In O'Leary JP (ed): *The Physiologic Basis of Surgery,* ed 2. Baltimore: Williams and Wilkins, 1996, pp 118–140.
3. Zuidema GD, Ritchie WP Jr (eds): *Shackelford's Surgery of the Alimentary Tract,* ed 4, vol II. Philadelphia: W.B. Saunders, 1996, pp 250–368.

6

Tubes and Drains

Tubes and drains are omnipresent in surgical patient areas, and familiarity with them will help the beginning surgical resident or clerk to become acclimated quickly. The use of tubes and drains often seems governed by habit and tradition rather than by sound surgical principles, but there are principles that do provide a guide to use of drains and tubes.

CASE 6–1

A Drain in Proximity to the Duodenal Stump

A 45-year-old alcoholic man underwent vagotomy and hemigastrectomy and Billroth II gastrojejunostomy for his third episode of massive upper gastrointestinal bleeding in 3 months' time. Seven days postoperatively, his temperature rose to 102°F. The next day he was found to have duodenal contents in the Jackson-Pratt drain that had been left in proximity to the duodenal stump.

The patient was given nothing by mouth and was placed on total parenteral nutrition and given broad-spectrum antibiotics. His fever subsided over the course of the next 3 days. Over the next 6 weeks the fistula drainage from the Jackson-Pratt drain decreased from 400 ml daily to nothing, and he never developed signs of peritonitis. He tolerated feeding well after the fistula drainage ceased, and he was discharged.

DISCUSSION OF CASE 6–1

Drains should be used when they serve a purpose, such as evacuating ongoing discharge from a hollow viscus. It is reasonable to place a drain near the duodenal stump after gastrectomy and Billroth II gastrojejunostomy, as the duodenal stump has a small but definite incidence of "blowout." If duodenal contents were allowed to flow freely into the peritoneal cavity, generalized peritonitis would ensue, necessitating immediate reoperation. If, however, the leak can be controlled (that is, if fluid exits the peritoneal cavity through the previously placed drain), peritonitis and reoperation *may* be avoided. Duodenal secretions can be minimized if the patient is kept NPO and fed by total parenteral nutrition; the leak may eventually close without reoperation. If, however, the patient develops evidence of peritonitis or of sepsis, reoperation and repair of the fistula must be performed. CT can be performed to ensure that there is no undrained collection of duodenal contents in the peritoneal cavity that could serve as a source of sepsis.

The *Jackson-Pratt drain* (Fig. 6–1) operates by virtue of the suction created when the bulb is compressed with the port unplugged. This setup not only creates effective drainage but provides a *closed system,* so that bacteria cannot use the drain as a portal into the wound. The *Penrose drain* (Fig. 6–2) is an old standard that relies on capillary action to function. It is a reasonably efficient drainage system but has the distinct disadvantage of providing a portal through which bacteria can enter the wound (i.e., it is a two-way street).

The *Hemovac drain* (Fig. 6–3) relies on a spring-activated evacuator for potential energy to provide suction to a wound, to evacuate serum and blood. The Hemovac drain, a closed system, minimized the possibility of its providing a source of infection. It has traditionally been used to evacuate serum from beneath mastectomy flaps, allowing the two flaps to become apposed so that healing can take place. The Hemovac drain can be removed from a mastectomy incision when drainage volume is less than 15 ml per 24-hour period. If it is removed while drainage is too voluminous, a seroma will form that requires aspiration.

In the past, placing a Penrose drain subcutaneously in the process of closing a laparotomy incision was common practice. This has largely been abandoned, as a drain is a foreign body; thus, fewer bacteria are required to produce an invasive infection in a wound so drained. Drains should be used only when there is fluid to be evacuated or the potential for fluid accumulation. In any event, drains

Figure 6–1. Jackson-Pratt drain provides a closed suction system that cannot serve as a portal by which bacteria can enter the wound or the peritoneal cavity. Compression of the bulb with the port opened generates the potential energy that provides the suction.

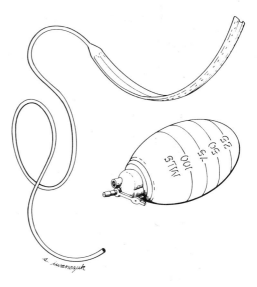

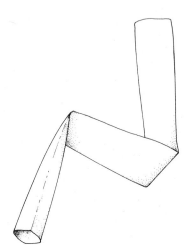

Figure 6–2. The Penrose drain evacuates fluid such as bile, blood, and serum by capillary action. This is an old standard, but it should not be used in most cases. It is a two-way street: that is, it also provides a portal of entry for bacteria into the wound.

Figure 6–3. The Hemovac drain provides a closed drainage system and is traditionally used after mastectomy. A spring provides the potential energy to generate the suction. This drain can evacuate blood and serum, which tend to accumulate between the mastectomy flaps and the chest wall. With it, a seroma is avoided and good apposition and healing are produced.

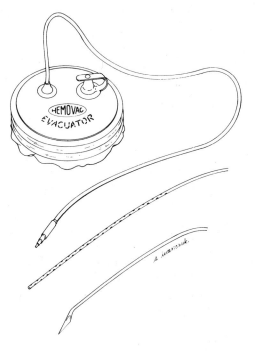

should not be brought directly out through the primary incision, as this increases the risk of wound infection and of incisional hernia. Placement of a closed drainage system in the hepatorenal space (Morrison's pouch) after cholecystectomy is often performed to evacuate blood and bile, the accumulation of which may predispose to subhepatic abscess. The necessity for drainage after "routine" cholecystectomy has been questioned, however. It is not done following laparoscopic cholecystectomy and few if any such patients suffer from lack of a drain.

CASE 6–2

Long-Tube Decompression

A 70-year-old woman was admitted with her seventh bout of intestinal obstruction since colectomy for perforated diverticulitis 10 years earlier. She had undergone three laparotomies with lysis of adhesions in the last 5 years for mechanical small bowel obstruction caused by adhesions. During her other three admissions the intestinal obstruction resolved spontaneously after the bowel was decompressed with a Cantor tube. Accordingly, a Cantor tube was placed in the emergency department, and the patient was admitted and hydrated. By the next morning, however, she reported localized tenderness in the left lower quadrant with fever and leukocytosis, and therefore underwent laparotomy. At surgery, a closed-loop strangulated obstruction was encountered, and a small bowel resection with end-to-end anastomosis was performed. After a stormy postoperative course, the patient recovered and was discharged.

DISCUSSION OF CASE 6–2

A *Cantor tube* (Fig. 6–4) is an example of a long intestinal tube that has a balloon on the end. A syringe is utilized to fill the balloon with mercury, and the balloon and tube are passed through the nostril into the stomach. Gravity (or fluoroscopy) is used to maneuver the balloon into the duodenum. If there is peristalsis, the balloon may pass into the intestine. The tube can then evacuate fluid and air and help decompress the obstruction. If the edema resolves, so may the obstruction. In many instances, however, operative intervention is required. In Case 6–2, the presence of localized tenderness, fever, and leukocytosis signaled the presence of gangrenous bowel, and prompt laparotomy was mandatory. Failure of an obstruction to resolve promptly with long-tube decompression is an indication for surgery.

The *Miller-Abbott tube* (Fig. 6–5) is another variant of the long tube. It has a double lumen, so that the balloon can be filled with mercury after it has passed into the stomach. This obviates the trauma of forcing the mercury-filled balloon through the nares.

The *Levin tube* (Fig. 6–6) is meant to be passed into the stomach. Since most intestinal gas is swallowed air, the Levin tube (*nasogastric*

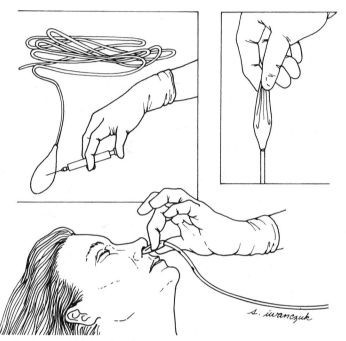

Figure 6–4. The Cantor tube is a long intestinal tube used for small bowel decompression of intestinal obstruction. Mercury is injected into the balloon with a needle and syringe, and the mercury-filled balloon is inserted through the patient's nostril and allowed to slip into the stomach. If peristalsis is present, the tip of the tube can migrate into the small intestines, sucking out fluid and gas. Long tubes require considerable time to pass and may not pass at all when peristalsis is absent. If expeditious surgery is anticipated, a Levin tube or Salem sump nasogastric tube may be preferable.

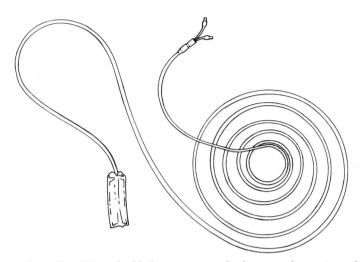

Figure 6–5. The Miller-Abbott double-lumen intestinal tube is another variant of the long tube. In this case, the balloon can be filled with mercury after it has been passed through the nostril into the stomach, obviating the discomfort of inserting the mercury-filled balloon through the nostril. The aim is to have the tube pass into the small intestines, accomplishing decompression.

Figure 6–6. The Levin tube is the standard naso-gastric tube that is passed into the stomach to prevent gastric dilatation and vomiting. It can be used in the event of ileus, as the major source of gas in the intestines is swallowed air. Many surgeons use it for mechanical intestinal obstruction, because aggressive management mandates early surgery and a long tube would not have time to pass in such a short period.

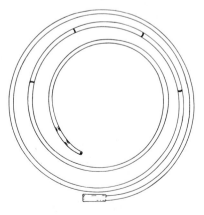

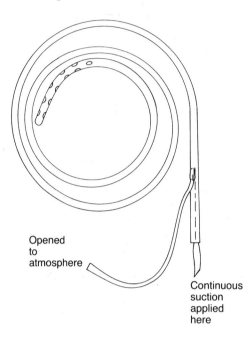

Opened
to
atmosphere

Continuous
suction
applied
here

Figure 6–7. The Salem sump, a variant nasogastric tube that has a double lumen. Suction is applied to one lumen, and the other provides a vent for entrance of air to break the vacuum, so that mucosa does not become invaginated into the tube. This prevents both occlusion of the tube and damage to the mucosa. A Salem sump can be connected to continuous suction, whereas a Levin tube must be connected to intermittent suction to prevent mucosa from occluding the tube.

tube) may prevent progression of distention by evacuating swallowed air from the stomach. The Levin tube has the advantage of direct placement into the stomach. Since aggressive surgical management of intestinal obstruction is often the safest course, there may only be enough time to pass a nasogastric tube. By the time the long tube would have been passed, surgery could already have been performed. The Levin tube is connected to low intermittent suction because, if continuous suction were used the mucosa of the stomach could be sucked into the tube and could occlude it, perhaps traumatizing the mucosa. The *Salem sump* (Fig. 6–7) has two lumens; one provides the suction and the other the air vent to break the vacuum when the contents of the stomach have been evacuated. This prevents the gastric mucosa from occluding the tube and allows more efficient suction. A Salem sump is connected to low continuous suction. Although nasogastric tubes are widely and routinely used after gastrointestinal operations, they cause significant patient discomfort, and studies show that they do not decrease the incidence of postoperative complications such as ileus, wound dehiscence, and breakdown of the anastomosis in colon surgery.

Tubes and drains are important tools of the surgeon. House staff and students must become familiar with the preferences of the attending staff, each of whom usually prefers a *"slightly different"* regimen. Understanding the underlying principles, however, will allow the novice to become comfortable with the use of tubes and drains.

Recommended Reading

1. Hochberg J, Murray GF: Principles of operative surgery: Antisepsis, technique, sutures, and drains. In Sabiston DC (ed): *Textbook of Surgery: The Biological Basis of Modern Surgical Practice,* ed 15. Philadelphia: W.B. Saunders, 1997, pp 253–263.
2. Saltzman DA, Snyder CL, Leonard AS: Intestinal intubation. In Zuidema GD, Ritchie WP Jr (eds): *Shackelford's Surgery of the Alimentary Tract,* ed 4, vol II. Philadelphia: W.B. Saunders, 1996, pp 33–41.
3. Adams GA, Bresnick SD: *On Call Surgery.* Philadelphia: W.B. Saunders, 1997, pp 355–393.

7

The Acute Surgical Abdomen

The acute surgical abdomen is a diagnostic and therapeutic challenge that requires all of the judgment and skills of the general surgeon. Its management is at the epicenter of the specialty of general surgery.

CASE 7–1

Acute Appendicitis

A 24-year-old soldier home on leave came to the emergency department with a 4-day history of abdominal pain.

Four days before admission, he developed vague periumbilical abdominal pain while on the bus home. Over the next 3 days, the pain became more severe and migrated to the right lower abdominal quadrant and he became anorexic. When nausea, vomiting, and a fever of 101°F developed his family insisted he come to the hospital. There was no antecedent history of gastrointestinal symptoms, and he had had no previous abdominal surgery. His last bowel movement was 3 days before admission, and there was no history of diarrhea or hematochezia.

Past medical history was negative for heart disease, diabetes, hypertension, and other serious medical illnesses. Family history was unremarkable. He did not drink or smoke and was taking no medications. Review of systems was negative for a recent upper respiratory infection, and there was no history of dysuria, frequency, nocturia, or hematuria.

Physical findings on admission included a pulse of 110 and a blood pressure of 110/60. His temperature was 101.4°F. There were no surgical scars and no abdominal distention. Bowel sounds were absent. There was no hepatosplenomegaly, the kidneys were not palpable, and no masses or incarcerated hernias were found. The patient's entire abdomen was diffusely tender, especially in the right lower quadrant. The abdomen was rigid and boardlike with generalized rebound tenderness and involuntary guarding. There was hyperesthesia of the skin near McBurney's point. Rectal examination revealed tenderness on the right. Psoas and obturator signs were negative.

Laboratory examination revealed a white blood cell count of 12,400 with 86 polys and 10 bands. The amylase and urinalysis were normal. Flat and upright abdominal x-rays revealed no free air under the diaphragm. There were air-filled loops of small and large bowel with occasional air-fluid levels. No fecalith, radiopaque gallstones, or urolithiasis could be appreciated.

The diagnosis of acute appendicitis was made; the patient was rehydrated aggressively; intravenous gentamicin, metronidazole, and ampicillin were administered; and a laparotomy was performed through McBurney's incision. A gangrenous appendix was removed, and cultures of the peritoneal fluid were obtained. The peritoneum and fascia were closed and the skin was packed open. The cultures of the peritoneal fluid ultimately grew *E. coli* and *Bacteroides fragilis.* Antibiotics were continued for 48 hours postoperatively. The incision was closed with Steri-Strips on the 3rd postoperative day, and the patient was discharged to home on the 5th postoperative day.

DISCUSSION OF CASE 7–1

The acute surgical abdomen requires emergency laparotomy. Some conditions exist, however, that mimic acute surgical abdomen but are often best treated nonoperatively. Diffuse tenderness, generalized rebound tenderness, and involuntary guarding with a rigid, boardlike abdomen are indicative of acute surgical abdomen and mandate surgery unless one of the medical conditions that resemble acute surgical abdomen is known to be present.

Diagnosis

History. The symptoms of the patient in Case 7–1 are rather typical of appendicitis. The pain often originates in the periumbilical area, since it is initially mediated by autonomic sensory receptors in the serosa of the appendix. The pain from autonomic nerve fibers is poorly localized; in the case of a midgut structure such as the appendix, the pain is felt in the periumbilical region. As the parietal peritoneum overlying the appendix becomes involved, somatic sensory receptors are stimulated and the pain is localized to McBurney's point, overlying the appendix. The nausea and vomiting are reflex in nature. Diarrhea is usually absent, but it occasionally occurs in appendicitis.

The examiner should attempt to elicit a history of a recent upper respiratory infection, as this can be associated with transient enlargement of mesenteric lymph nodes, which can cause abdominal pain and thus mimic appendicitis. Mesenteric adenitis is essentially a diagnosis of exclusion. In this situation the surgeon may be tempted to perform appendectomy, to avoid delaying early diagnosis of appendicitis. Early diagnosis and treatment of the acute abdomen are important if complications are to be minimized, and a negative laparotomy usually has fewer untoward consequences than delayed treatment of a septic focus.

One must try to elicit the symptoms of dysuria and frequency, as they might indicate a urinary tract infection. This could mimic appendicitis and result in an operation that could otherwise be avoided. One can be reasonably sure of the diagnosis by history alone in a significant percentage of patients with acute surgical abdomen.

The determination that acute surgical abdomen is present and that surgery is required is more important than preoperative diagnosis of the exact cause of the acute abdomen. Nevertheless, an attempt should be made to provide the correct preoperative diagnosis, to properly counsel the patient and to plan the incision. Moreover, intellectual standards demand that one try to make the exact diagnosis preoperatively, even though this often is not possible and does not affect the outcome.

Physical Examination. As previously mentioned, diffuse tenderness, generalized rebound, and involuntary guarding with a rigid, boardlike abdomen suggest peritonitis resulting from an acute surgical abdomen. Bowel sounds are likely to be absent, as peritonitis causes ileus. Distention may ultimately occur and in the elderly may be the only indication of an intraabdominal catastrophe. Tenderness on rectal examination suggests the presence of appendicitis or pelvic abscess. Sinus tachycardia and hypotension may occur because of fluid lost from the intravascular compartment into the peritoneal cavity and into the intestinal lumen and because of cytokines released in the systemic inflammatory response syndrome (SIRS). The patient's demeanor may help the surgeon make the diagnosis. The patient with peritonitis usually lies completely still on the examining table, as any movement elicits pain, whereas the patient with an obstructed tubular structure such as a ureter is usually writhing in pain, unable to lie still.

Laboratory Studies. Leukocytosis suggests the presence of an inflammatory process. Anemia in a patient suspected of having appendicitis should be a warning that the patient may actually have Crohn's disease, which can result in anemia of chronic illness. Carcinoma of the cecum or gastric cancer can result in iron deficiency anemia, and these entities can produce an acute surgical abdomen if they cause perforation. An elevated serum amylase reading suggests pancreatitis, a medical condition that can imitate an acute surgical abdomen. However, intestinal obstruction, perforated ulcer, and mesenteric ischemia can all elevate the amylase level, and, in contradistinction to pancreatitis, these conditions mandate emergency surgery.

Imaging. Flat and upright abdominal x-rays and an upright chest x-ray may prove helpful. Free air under the diaphragm suggests a ruptured hollow viscus and indicates that expeditious surgery is required to prevent further peritoneal contamination from gastrointestinal contents with resultant sepsis. A distended loop of small bowel that seems to have lost its normal contour suggests a strangulated closed-loop obstruction that may be the cause of the acute surgical abdomen.

Calcifications in the wall of the aorta may help the surgeon to make the diagnosis of a ruptured abdominal aortic aneurysm in a patient with abdominal tenderness. A fecalith in the appendix may be visible on flat plate (KUB—kidneys, ureters, bladder) view and may enable the surgeon to diagnose appendicitis with near certainty. Although only 15% of gallstones are radiopaque, when they are visible on abdominal x-ray in a patient with marked right upper quadrant abdominal tenderness, acute cholecystitis must be high on the list of suspected causes of the acute abdomen. Eighty-five percent of stones of urolithiasis are radiopaque, and their presence may suggest a genitourinary cause for the abdominal pain. The chest x-ray is important, as right lower lobe pneumonia can mimic acute abdomen. Ultrasonography (US) and computed tomography (CT) have some utility in the diagnosis of acute surgical abdomen. These studies can be helpful when the diagnosis or the need to operate is in question. Ultrasonography and CT can demonstrate an appendicolith or thickened appendix that is not apparent on KUB films. CT has the advantage of not being obscured by overlying bowel gas. Small amounts of free air under the diaphragm or an intraabdominal septic process too small to be visualized on plain film can be visualized on CT. Doppler studies of the mesenteric vessels may demonstrate occlusion, suggesting intestinal infarction. Laparoscopy has gained some acceptance in the management of acute surgical abdomen.

Electrodiagnostic Study. The ECG is helpful, because an acute myocardial infarction can cause abdominal pain. One must remember, however, that gallbladder disease can also cause changes on ECG. Moreover, peritonitis, with its accompanying fluid shifts and other hemodynamic derangements, can precipitate myocardial infarction in a patient with underlying coronary artery disease.

Treatment

Before definitive surgical treatment can be undertaken, aggressive fluid resuscitation must be accomplished with a physiologic saline solution such as Ringer's lactate or normal saline. The latter is required if the patient has alkalosis from persistent vomiting. Broad-spectrum antibiotics are often required to treat established sepsis. Respiratory failure requiring intubation and mechanical ventilation can result from intraabdominal sepsis. In fact, when respiratory failure occurs without an obvious cause, one must suspect occult intraabdominal sepsis.

Acute appendicitis is treated by appendectomy (Fig. 7–1). When the surgeon is sure that appendicitis is responsible for the acute surgical abdomen, an operation can be performed through a *muscle-splitting incision (McBurney's incision)* in the right lower quadrant. This has the advantage of a low incidence of wound complications such as incisional hernia and wound dehiscence, but it has the disadvantage of limited exposure, making difficult the more extensive surgery often required for acute surgical abdomen of some other causes. Laparoscopic appendectomy is performed in many centers.

Postoperatively, the patient's fluid requirements must be met with intravenous fluids until gastrointestinal function has returned and the patient is allowed to eat. Atelectasis must be prevented, as breathing is painful after an abdominal operation and can severely compromise respiratory function.

One must be vigilant for the evolution of a postoperative wound infection, as this is common in dirty cases (those with preestablished infection such as appendicitis or perforated diverticulitis). A postoperative pelvic abscess may be manifested by diarrhea and fever and is characterized by a tender mass on rectal examination. It may be

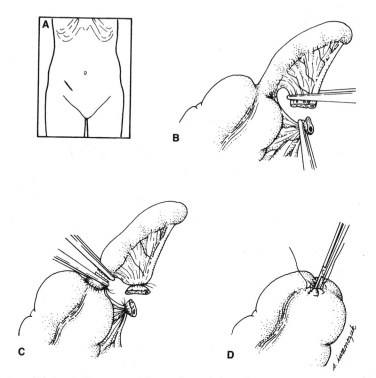

Figure 7–1. *(A)* Appendectomy can be performed through *McBurney's incision* when the surgeon is reasonably sure the diagnosis is acute appendicitis. *(B)* The mesoappendix is serially clamped, transected, and ligated. *(C)* The base of the appendix is clamped, transected, and ligated. *(D)* The stump can then be inverted with a pursestring suture, although this last step is not universally considered necessary, or even desirable.

drained through the rectum with ultrasound guidance. A subphrenic abscess may occur after surgery for acute surgical abdomen, since the lymphatics that clear bacteria from the peritoneal cavity course through the diaphragm. A subphrenic abscess may be demonstrated by an abnormal air-fluid level in the abdomen on upright film or by evidence of a pleural effusion on chest x-ray, by ultrasonography, or by CT. One must have a high degree of suspicion to avoid overlooking it, and one must pay attention to the adage, "Pus somewhere, pus nowhere, pus under the diaphragm." A subphrenic abscess may be drained extraserously through the bed of the 11th rib or through a subcostal incision, or it can be drained percutaneously under CT or ultrasonographic control.

DIFFERENTIAL DIAGNOSIS OF THE ACUTE SURGICAL ABDOMEN

To reiterate, the most important determination is that an acute surgical abdomen is present and that surgery is necessary. An accurate preoperative diagnosis nevertheless aids in planning the operation and helps to determine its urgency. For instance, when the abdominal tenderness is due to a ruptured abdominal aortic aneurysm, the patient must be brought immediately to the operating room without waiting for any tests whatsoever; however, when acute cholecystitis is the cause of the acute surgical abdomen, parenteral antibiotics may be tried preoperatively to see whether the acute condition will "quiet down" so that the operation can be performed on a less urgent basis.

The causes of acute surgical abdomen and the typical sites of the associated pain are listed in Figure 7–2. These are not engraved in stone, and the figure is merely intended to suggest some of the more likely causes of pain and tenderness in each site.

Pain and tenderness in the right upper abdominal quadrant suggest acute cholecystitis and may be associated with a mass. If the pain radiates to the right subscapular region and is associated with nausea and vomiting, the diagnosis of acute cholecystitis is even more likely. If

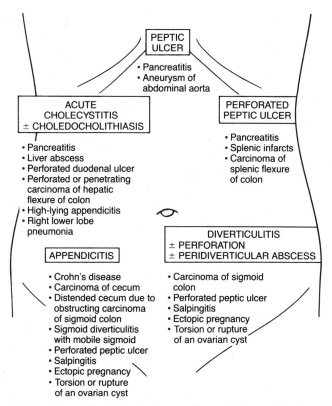

Figure 7–2. The location of the abdominal pain, along with a working knowledge of the diagnostic possibilities, give the surgeon a head start in making an accurate diagnosis and instituting proper treatment.

there is a history of dark urine and clay-colored stools, choledocholithiasis is probably also present. Elevated amylase levels suggest associated gallstone pancreatitis. An ultrasonographic examination revealing gallstones and an HIDA scan showing an obstructed cystic duct almost clinch the diagnosis. One must remember, however, that liver abscess, perforated duodenal ulcer, carcinoma of the hepatic flexure of the colon, and even appendicitis in a high-lying appendix can cause right upper quadrant abdominal pain, as can right lower lobe pneumonia.

Pain and tenderness in the right lower abdominal quadrant suggest appendicitis. If nausea, vomiting, and anorexia are present with tenderness on rectal examination, along with fever and leukocytosis, appendicitis is the likely diagnosis. Crohn's disease, carcinoma of the cecum, and a distended cecum due to obstructing carcinoma of the left colon can cause right lower quadrant abdominal tenderness. A mobile sigmoid colon can actually lie in the right iliac fossa, so that diverticulitis in such a sigmoid colon can cause right lower quadrant tenderness, as can diverticulitis in a solitary congenital true diverticulum of the right colon. Gastrointestinal contents from a perforated gastric or duodenal ulcer can flow in a track down the right colic gutter, causing right lower quadrant tenderness.

Left lower quadrant abdominal pain and tenderness are frequently due to diverticulitis. If peritoneal signs are present, perforated sigmoid diverticulitis is likely. Carcinoma of the sigmoid colon can cause left lower quadrant tenderness as well. A perforated peptic ulcer can cause left lower quadrant tenderness when gastrointestinal contents drain down the left colic gutter.

Left upper quadrant tenderness is uncommon but can be caused by perforation of a peptic ulcer, a splenic infarct, or carcinoma of the splenic flexure of the colon. *Epigastric tenderness is caused by lesions of the foregut* such as pancreatitis, penetrating or perforated peptic ulcer, and even acute cholecystitis. Carcinoma of the pancreas may cause epigastric pain in association with back pain, but the stigmata of peritonitis are absent. Abdominal aortic aneurysm can cause epigastric pain and tenderness, the former radiating to the back.

Strangulated closed-loop intestinal obstruction can cause pain and tenderness anywhere in the abdomen, depending on the location of the strangulated segment. In females, gynecologic problems such as torsion or rupture of an ovarian cyst, pelvic inflammatory disease, and ectopic pregnancy can cause lower abdominal pain and tenderness, usually without associated gastrointestinal complaints such as nausea, vomiting, and anorexia. Mesenteric infarction can cause periumbilical pain without much tenderness.

The acute surgical abdomen is a potentially fatal entity if not promptly diagnosed and treated. For a patient with acute abdomen it is better to perform a laparotomy that turns out to be negative than to delay operation. Patients who are obese, who are taking steroids, or who are elderly may harbor an intraabdominal catastrophe without exhibiting the full set of signs and symptoms usually apparent in others. Very young patients also pose difficulties in diagnosis because of their inability to describe their complaint. Signs of an acute abdomen may be more subtle in a diabetic, perhaps because of diabetic neuropathy.

There are diseases that mimic the acute surgical abdomen; that is, they *seem* to require emergency surgery even though they do not. Examples of these conditions are pancreatitis, diverticulitis without perforation, terminal ileitis without associated complications, pyelonephritis, diabetic ketoacidosis, porphyria, gastroenteritis, sickle cell crisis, lead poisoning, mesenteric adenitis, salpingitis, and black widow spider bite. We try to avoid surgery for these entities, but since they can cause generalized abdominal pain with rebound and guarding, nonoperative therapy may not always be safe. To repeat, it is far better to perform laparotomy and find no surgically correctable disease than to delay operative treatment of catastrophic intraabdominal lesion with peritonitis. Skillful management of this treacherous problem is one of the major tasks of the general surgeon.

Recommended Reading

1. Silen W: *Cope's Early Diagnosis of the Acute Abdomen,* ed 19. New York: Oxford University Press, 1996.
2. Diethelm AG, Stanley RJ, Robbin ML: The acute abdomen. In Sabiston DC (ed): *Textbook of Surgery: The Biological Basis of Modern Surgical Practice,* ed 15. Philadelphia: W.B. Saunders, 1997, pp 825–846.
3. McFadden DW, Abdominal pain. In Zinner MJ, Schwartz SI, Ellis H: *Maingot's Abdominal Operations,* ed 10. Stamford, CT: Appleton & Lange, 1997, pp 351–360.

8

Intestinal Obstruction

Intestinal obstruction is an important part of the core of general surgery. Proper management requires a thorough understanding of its various causes, their natural history, and the best method of treatment. Understanding intestinal obstruction is critical for the general surgeon.

Many classifications can be applied to intestinal obstruction. The classifications are not mutually exclusive, and each one further delineates the exact pathophysiology of a given lesion. The obstruction can be mechanical or can be an adynamic ileus. The patient can have large bowel obstruction or small bowel obstruction. The obstruction can be simple or closed-loop and it may be extrinsic, intramural, or intraluminal (Table 8–1). These distinctions are further elucidated later in this chapter.

CASE 8–1

Extrinsic Obstruction; Small Bowel Obstruction
Due to Adhesions

A 55-year-old man was admitted with the chief complaint of cramping abdominal pain of 3 days' duration.

Six years before admission, the patient underwent appendectomy for a perforated appendicitis. He had a stormy postoperative course with high fevers and diarrhea, and a pelvic abscess was drained through the rectum under ultrasound guidance. Four years before admission he was admitted to the hospital with signs and symptoms of small bowel obstruction. He was hydrated and kept NPO; a Cantor tube was placed, and his intestinal obstruction resolved spontaneously. He had had a similar episode 2 years before admission, which again had resolved without surgery. Three days before the latest admission he began to notice cramping midabdominal pain followed by nausea and vomiting. He was anorexic and had last had a bowel movement 2 days before admission. He was instructed by his internist to come to the emergency department, and the surgeon was called in consultation.

Past medical history includes angina pectoris, well-controlled on medical therapy. His only previous surgery was as outlined.

Physical examination revealed the pulse to be 110 and regular. It was thin and thready. The blood pressure was 100/60 mm Hg. The mucous membranes were dry. Examination of the heart and lungs

Table 8–1. Classification and Common Causes (or Etiologies) of Intestinal Obstruction

I. Nonobstructive ileus
   A. Hypokalemia
   B. Peritonitis
   C. Ischemia of intestines
   D. Hemoperitoneum
   E. Retroperitoneal hematoma
II. Mechanical obstruction
   A. Small bowel obstruction
      1. Extrinsic
         a. Adhesions
         b. Incarcerated hernia
         c. Encasement by tumor (metastatic)
         d. Incorporation of bowel into abscess cavity
         e. Obstruction from metastatic implants
      2. Intramural
         a. Crohn's disease
         b. Lymphoma or primary carcinoma (rare)
         c. Stenosis from radiation enteritis
      3. Intraluminal
         a. Gallstone "ileus"
         b. Intussusception
   B. Large bowel obstruction
      1. Extrinsic
         a. Encasement in "frozen pelvis"
      2. Intramural
         a. Colon carcinoma
         b. Colon volvulus
         c. Stricture from
            i. Diverticular disease
            ii. Crohn's disease (granulomatous colitis)
            iii. Ischemic colitis
            iv. Radiation enteritis
            v. Lymphogranuloma venerum
      3. Intraluminal
         a. Fecal impaction

was otherwise unremarkable. Examination of the abdomen revealed it to be moderately distended with a tender mass in the middle. There was no generalized rebound or involuntary guarding. Bowel sounds were hypoactive. Rectal examination revealed no masses or tenderness.

The hematocrit was 55% and the white blood cell count was 14,300, with 86 polymorphonuclear leukocytes and 10 bands. The amylase was normal. The flat and upright abdominal x-rays showed multiple loops of distended small bowel with multiple air-fluid levels. There was in the midabdomen a loop of small intestine that was especially dilated and seemed to have lost its normal architecture. No air was visible in the large intestines.

On arrival in the emergency department, a large-bore intravenous line was inserted as the laboratory samples were drawn. The patient's blood was typed and cross-matched for 2 units of packed cells, and 2 L of normal saline was rapidly infused. A nasogastric tube was inserted, yielding 900 ml of feculent material. A Foley catheter was inserted, and 15 ml of dark urine drained. After administration of 2 L of normal saline, urine output was still minimal, so a central venous pressure line was inserted through the right subclavian vein. A chest x-ray showed no pneumothorax and showed the line to be in the superior vena cava at the junction with the right atrium. Central venous pressure was still 2 cm H_2O, and there was no vascular congestion on the film, so another liter of normal saline was instilled. Fifty cubic centimeters of urine flowed into the urometer, and there was more in the tubing. The pulse decreased to 90 and the blood pressure increased to 130/70. The central venous pressure increased to 7 cm H_2O, and the patient was brought to surgery.

At surgery, a closed-loop obstruction caused by adhesions was encountered. The obstructed loop of small bowel was gangrenous. Small bowel resection with end-to-end anastomosis was performed. In the recovery room, the urine output was again found to be marginal, and another liter of normal saline was infused. At this point, the patient developed respiratory distress, with rales halfway up both lung fields, along with a ventricular diastolic gallop; chest x-ray revealed pulmonary edema.

The central venous pressure line was replaced over a guidewire by a Swan-Ganz catheter. The pulmonary capillary wedge pressure was found to be 24 mm Hg, and the cardiac output 3.2 liters. Dopamine was given—4 μg/kg per minute, and the cardiac output increased to 5.5 L per minute, the wedge pressure decreased to 18 mm Hg, and urine output increased to 40 ml per hour.

By the next day the patient had been weaned from dopamine, and it was discontinued. The wedge pressure was 16 mm Hg. Cardiac output was 4.5 L per minute with adequate urine output. The patient was extubated, and the Swan-Ganz catheter was discontinued over the next 36 hours. The patient continued to be afebrile and his incision healed per primum. He was eating a regular diet and having bowel movements at discharge from the hospital on the ninth postoperative day.

DISCUSSION OF CASE 8–1

Diagnosis

CC. Patients with mechanical small bowel obstruction often complain of cramping abdominal pain. The pain is usually poorly localized because it is mediated by stretch receptors in the visceral peritoneum innervated by the autonomic nervous system. If the obstruction is low in the small bowel, the entire small intestine can fill with gas and fluid before vomiting occurs, and abdominal distention can precede nausea and vomiting. This is not always true even of a distal obstruction, however, since vomiting can occur early as a reflex.

HPI. The history of this present illness begins at the time of appendectomy 6 years earlier. Lower abdominal surgery is a frequent cause of postoperative adhesions, and adhesions are the most common cause of mechanical small bowel obstruction in a patient who has had previous surgery. The presence of peritonitis at the time of appendectomy would further predispose to the development of adhesions.

Two episodes of small bowel obstruction were treated nonoperatively by keeping the patient NPO, administering intravenous fluids, and instituting gastrointestinal decompression with a long tube such as a Cantor tube. Nonoperative treatment is sometimes acceptable when the patient is thought to have adhesions that are causing the obstruction and when there is no fever, tachycardia, abdominal tenderness, or leukocystosis.

Since adhesions tend to re-form, this nonoperative approach is sometimes employed to spare the patient multiple operations for lysis of adhesions. It must be remembered, however, that, once strangulation of the bowel has occurred, mortality and morbidity risks are increased substantially, and when any one of the previously mentioned ominous findings occurs, expeditious laparotomy is necessary. Constipation and obstipation (failure to pass flatus) may occur after the bowel distal to the obstruction has had time to empty.

PMH. It is important to obtain a past medical history, as this can affect perioperative management and can contribute to the diagnosis of the present illness. In this case, the history of atherosclerotic cardiovascular disease suggests that the Swan-Ganz catheter will be useful in management of this case. Since atherosclerosis is a generalized process, the presence of atherosclerotic cardiovascular disease might lead one to suspect mesenteric infarction from atherosclerotic narrowing of the visceral vessels. Mesenteric infarction can also be caused by a low-flow state secondary to decreased cardiac output. Mesenteric infarction could have caused this constellation of findings, but it turned out not to be the problem here.

Physical Examination. The tachycardia, hypotension, and thin, thready pulse are suggestive of hypovolemia. Volume depletion is often present when intestinal obstruction occurs, as bowel obstruction increases secretion of fluid into the bowel lumen and decreases reabsorption of fluid out of it. When strangulation is present, peritonitis ensues and fluid is lost into the peritoneal cavity, contributing to hypovolemia. Cytokines released by the septic process can cause further hemodynamic derangements.

Swallowed air accounts for the greatest percentage of intestinal gas, and this contributes to intestinal distention if it cannot pass aborad. The increased tension on the bowel wall first compromises lymphatic drainage, increasing the edema until venous pressure is exceeded, when outflow is further compromised. Finally, arterial inflow is compromised by the increase in pressure, and strangulation and gangrene occur. It can easily be seen that this occurs more quickly with a closed-loop obstruction than with a simple one (Fig. 8–1). Although the small intestine is usually relatively free of colon flora, obstruction causes proliferation of enteric bacteria, and this is the cause of feculent vomiting. When strangulation occurs, the intestinal wall loses its integrity and allows bacteria and their toxins to enter the blood, with resulting bacteremia and endotoxemia. Peritonitis also ensues.

Abdominal distention develops when the small bowel fills with fluid and gas. In a high intestinal obstruction, abdominal distention

SIMPLE OBSTRUCTION

CLOSED LOOP
OBSTRUCTION

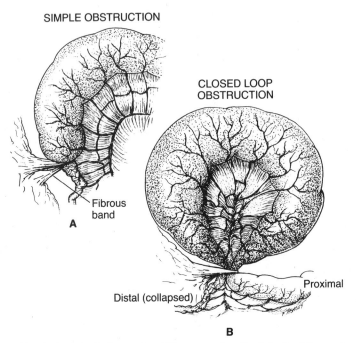

Fibrous
band

A

Proximal

Distal (collapsed)

B

Figure 8–1. Simple intestinal obstruction *(A)* occurs when the intestinal lumen is occluded in one place only. The entire bowel above the blockage may fill with fluid and gas before arterial pressure is exceeded and gangrene occurs. A closed-loop obstruction *(B)* occurs when the intestinal lumen is obstructed in two places. The intraluminal pressure can build up quickly, and gangrene of the bowel can occur early in the course of the closed-loop obstruction. A closed-loop obstruction may be impossible to see on plain abdominal films when the liquid contents displace all the gas.

may be absent, since fluid and air cannot pass into the distal gut. In this case, vomiting would be expected to be an early finding.

The tender mass is suggestive of a strangulated closed-loop obstruction and argues for expeditious surgery. By the absence of generalized rebound tenderness and involuntary guarding it can be inferred that generalized peritonitis has not yet occurred. Perforation of the gangrenous bowel into the free peritoneal cavity further exacerbates systemic sepsis—and fluid loss into the abdominal cavity (third-space loss). Bowel sounds are usually hyperactive early in intestinal obstruction, while the bowel is attempting to overcome the obstruction. When strangulation occurs, the intestines become adynamic and the bowel becomes silent. A negative rectal examination argues against a "frozen pelvis" or Bloomer's shelf from transcoelomic (across the peritoneal cavity) spread of carcinoma. This is helpful because intraabdominal carcinomatosis is one of the many possible causes of intestinal obstruction.

Laboratory Examination. Although no single laboratory examination can completely rule out strangulation or verify its presence, laboratory data can provide much useful information. The elevated hematocrit in this case is due to hemoconcentration. A patient with intestinal obstruction may be anemic, however, when the obstruction is caused by Crohn's disease or gastrointestinal malignancy. The leukocytosis with a left shift suggests that strangulation obstruction is occurring, and it usually would be wrong to treat such a patient nonoperatively. The amylase value may be normal, but elevation of the amylase level can occur with intestinal obstruction and one cannot assume that it implies pancreatitis. This point is important because the latter entity is often treated nonoperatively.

Diagnostic Imaging. The flat and upright abdominal x-rays are a cornerstone of diagnosis of intestinal obstruction. In small bowel obstruction, multiple loops of small bowel distended with gas are usually present, along with air-fluid levels in the small intestine. Usually, not much gas is found in the large bowel. The upright film is required to demonstrate air-fluid levels and to demonstrate free air if it exists from an associated condition such as a perforated duodenal ulcer or perforated sigmoid diverticulitis.

These conditions can mimic intestinal obstruction by virtue of the fact that the associated peritonitis may cause adynamic ileus, which gives the appearance of small bowel obstruction. The small intestines may be incorporated in an abscess caused by diverticulitis and may become obstructed from extrinsic pressure, a picture resembling small bowel obstruction. In any event, these entities require laparotomy, as does mechanical small bowel obstruction. Thus, it is not absolutely critical that they be specifically diagnosed preoperatively. A closed-loop obstruction may not be visible on plain abdominal films when all air in the obstructed loop is displaced by fluid.

Upright chest x-ray may give a better view of the diaphragm than upright abdominal film. Some patients are too sick to assume the upright position. For them, the left lateral decubitus view of the abdomen (also called the "right-side-up decubitus position") may be required to elicit the finding of pneumoperitoneum (free air in the abdominal cavity, usually indicating a ruptured hollow viscus).

With large bowel obstruction, the usual finding is a massively dilated colon. Perforation is impending when the cecum reaches 8 to 10 cm in diameter. With large bowel obstruction the small bowel may also be dilated if the ileocecal valve is incompetent. Adynamic ileus, such as may be seen postoperatively or with hypokalemia, peritonitis, or ischemia, causes the x-ray picture of multiple loops of air-filled small *and* large bowel.

Since the picture of large bowel obstruction can be caused by Ogilvie's syndrome (pseudoobstruction of the colon associated with old age, extended bed rest, and chronic cathartic abuse, among others) and since this syndrome of colonic ileus is sometimes treated nonoperatively by colonoscopic decompression, barium enema may be indicated to demonstrate mechanical obstruction of the colon. When this study is done, it should be performed with careful fluoroscopic monitoring to avoid instilling too much barium above a point of large bowel obstruction. The importance of this lies in the fact that the colon absorbs copious amounts of water, so that barium above a colon obstruction may become inspissated and convert a partial obstruction into a complete one. For the same reason, barium should not be given by mouth in the performance of an upper gastrointestinal series and small bowel series if colonic obstruction is suspected. When there is concern that a perforation may be present, a Gastrografin enema can replace a barium enema. Although barium gives more detail, the effects of Gastrografin are not so deleterious should extravasation into the free peritoneal cavity occur.

When the surgeon is faced with a partial small bowel obstruction and would like to localize the area of narrowing to help decide between nonoperative and surgical treatment, a small bowel series with barium may be helpful. It can localize the transition from dilated proximal to collapsed distal bowel and help to quantitate the grade of obstruction. The large amount of fluid (succus entericus) in the small intestine should dilute the barium thus administered and prevent it from obstructing the remaining lumen, if there is one (that is, if the obstruction is partial rather than complete).

TREATMENT OF MECHANICAL SMALL BOWEL OBSTRUCTION

As in other critical illnesses, resuscitation and definitive diagnosis must occur concurrently. The ABCs must be followed (establish an *a*irway, be sure the patient is *b*reathing effectively, and maintain *c*irculation). Once ventilation is found to be adequate, the circulation must be supported with a solution that approximates the electrolyte content of plasma. Physical examination and diagnostic tests are initiated as soon as the initial resuscitation is under way.

Preoperative Management

If the obstruction is high in the small intestines, the fluid lost from vomiting may be similar to gastric juice, with its high sodium, chloride, and hydrogen ion content. Thus, normal saline should be utilized for resuscitation, to help treat the expected hypokalemic, hypochloremic metabolic alkalosis. Once the patient's renal function is found to be adequate by demonstration of good urine output, potassium chloride can be added to the infusion to counterbalance the potassium lost in the urine owing to increased activity of the aldosterone pump. When the small bowel obstruction is caudad in the small intestine, Ringer's lactated solution may be used for resuscitation. At the time the large-bore intravenous line is inserted, blood can be drawn for laboratory investigation and for typing and cross-matching, as blood transfusion may be required if resection of intestine is necessary.

A nasogastric tube may be inserted to decompress the stomach, lessening the probability of vomiting and aspirating gastric contents into the lungs. The nasogastric tube prevents swallowed air from further distending the bowel. A nasogastric tube with two lumens (such as the Salem sump) may drain nasogastric contents more efficiently than a one-lumen nasogastric tube. A long tube with a mercury-weighted balloon at the end can be inserted into the stomach and passed into the duodenum under fluoroscopic guidance. This tube has the advantage of being carried into the small bowel by peristalsis, if it is still present, but it has the disadvantage of taking time to progress into the intestines. Thus, its use may not be practical if expeditious laparotomy is indicated. In Case 8–1, the nasogastric drainage is feculent because the obstruction has caused the small bowel to be colonized by colon flora.

The Foley catheter was inserted because hourly monitoring of urine output is an excellent way of keeping track of cardiac output and tissue perfusion. The sympathetic response to a low-flow state due to hypovolemia or left ventricular failure causes oliguria as one of its earliest manifestations. The central venous pressure line is an imperfect indicator of state of hydration because the compliance is so great on the right side of the circulation. Accordingly, the patient can be in left ventricular failure without a greatly elevated central venous pressure. In addition, hypoxia can cause pulmonary arteriolar constriction and pulmonary hypertension with an increased central venous pressure in the absence of left ventricular failure. However, a very low central venous pressure argues against fluid overload. A central line therefore can be used to gain some information during resuscitation in addition to serving as a route of venous access. Patients with several risk factors, such as obesity, malignant disease, previous venous thromboembolic event, age over 40, congestive heart failure, hypercoagulable state, and anticipated prolonged operation, should undergo prophylactic measures against deep vein thrombosis. This can be accomplished with low-dose subcutaneous heparin begun 2 hours preoperatively or with external pneumatic compression devices.

Surgery

The timing of surgical intervention is critical, since it is dangerous to administer anesthesia to an incompletely resuscitated patient. However, it may not be possible to restore hemodynamic stability to a patient with intraabdominal sepsis until the source has been surgically extirpated. Thus, the risk of delay may outweigh the risk of operating on a patient whose condition is unstable. Accurate judgment is vital here.

At laparotomy, a strangulated closed-loop obstruction was encountered. This necessitated segmental resection of the gangrenous small bowel and end-to-end anastomosis (Fig. 8–2). If surgery had been performed earlier, when the intestinal loop was still viable, lysis of adhesions—merely cutting the adhesive band(s)—might have sufficed. A simple obstruction is less likely to strangulate so early in its course, and lysis of adhesions (enterolysis) is more likely to suffice as treatment (Fig. 8–3).

Unfortunately, adhesions are likely to re-form, and the patient remains at risk for recurrent obstruction later. Because of this, it is not advisable to lyse all the adhesions in the abdominal cavity but only those that need to be lysed to relieve the obstruction. It is important, however, to ascertain that a second point of obstruction is not present, as leaving it untreated obviously would result in failure. Adhesions are a cause of extrinsic mechanical obstruction of the small bowel and, in fact, are the most common cause in a patient

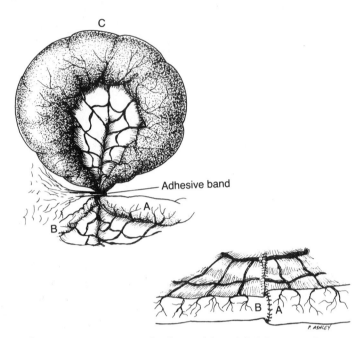

Figure 8–2. Gangrene can occur in the loop of bowel (C) between the two points of obstruction (A, B), which may be caused by one adhesive band. Treatment consists of resecting the gangrenous loop and anastomosing to each other the proximal and distal ends of healthy intestine (A, B). The vessels in the mesentery must be serially clamped, transected, and ligated in the process of resecting the dead segment of bowel.

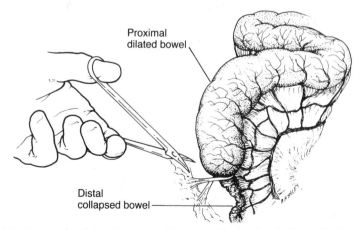

Figure 8–3. In simple obstruction caused by an adhesive band. Typically the proximal bowel is dilated and the distal bowel collapsed. When no devitalized intestine is encountered, treatment consists of cutting the obstructing adhesion. This operation is called *lysis of adhesions,* or *enterolysis.*

with a history of surgery. Hernia, tumor (by direct extension or by metastasis), and compression by abscess formation are other extrinsic causes of obstruction.

Postoperative Care After Lysis of Adhesions

Meticulous attention to the state of hydration is necessary, since fluid continues to be sequestered in the bowel lumen and in the peritoneal cavity for several days after surgery. Pulse, blood pressure, urine output, and central venous pressure or pulmonary capillary wedge pressure help in the assessment of volume status. A healing abdominal incision is painful and can interfere with coughing and deep breathing, predisposing to atelectasis and retained secretions; thus, aggressive pulmonary toilet—coughing, deep breathing, incentive spirometry—and ambulation must be encouraged. When peristalsis returns, as signaled by the return of bowel sounds and the passage of flatus and feces, the nasogastric tube can be removed and oral intake begun.

CASE 8–2

Intestinal Obstruction Due to Incarcerated Hernia

An 87-year-old man was admitted via the emergency department with a 3-day history of nausea, vomiting, and cramping abdominal pain.

Six years before admission, he first noticed a left inguinal hernia, for which a truss was prescribed by his family physician, who made the judgment that the patient's advanced age militated against herniorrhaphy. The patient had no further difficulties until 2 days before admission, when he developed some discomfort in the left groin and inability to reduce the hernia. One day before admission he began to experience cramping abdominal pain, and he came to the hospital after vomiting. His last bowel movement had been 2 days before admission.

Past medical history included osteoarthritis but was otherwise unremarkable.

Physical examination revealed sinus tachycardia with normal blood pressure. The mucous membranes were dry. The abdomen was moderately distended, with mild left lower quadrant tenderness but no guarding or rebound tenderness. Bowel sounds were absent. Rectal examination revealed no masses or tenderness. There was no stool on the examining glove. In the left groin, was a large, tender, erythematous bulge with edema of the overlying skin.

The white blood cell count was 13,000 with 86 polymorphonuclear leukocytes and four bands. The amylase reading was normal. The flat and upright abdominal x-rays revealed multiple loops of distended small bowel with multiple air-fluid levels. There were minimal air and feces in the colon. A loop of small bowel could be seen in the left inguinal hernia.

A left groin incision was made, the aponeurosis of the external oblique muscle was incised in the direction of its fibers, and the external inguinal ring was bisected, relieving the constriction around the bowel within the hernia sac. The sac was dissected free and opened, and a gangrenous segment of small bowel was delivered into the wound. This segment was resected, and intestinal continuity was reestablished with an end-to-end anastomosis. The small bowel was returned to the peritoneal cavity. Hernia repair was achieved by high ligation of the sac and by approximating the medial leaf of transversalis fascia and the conjoined tendon to the lateral leaf of transversalis fascia and the shelving edge of the ligamentum inguinale (Poupart's ligament). The patient had an unremarkable postoperative course and was discharged home on the 7th postoperative day.

DISCUSSION OF CASE 8–2

Hernia is the most common cause of small bowel obstruction in a patient with no history of surgery. (It is, of course, a common cause as well in patients with a history of surgery.) The potential for incarceration and strangulation is the principal rationale for prophylactic hernia repair. The age and life expectancy of the patient must be taken into consideration, however, since a patient with only a short time to live may have little likelihood of developing strangulation and may be a poor operative risk, even for relatively minor surgery. Inguinal and femoral hernias can be the cause of intestinal obstruction, as can umbilical, epigastric, and incisional hernias. Internal hernias occur when a hollow viscus protrudes through an intraabdominal defect; they can occur when a tear is inadvertently left unrepaired in the mesentery after small bowel resection (enterectomy) or when a space is left between an end sigmoid colostomy and the lateral abdominal wall. Incarcerated internal hernia can cause mechanical small bowel obstruction.

A known hernia can facilitate diagnosis of incarcerated hernia as the cause of intestinal obstruction; however, such a history may be absent, and incarceration and strangulation may be the first manifestations of a hernia. Tenderness, erythema, or edema in an abdominal wall hernia suggests strangulation and is an indication for emergency surgery. The signs and symptoms and radiologic manifestations of intestinal obstruction mandate expeditious surgery, as does the mere presence of a newly incarcerated hernia.

When a gangrenous segment of bowel is encountered, it can often be resected through the groin incision (Fig. 8–4). If the incarcerated segment of intestine appears viable after the tight ring is incised, it can be placed back into the peritoneal cavity and the hernia repaired without resection. If the hernia reduces during the induction of anesthesia and bloody fluid is encountered when the sac is opened, laparotomy is indicated to ensure that a necrotic loop of bowel is not present in the peritoneal cavity. An exception is when the loop that was incarcerated can be delivered into the wound with a Babcock clamp for inspection and when on inspection it is found to be viable.

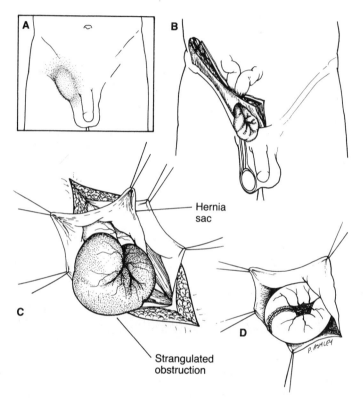

Figure 8–4. *(A)* An erythematous, warm, tender bulge in the groin suggests a strangulated inguinal or femoral hernia. *(B)* In the case of a strangulated inguinal hernia, the external ring provides the incarcerating "noose." In a femoral hernia, the lacunar ligament, the femoral sheath, Poupart's ligament, and the pubic bone incarcerate the hernia. *(C)* The strangulated loop of intestine can usually be grasped and delivered into the hernia incision once the sac has been opened. A small bowel resection and end-to-end anastomosis can be performed right through the hernia incision. The anastomosed bowel can be replaced into the abdominal cavity *(C, D)* and the hernia repaired in the usual fashion.

CASE 8–3

Intestinal Obstruction Due to an Intramural Cause: Crohn's Disease

A 23-year-old woman with Crohn's disease was referred to the surgeon for possible bowel resection.

Nine years before admission the patient underwent appendectomy for what turned out to be regional enteritis. Although she recovered and left the hospital, she remained chronically ill with intermittent cramping abdominal pain associated with nausea, vomiting, and anorexia. She had seven to ten loose bowel movements daily. She was treated with prednisone and a 5-ASA preparation, to no avail, and a small bowel series revealed partial obstruction in the terminal ileum. At surgery performed 3 months after the appendectomy, Crohn's disease involving the terminal ileum and ascending colon was discovered; accordingly, the patient underwent ileocolic resection. Postoperatively, she did well and was asymptomatic for the ensuing 9 years, until nausea, vomiting, and cramping abdominal pain recurred.

Barium enema and colonoscopy again showed recurrent narrowing in the ileum just proximal to the previous anastomosis and extending 20 cm into the remaining colon. Repeat ileocolic resection was performed. After 2 years' follow-up, she remained relatively asymptomatic, with only two loose bowel movements per day.

DISCUSSION OF CASE 8–3

Crohn's disease is *transmural* and, accordingly, has a propensity for obstructing the bowel lumen, in contradistinction to ulcerative colitis, which is *mucosal* and does not cause mechanical obstruction unless colon carcinoma supervenes (Fig. 8–5). Crohn's disease can affect the gastrointestinal tract in any site from mouth to anus. Thus, it can cause large bowel obstruction in the case of granulomatous colitis (Crohn's disease involving the colon) or small bowel obstruction in the case of small bowel involvement (regional enteritis, terminal ileitis).

In Case 8–3, Crohn's disease mimicked appendicitis at presentation. This is not uncommon, and appendectomy is indicated when the cecum does not appear to be involved at laparotomy performed inadvertently for terminal ileitis (Fig. 8–6) because the preoperative diagnosis was appendicitis. The advantage of doing the appendectomy instead of merely closing the abdomen is that, should symptoms recur, the diagnosis of appendicitis need no longer be considered. The disadvantage is that the complication of enterocutaneous fistula can occur if the appendix is removed from a patient with Crohn's disease. This patient did not develop a fistula but did remain sick after appendectomy. In the presence of partial obstruction, medical

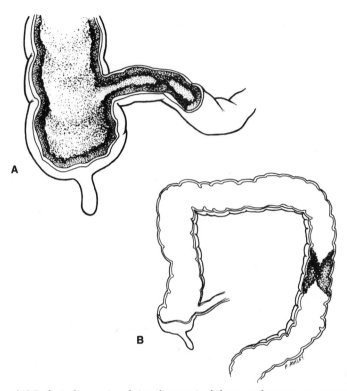

Figure 8–5. *(A)* Crohn's disease involving the terminal ileum and cecum can cause mechanical small bowel obstruction, as can Crohn's disease confined to the small bowel. The transmural nature of Crohn's disease predisposes to intestinal obstruction. Resection and end-to-end anastomosis is the treatment of choice. In this case, the terminal ileum and ascending colon require resection, and end-to-end anastomosis would be performed between the ileum proximally and the ascending colon distally. *(B)* Ulcerative colitis is a mucosal disease and does not cause colonic narrowing unless colon cancer is also present. This situation is not uncommon, however, since ulcerative colitis predisposes to colon cancer.

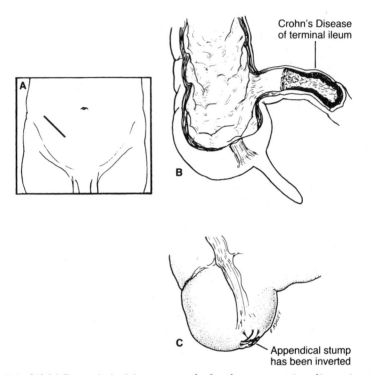

Figure 8–6. *(A)* McBurney's incision was made for the presumptive diagnosis of acute appendicitis. *(B)* At surgery, Crohn's disease involving the terminal ileum was discovered. *(C)* Since the cecum was not involved with disease, appendectomy was performed so that the diagnosis of appendicitis would never need to be considered again if the patient developed recurrent gastrointestinal symptoms from Crohn's disease. The segment of ileum was left in situ because there was no indication for resection, as no obstruction, perforation with abscess formation, bleeding, or fistulization could be attributed to that segment. Resection of areas involved with disease but devoid of complications would merely increase the chances of short-gut syndrome without preventing recurrence. Be that as it may, failure to thrive in spite of good medical therapy often necessitates surgery. This latter indication is less clearly defined than the others but is a common indication nonetheless.

treatment with prednisone and other agents is unlikely to be helpful and resection of the diseased segment usually is necessary (Fig. 8–7).

The patient in Case 8–3 had a recurrence of Crohn's disease 8 years later, as do a substantial percentage of Crohn's patients. For reasons that are unclear the typical site of recurrence is just proximal to the suture line. Because the recurrence was obstructing, repeat resection was indicated (Fig. 8–8). Because of the tendency of Crohn's disease to recur after surgery, its mere presence is not an indication for operation, as repeated small bowel resections could produce *short-gut syndrome,* the result of the absorptive surface being too small to sustain adequate nutrition. Thus, surgery is indicated for complications of Crohn's disease such as obstruction, sealed-off perforation with abscess formation, fistulization, and bleeding. Surgery is also sometimes necessary for persistent, severe symptoms refractory to good medical therapy. So-called skip areas, which are segments of diseased bowel apparent to the surgeon at the time of operation but that are separate from the segment causing the problem, should not be resected unless they are responsible for a complication. Their sacrifice could also ultimately lead to short-gut syndrome.

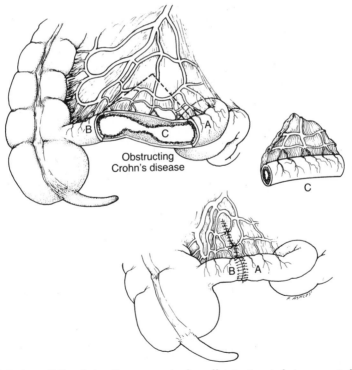

Figure 8–7. A partially obstructing segment of small intestine is being resected. Such a segment may be responsible for cramping abdominal pain, nausea, vomiting, and intractable diarrhea. Medical treatment is unlikely to be effective in the presence of such an anatomic abnormality.

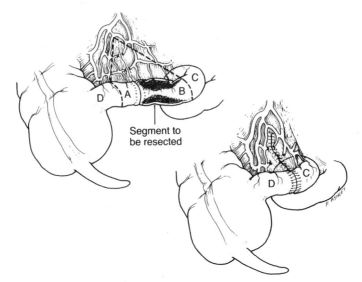

Figure 8–8. A recurrence of Crohn's disease just proximal to the previous anastomosis. This is the typical pattern. Repeat resection and end-to-end anastomosis are indicated.

Stenosis in a skip area can sometimes be treated without resection, by stricturoplasty. Stricturoplasties are analogous to pyloroplasties (see Fig. 9–3). Skip areas may sometimes be resected if they are in very close proximity to the area of major involvement, thus necessitating resecting of little additional intestine.

CASE 8–4

Intraluminal Cause of Mechanical Small Bowel Obstruction: Gallstone Ileus

An 88-year-old woman was admitted via the emergency department with a week-long history of cramping abdominal pain, nausea, and vomiting. Her last bowel movement was 3 days before admission.

Past medical history included insulin-dependent diabetes mellitus, hypertension treated with diuretics, and myocardial infarction 3 years before admission.

Abdominal examination on admission revealed a moderately distended abdomen and high-pitched bowel sounds. There was no abdominal tenderness, rebound, or guarding. Rectal examination was negative.

The hematocrit was 43 and the white blood cell count was 8000. Bilirubin and alkaline phosphatase levels were within normal limits. Flat and upright abdominal x-rays revealed air-filled loops of small bowel with multiple air-fluid levels. Air could be seen in the biliary tree. No radiopaque gallstones were detected.

A diagnosis of gallstone ileus was made. At surgery, a 4-cm gallstone was found to be obstructing the distal ileum, and enterolithotomy was performed (Fig. 8–9). There were dense adhesions in the right upper abdominal quadrant, where a cholecystoduodenal fistula was believed to be present. The surgeon decided against "lysing" the adhesions or attempting to deal with the biliary-enteric fistula, and the operation was terminated. The patient had an unremarkable postoperative course and was asymptomatic until 3 years later, when she had a massive cerebrovascular accident and died.

DISCUSSION OF CASE 8–4

Diagnosis

History. The symptoms of gallstone ileus are really those of mechanical small bowel obstruction; *ileus* is a misnomer here. The symptoms include nausea, vomiting, and cramping abdominal pain.

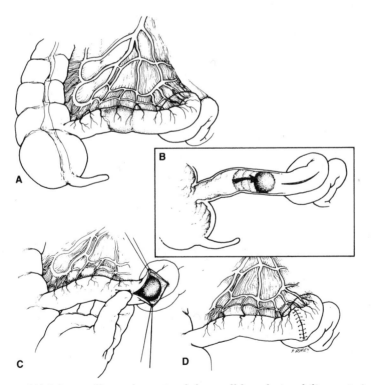

Figure 8–9. *(A)* A large gallstone has entered the small bowel via a biliary-enteric fistula (usually a cholecystoduodenal fistula caused by acute cholecystitis with a gallstone eroding through both the gallbladder and duodenal wall). It becomes lodged in the distal ileum, causing intrinsic mechanical small bowel obstruction. *(B)* The calculus is milked proximally to a healthier segment of bowel that has not been traumatized by the stone, and it is removed via a longitudinal incision (enterolithotomy). The incision is closed transversely to prevent narrowing *(C, D)*.

The pain may be intermittent, owing to the "tumbling phenomenon" (the stone lodges and then dislodges at several places in the small bowel until it comes to rest in the ileum, where the obstruction becomes permanent). The initially intermittent nature of the symptoms may cause the patient to delay seeking medical attention and the physician to delay advising surgical intervention.

The patient in Case 8–4 is typical of those with gallstone ileus in that she had several associated medical conditions that made her a poor operative risk. That no antecedent history of gallstone disease could be elicited is not uncommon.

Physical Examination. Abdominal distention and hyperactive, high-pitched bowel sounds are typical of mechanical obstruction. The absence of generalized tenderness, rebound tenderness, and involuntary guarding and the presence of bowel sounds suggest that strangulation had not yet occurred. Jaundice is usually absent in these patients, since the biliary-enteric fistula provides egress for bile into the gut, even in the presence of common bile duct obstruction from choledocholithiasis.

Laboratory and X-Ray Examinations. The white blood cell count can be normal if gangrene of the intestines from mechanical obstruction has not yet developed. It may be elevated, however, if there is an element of acute cholecystitis or obstructive cholangitis. The liver function tests may be normal, since the fistula has relieved the biliary obstruction. The abdominal films show the pattern of mechanical small bowel obstruction. Air in the biliary tree (outlining the bile ducts), when present, suggests gallstone ileus. Although only 15% of gallstones are radiopaque, a large, calcified gallstone identified in the right lower quadrant on x-ray in the presence of intestinal obstruction is pathognomonic for gallstone ileus.

Surgical Treatment

Because patients tend to be elderly and poor surgical risks owing to many serious associated medical problems, and because many of them have no symptoms referable to their cholecystoduodenal fistula after relief of intestinal obstruction by enterolithotomy, definitive biliary surgery generally is not performed at laparotomy. However, when the patient is febrile or jaundiced or has evidence of inflammation in the right upper abdominal quadrant at the time of the original operation, cholecystectomy and closure of the duodenum may be necessary (Fig. 8–10). Recurrent intestinal obstruction in the early postoperative period can be due to a second large stone that was already in the intestine but was missed at the first operation; the small bowel must be carefully examined at the initial operation to prevent this. In a small number of cases, a definitive biliary operation is required later.

CASE 8–5

Mechanical Large Bowel Obstruction

A 63-year-old man was admitted with a history of obstipation of 1 week's duration.

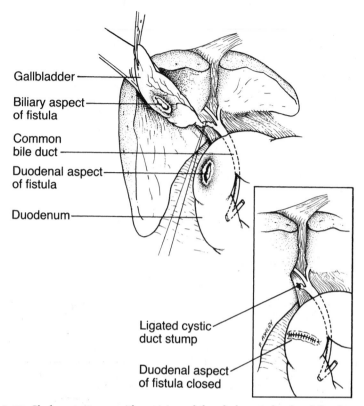

Gallbladder

Biliary aspect
of fistula

Common
bile duct

Duodenal aspect
of fistula

Duodenum

Ligated cystic
duct stump

Duodenal aspect
of fistula closed

Figure 8–10. Cholecystectomy with excision of the cholecystoduodenal fistula and repair of the duodenum in a patient who had undergone enterolithotomy for gallstone ileus. This definitive biliary tract surgery generally should be avoided in these patients, as they are usually elderly—and poor operative risks because of associated illnesses. Moreover, many can be expected to have no further sequelae of the biliary tract disease. When, however, the patient is jaundiced or appears to have cholangitis, definitive biliary tract surgery may be required during the initial operation, or later. Concomitant common bile duct exploration might be required.

Six months earlier, the patient began to notice blood streaked on the outside of his stool. He attributed this to hemorrhoids. One month before admission he had begun to notice a decrease in caliber of stool, and he had not had a bowel movement or passed flatus for approximately a week before admission. On the day of admission, he noticed severe right lower quadrant abdominal pain associated with nausea and vomiting of feculent material.

Physical examination revealed a temperature of 98.6°F. The pulse was 110 and thready. Mucous membranes were dry. The abdomen was markedly distended, with right lower quadrant tenderness. There was no involuntary guarding or generalized rebound tenderness. Bowel sounds were present. Rectal examination was negative.

The white blood cell count was 10,000 without a leftward shift.

Abdominal x-rays showed a markedly dilated colon with a cecum 10 cm in diameter. Upright chest x-ray revealed no free air under the diaphragm.

The patient was resuscitated with infusion of Ringer's lactate solution. A nasogastric tube was inserted, and 1000 ml of feculent material was aspirated. A Foley catheter was inserted, and after the initial fluid replacement, urine began to flow. Sigmoidoscopy to 25 cm revealed no intrinsic lesion. Barium enema was performed under careful fluoroscopic control, and an annular, constricting carcinoma was visualized 30 cm from the anal verge, obstructing the retrograde flow of barium. The patient was brought to surgery and a transverse colostomy was performed (Fig. 8–11). One week later, a bowel preparation was given, and sigmoid resection with end-to-end anastomosis was performed (Fig. 8–12). Six weeks later, the transverse colostomy was closed.

DISCUSSION OF CASE 8–5

Large bowel obstruction is discussed further in Chapter 11. It should be noted, however, that when the cecum approaches 8 to 10 cm, perforation may be imminent and prompt intervention is often re-

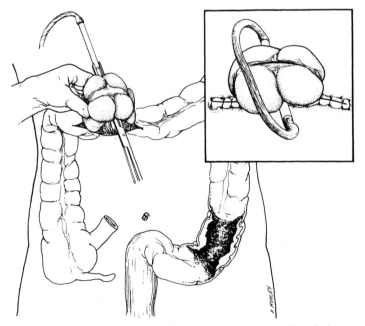

Figure 8–11. Annular carcinoma of the left colon is causing large bowel obstruction. The cecum tends to distend most and is at greatest risk for perforation. As the first stage this patient had a transverse colostomy to relieve the obstruction.

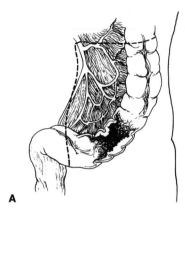

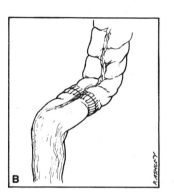

Figure 8–12. *(A, B).* The transverse colostomy was followed 1 week later with resection of the left colon and end-to-end anastomosis. The previous transverse colostomy relieved the obstruction and allowed the bowel to be prepped before the left colon resection. The third stage consisted of closing the transverse colostomy several weeks later.

quired. Rigid sigmoidoscopy may identify an obstructing lesion within 25 cm of the anal verge. If not, barium enema may identify a mechanical obstruction of the left colon, but this study must be done under careful fluoroscopic control and instillation of barium stopped as soon as the lesion has been indentified, since barium above a colon lesion can convert a partial obstruction to a complete one when the colon absorbs the water from its lumen. Furthermore, the barium may cause contamination if emergency colectomy is chosen. If there is concern about the possibility of perforation, a Gastrografin enema may be safer.

Prolonged bed rest or the presence of multiple medical problems can cause colonic pseudoobstruction (Ogilvie's syndrome), which can sometimes be treated by colonoscopic decompression. The presence of marked dilatation on x-ray, of tenderness, or of leukocytosis can be a strong indication for expeditious surgery without barium enema. Chapter 11 describes other approaches to large bowel obstruction and discusses other lesions involving the colon.

Recommended Reading

1. Tito WA, Sarr MG: Intestinal obstruction. In Zuidema GD, Nyhus LM (eds): *Shackelford's Surgery of the Alimentary Tract,* ed 4, vol 5. Philadelphia: W.B. Saunders, 1996, pp 375–416.
2. Jones RS: Intestinal obstruction. In Sabiston DC (ed): *Textbook of Surgery: The Biological Basis of Modern Surgical Practice,* ed 15. Philadelphia: W.B. Saunders, 1997, pp 915–922.
3. Ott DJ: Radiographic examination of the small bowel and colon. In Mazier WP, Levien DH, Luchtefeld MA, Senagore AJ (eds): *Surgery of the Colon, Rectum, and Anus.* Philadelphia: W.B. Saunders, 1995, pp 98–130.

9

Gastric Surgery

Elective gastroduodenal surgery has become less common over the past few decades. This has often been attributed at least partially to the development of effective antiulcer medications such as histamine H2 blockers, proton pump inhibitors, and antibiotic eradication of *Helicobacter pylori*. The surgical trainee must nevertheless be familiar with the principles of gastric surgery to effectively manage patients whose conditions are refractory to medical treatment and those who develop a complication of peptic ulcer disease. The case discussions in this chapter cover gastric and duodenal ulcers and their treatment, followed by a discussion of gastric carcinoma. Surgical clerks and surgical residents will find that familiarity with the fundamentals of gastroduodenal surgery will give them an area of common ground by which to converse with their mentors.

CASE 9–1

Perforated Duodenal Ulcer

A 37-year-old man presented to the emergency department with a 2-hour history of severe epigastric pain associated with nausea and diaphoresis. He stated that the pain began at exactly 8:00 PM and that he thought he was going to die. He had been experiencing some epigastric distress for the last year, exacerbated by hunger, spicy foods, and alcohol. He attributed this to the stress he was under at work and usually took proprietary antacid for relief. He had had no previous abdominal surgery.

Past medical history was negative for serious medical illnesses, and there were no known allergies and no bleeding tendencies.

Temperature on admission was 101°F and pulse was 120. His blood pressure was 100/50 mm Hg, and he was lying absolutely still on the stretcher, in obvious distress.

Examination of the heart and lungs was normal except for the sinus tachycardia and possible mild hypotension. He had a rigid, boardlike abdomen with diffuse tenderness, generalized rebound tenderness, and involuntary guarding. Bowel sounds were absent. Rectal examination was negative.

The hematocrit was 48 and the white blood cell count was

14,000, with a left ward shift. The electrolytes, BUN, blood sugar, and amylase levels were normal.

The flat and upright abdominal films and upright chest x-ray revealed multiple loops of air-filled small bowel with occasional air-fluid levels and with air and faces in the colon (ileus pattern). There was, however, free air under the diaphragm.

A large-bore intravenous line had been inserted on admission to the emergency department, and fluid resuscitation was instituted even before the laboratory and x-ray evaluations were begun. A Foley catheter was inserted to monitor the urine output. Treatment with broad-spectrum antibiotics was begun. The diagnosis of a perforated hollow viscus, probably perforated peptic ulcer, was made, and the patient was brought speedily to the operating room.

At surgery, a 4-mm perforation was identified on the anterior aspect of the duodenum, and approximately 1 L of bilious fluid was free in the abdomen. The perforation was closed with interrupted gastrointestinal suture, and an omental patch was placed. The peritoneal cavity was irrigated with warm saline and the incision was closed.

The patient was given an H2 blocker. The intravenous fluids were continued until the patient began to tolerate food on the 4th postoperative day, when they were discontinued. The incision healed per primum, and the patient was discharged on H2 blocker on the 8th postoperative day. After full recovery, the patient underwent upper endoscopy, and the presence of *H. pylori* was documented. The organisms were eliminated with a regimen that included bismuth and antibiotics.

CASE 9–2
Obstructing Duodenal Ulcer

A 47-year-old man was admitted to the hospital with a 1-week history of nausea and vomiting of undigested food. He had been diagnosed 15 years before admission as having peptic ulcer disease. His symptoms became worse every spring and fall but were usually controlled by avoiding spicy foods, alcohol, tobacco, and hunger. He originally had been treated with antacids—more recently with H2 blocker. His upper gastrointestinal series had been repeated on multiple occasions over the past 15 years. On some occasions it had revealed an active ulcer crater and at other times it had demonstrated complete healing. More recently, a scarred duodenal bulb was demonstrated. His last esophagogastroduodenoscopy revealed only scarring of the duodenal bulb. *H. pylori* had been treated with antibiotics and multiple subsequent tests suggested its complete eradication. He had been urged to stop smoking and to refrain from excessive alcohol, aspirin, and NSAIDS. He had been urged to consider surgery during his last exacerbation but had declined.

Past medical history included mild hypertension and a 30–pack-year history of smoking, although he stated he had "cut down" recently.

Physical examination on admission revealed a pulse of 110 and a blood pressure of 160/90 mm Hg. He vomited during the course of the examination. Examination of his lungs revealed breath sounds to be distant, and there were a few scattered rhonchi. Except for the sinus tachycardia, cardiovascular examination was unremarkable. Examination of the abdomen revealed it to be slightly tympanitic, especially in the left upper quadrant, and there was a succussion splash. There were no masses and no hepatosplenomegaly. Rectal examination was negative.

Laboratory examination on admission revealed hematocrit of 50 and sodium of 146 mEq/pr L, potassium of 3.4, chloride of 90, and CO_2 of 33. The BUN was 26. Abdominal x-rays revealed a markedly dilated stomach.

At admission he was kept NPO and a nasogastric tube was inserted. Intravenous fluids were begun. Over the next week, 2 L of nasogastric juice per day drained from the nasogastric tube. Endoscopy was performed, but the gastroscope could not be advanced into the duodenum. An upper GI series showed complete gastric outlet obstruction, believed to be the result of a duodenal ulcer.

A surgical consultation was called. By the time the patient was seen by the surgeon, the potassium value was 2.9, chloride was 80, and CO_2 was 40. The surgical consultant recommended correction of the hypokalemic, hypochloremic metabolic alkalosis with infusion of large amounts of normal saline and potassium chloride and institution of total parenteral nutrition. When the fluid and electrolyte derangements had been corrected, the patient underwent truncal vagotomy and antrectomy. The patient continued to produce large amounts of nasogastric tube drainage postoperatively. This was replaced with normal saline and small amounts of potassium chloride, and nutritional support was continued parenterally. On the 10th postoperative day the nasogastric output diminished and the patient began to have bowel movements. The nasogastric tube was removed, and a diet was instituted per os. The intravenous lines were discontinued, and the patient was discharged to home on the 16th postoperative day.

CASE 9–3

Surgery for Intractable Duodenal Ulcer

A 37-year-old man was referred to the surgeon's office with a long history of duodenal ulcer refractory to medical therapy.

While a freshman in college, the patient was admitted to a local hospital with syncope and black, tarry stools. He was treated with blood transfusions, and an upper gastrointestinal series at that time revealed a duodenal ulcer. He was treated further with antacids, bland diet, and phenobarbital. The patient discontinued the latter because it interfered with his studies. The patient would go for long periods without symptoms but would develop epigastric pain each fall and spring, although he never had another episode of bleeding. Five years before admission he came under the care of a gastroenterologist who demonstrated an active duodenal ulcer on esophagogastroduodenoscopy. He was treated with an H2 blocker, initially with good results. For the last 2 years, however, he had had frequent bouts of epigastric distress that occurred despite H2 blocker treatment, proton pump inhibitors, and treatment for *H. pylori.* Repeat upper G1 endoscopy revealed a duodenal ulcer crater, and the patient requested surgical treatment of his long-standing duodenal ulcer.

Past medical history was negative for heart disease, diabetes, and other serious medical illness. There were no bleeding tendencies and no known allergies. The patient drank two cans of beer per night and smoked one pack of cigarettes per day, in spite of the admonitions of his gastroenterologist.

Physical examination revealed a thin, white male in no acute distress. The vital signs were stable. The abdomen was scaphoid. There were no masses or organomegaly, and rectal examination was negative.

Laboratory examination, including hematocrit and hemoglobin, was entirely within normal limits.

The patient was admitted to the hospital and a highly selective vagotomy was performed, followed by an unremarkable postoperative course. By the third postoperative day, the patient had resumed a regular diet, and he was discharged on the 7th postoperative day. Six months postoperatively, in spite of resumption of maximal medical therapy, the patient remained symptomatic and repeat upper endoscopy revealed an active duodenal ulcer but no *H. pylori.* Further steps being contemplated by the gastroenterologist included determining whether the vagotomy was complete, ruling out gastrinoma (Zollinger-Ellison syndrome), and referring the patient for additional surgery (re-vagotomy and antrectomy).

DISCUSSION OF CASES 9–1, 9–2, AND 9–3

Surgery for peptic ulcer disease is surgery for its complications or for intractability. As medical therapy with H2 blockers, proton pump inhibitors, and antibiotics to eliminate *H. pylori,* and avoidance of smoking, aspirin, and NSAIDS is becoming more effective, refractory disease is becoming a less frequent indication for surgery, but it can be a marker of more aggressive ulcer disease and can make surgical success more difficult to achieve. Complications include bleeding, perforation, and obstruction. Bleeding peptic ulcer is covered both in this chapter and in Chapter 10 on gastrointestinal hemorrhage, whereas the indications of perforation, obstruction, and intractability are illustrated in these case histories and further elucidated in the discussion to follow.

Physiology

Before the surgical treatment of peptic ulcer disease is outlined, a short discussion on gastric physiology is in order. The gastric glands reside in the body and fundus of the stomach. They contain parietal cells, which secrete hydrochloric acid, and chief cells, which secrete the proteolytic enzyme pepsin. This enzyme requires an acid environment to be active. The G cells in the antrum of the stomach secrete gastrin, which causes release of hydrochloric acid from the parietal cells. A negative feedback system helps to maintain homeostasis, whereby a low pH (high acid concentration) shuts off gastrin secretion. Mucus secreted by glands in the body, fundus, cardia, and antrum may help to prevent peptic ulceration by protecting the gastroduodenal mucosa from the deleterious effects of acid and pepsin, although this is only one facet of gastric cytoprotection. Other protective factors include tight junctions between cells, blood flow to the stomach, local secretion of bicarbonate, cell replication, and resistance to back-diffusion of hydrogen ion.

Gastric Secretion. Gastric secretion is classically divided into three phases: cephalic, gastric, and intestinal. The *cephalic phase* is mediated by parasympathetic stimulation of the vagus nerves and is akin to the salivation observed in Pavlov's dogs in response to the sight or smell of food. In humans, the thought, sight, or smell of food causes increased gastric acid secretion as a result of vagal stimulation.

The *gastric phase* of gastric secretion occurs in response to distention from food in the antrum and in response to substances called secretagogues, such as peptides, amino acids, caffeine, and alcohol, which are known to increase gastric acid secretion when they come into contact with gastric mucosa. The gastric phase is mediated by the hormone gastrin. This hormone is released into the blood in response to secretagogues or antral distention and causes the parietal cells to secrete hydrochloric acid. Interestingly, vagal stimulation not only stimulates gastric acid secretion directly, but also plays a role in gastrin release, indirectly stimulating hydrochloric acid liberation. In addition, histamine causes gastric acid secretion because of interaction with H2 receptors. This is prevented by the class of antiulcer medications called H2 blockers. Proton pump inhibitors block a common pathway involved with acid secretion.

The *intestinal phase* of gastric secretion is probably least important. Its name refers to the fact that, even when food passes into the small intestine, it can cause release of hormones that stimulate gastric acid release.

Gastric Motility. It should be mentioned at this point that normal gastric motility is dependent on the vagus nerves. These nerves stimulate the antral pump to propel food through the pyloric sphincter and cause reflex relaxation of the pylorus. When the vagus nerves are cut during the course of an ulcer operation, the pylorus must be bypassed, resected, or rendered incompetent if gastric outlet obstruction is to be avoided. This is discussed further in conjunction with the technical aspects of ulcer surgery.

Diagnosis

Symptoms. Abdominal pain, usually epigastric, is a symptom of peptic ulcer disease. It is often *precipitated* by hunger or eating spicy foods or drinking alcohol; *palliation* may be achieved by eating or taking antacids. The quality of the pain is often described as gnawing, and radiation may be to the back if the duodenal ulcer is penetrating posteriorly into the pancreas. *Severity* is variable. Determination of the *timing* of the pain may prove helpful in the diagnosis of peptic ulcer disease, as it may be episodic, with exacerbations in the spring and fall. During the course of each episode the pain may occur between meals, when the patient is hungry, if duodenal ulcer is the cause. At night it often awakens the patient from sleep. Contrariwise, the pain from gastric ulcer may be exacerbated by eating.

Associated symptoms can include nausea, vomiting, and early satiety if the ulcer is causing gastric outlet obstruction, and melena or hematemesis if the ulcer is bleeding. If the ulcer has perforated, the pain may be severe and of sudden onset. The letters *PPQRST* and *A* constitute a device for remembering the adjectives used to describe the symptom of pain whenever it is encountered. If these adjectives are used to describe the symptom of pain elicited by the surgeon from the patient, they can contribute to early and accurate diagnosis. It must be recognized that the "classic" symptoms may not be present, and some ulcers are asymptomatic. The first manifestation can be a complication such as upper gastrointestinal bleeding or perforation and peritonitis.

Signs. There may be no signs (physical findings) referable to peptic ulcer disease; however, if the ulcer has perforated, the signs of peritonitis are likely to be present. These include generalized tenderness, rebound tenderness, involuntary guarding, a rigid, board-like abdomen, and hypoactive or absent bowel sounds. If the patient has upper gastrointestinal bleeding from a peptic ulcer, his only physical findings may be those of hypovolemia, such as tachycardia, a thin, thready pulse, and hypotension. There may be guaiac-positive, black, or maroon stool on the examining glove at rectal examination. An obstructing duodenal ulcer can result in tympany over the stomach in the left upper abdominal quadrant and can also result in the signs of hypovolemia if the patient has been vomiting frequently. A *succession splash* is the sound audible when fluid in a distended, obstructed stomach shifts as the patient moves. The patient may appear malnourished because of early satiety.

Laboratory Evaluation. Abnormal laboratory values in a patient with a perforated gastric or duodenal ulcer may include leukocytosis with shift of the differential to the left. Metabolic acidosis (low bicarbonate concentration) may be present if peritonitis has resulted in inadequate cardiac output and poor tissue perfusion, with increased lactic acid production. The BUN may be elevated because of hypovolemia (prerenal azotemia). A patient with a bleeding peptic ulcer may have low hematocrit and hemoglobin values, although it must be remembered that, even with massive blood loss, the hemoglobin and hematocrit can initially be normal, even though the intravascular compartment is markedly contracted and the patient is hypotensive, tachycardic, and oliguric. Over time, fluid from the interstitium returns to the vascular compartment as an important defense mechanism to support intravascular volume and maintain cardiac output and tissue perfusion. It is only then that hemodilution with a resultant drop in hematocrit occurs. Blood loss combined with intravenous chrystalloid infusion will also cause hemodilution and a fall in hematocrit.

An obstructing duodenal ulcer can cause profound fluid and electrolyte derangements because of either copious vomiting or massive drainage of gastric juice if a nasogastric tube has been inserted.

The typical abnormality caused by large losses of gastric juice is *hypokalemic, hypochloremic metabolic alkalosis.* The pathogenesis of this derangement is as follows: Large amounts of sodium, chloride, and hydrogen ions are lost in the gastric juice. (Potassium has a relatively low concentration in gastric drainage as compared with sodium.) Accordingly, the juxtaglomerular apparatus and macula densa of the nephron "sense" a contracted volume and decreased sodium load, respectively, activating the renin-angiotensin system to increase aldosterone secretion by the adrenal glands. This causes reabsorption of sodium in the tubules, but at the expense of potassium and hydrogen ion excretion; thus, the hypokalemic, hypochloremic metabolic alkalosis. The urine is acid, in spite of the metabolic alkalosis, and this phenomenon is called *paradoxical aciduria.* This abnormality can usually be corrected by infusion of sodium chloride and potassium chloride, although rarely infusion of dilute hydrochloric acid is required. The BUN may also be elevated owing to hypovolemia from gastric losses.

Imaging. Radiologic evaluation may be helpful in the diagnosis of peptic ulcer disease. When a perforated ulcer is present there may be free air under the diaphragm (pneumoperitoneum) on upright abdominal or chest films, although it is possible to have a perforation without visible free air on upright films. If a patient is so ill that he is unable to stand, a left lateral decubitus film may demonstrate free air. An upper GI series is performed by having the patient swallow barium and air and then viewing the esophagus, stomach, and duodenum under fluoroscopy, taking appropriate permanent films. A gastric or duodenal ulcer may be apparent as a crater that appears consistently on several films or as a retained fleck of barium. A scarred duodenal bulb, pseudodiverticulum, and an eccentric lumen may be seen. Gastric outlet obstruction would be suspected if barium failed to pass through the pylorus into the duodenum. The use of barium and air (double-contrast radiography) improves accuracy.

Esophagogastroduodenoscopy. Fiberoptic endoscopy has added a great deal to the management of gastric and duodenal ulcers. The gastroscope is passed per os through the esophagus and stomach and into the duodenum, and abnormalities affecting the mucosal surface are identified. A gastric ulcer requires that multiple biopsies be obtained because of the ever present risk that the ulcer represents carcinoma of the stomach. Carcinoma of the duodenum is uncommon, but it does occur. Bleeding of a gastric or duodenal ulcer can often be identified at endoscopy. An obstructing duodenal ulcer can prevent passage of the scope into the duodenum. Bleeding duodenal ulcers can be treated endoscopically with a heater probe or injection of epinephrine. It must be emphasized that, after medical treatment, healing of a gastric ulcer on esophagogastroduodenoscopy does not confirm that the lesion was benign, as even ulcers that are gastric cancers can "heal" temporarily. At the time of endoscopy, multiple biopsies and possible brush cytology of gastric ulcers must be taken to exclude gastric cancer.

Types of Treatment

Severely restrictive diets are no longer recommended, as they confer minimal (if any) benefit and can even make matters worse by increasing a patient's anxiety. Hunger should be avoided. Anticholinergic agents such as propantheline bromide (Pro-Banthine) are no longer used, because, among other side effects, they can cause gastric outlet obstruction by interfering with gastric motility and, given in doses that are practical, they do not really reduce gastric secretion. Antacids such as Mylanta may promote healing of a duodenal ulcer by raising the pH of the stomach, inactivating pepsin. H2 blockers have proved effective in promoting ulcer healing. Omeprazole can be used to block the proton pump, and sucralfate may be effective by coating the ulcer and mucosa. Patients are instructed to avoid NSAIDS, stop smoking, and limit alcohol consumption. The importance of eliminating *H. pylori* can not be overstated.

Surgery for duodenal ulcer is performed for *intractability* (failure of medical therapy), but the more concrete indications are really complications of peptic ulcer disease: obstruction, perforation, and GI bleeding. Before discussing the particular operation to be performed for each indication, I will briefly describe the various ulcer operations. Although detailed analysis of the different procedures is beyond the scope of this book, a basic understanding of the operations will provide a framework upon which the surgical trainee can build. Historically, *subtotal (75%) gastrectomy* was performed for peptic ulcer disease (Fig. 9–1). The rationale for this procedure was that gastric acid could be reduced by removing the G cells in the antrum and by removing much of the parietal cell mass (acid- and pepsin-producing cells). Although this operation was relatively effective, it was a major procedure that had a significant recurrence rate. In addition, there were significant complications such as weight loss because of early satiety from the decreased size of the reservoir. It is now safe to say that no definitive operation for duodenal ulcer is complete without some form of vagotomy.

Truncal vagotomy (Fig. 9–2) is the standard with which other types of vagotomy are compared. The left vagus nerve, on leaving the

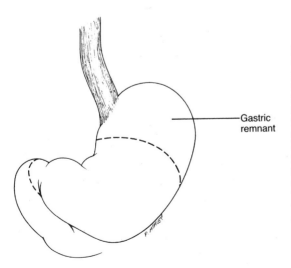

Gastric remnant

Figure 9–1. Subtotal gastrectomy was one of the earlier operations performed for duodenal ulcer. It consisted of resecting the distal 75% of the stomach, leaving a small gastric remnant. Its advantage was that it removed not only the G cells in the antrum but also much of the parietal cell mass. However, the small gastric remnant produced early satiety and weight loss, especially in thin women. Moreover, failure to include vagotomy neglected an important stimulus to gastric secretion.

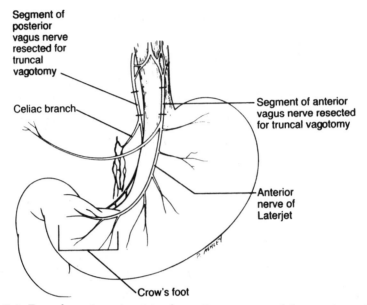

Figure 9–2. Truncal vagotomy consists of resecting segments of the anterior and of the posterior vagus nerve. The site of transection is above the hepatic and celiac nerves and interrupts the nerves of Laterjet. The latter fact necessitates a drainage procedure if functional gastric outlet obstruction is to be avoided. Interruption of the hepatic branch may contribute to bile stasis and gallstone formation, and interruption of the celiac branch to postvagotomy diarrhea.

chest and entering the abdomen, becomes the anterior vagus, and the right vagus rotates and becomes the posterior vagus nerve when it enters the abdomen. In a truncal vagotomy (or, more properly, *vagectomy*), segments of the anterior and posterior vagus nerves are resected between metal clips along their course in proximity to the abdominal esophagus. Truncal vagotomy not only decreases gastric acid secretion, which is helpful in the treatment of duodenal ulcer, but also interferes with gastric motility. A functional gastric outlet obstruction would develop if the competence of the pylorus were allowed to remain intact. Accordingly, truncal vagotomy must be accompanied by some form of drainage procedure, such as pyloroplasty (Fig. 9–3), gastroenterostomy (Fig. 9–4), or antrectomy (Fig. 9–5). Antrectomy, also called partial gastrectomy, destroys the competence of the pylorus by resecting it.

A truncal vagotomy results in interruption of the celiac and hepatic branches of the vagus nerve. Interruption of the former has the disadvantage of contributing to postvagotomy diarrhea, and interruption of the latter may contribute to denervation of the gallbladder, leading to biliary stasis and gallstones. To avoid these disadvantages, the technique of *selective vagotomy* was developed (Fig. 9–6). This entails cutting the vagus nerves below the takeoff of the celiac and hepatic branches. Both truncal and selective vagotomy interfere with

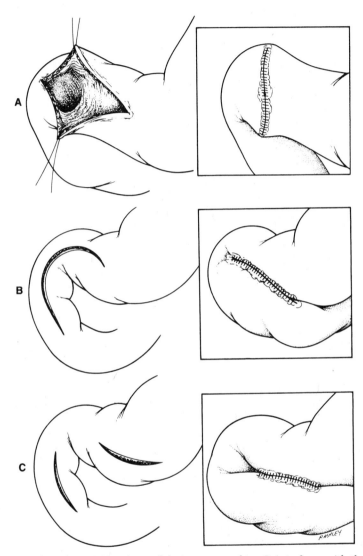

Figure 9–3. Pyloroplasty is one form of drainage procedure. It interferes with the competence of the pylorus, so that truncal or selective vagotomy does not cause gastric outlet obstruction. *(A)* Heineke-Mikulicz pyloroplasty entails opening the distal stomach and proximal duodenum longitudinally and closing them transversely, thus widening the pylorus Finney pyloroplasty *(B)* and *(C)* Jaboulay pyloroplasty destroy the competence of the pylorus, essentially by bypassing it; they are basically forms of gastroduodenostomy.

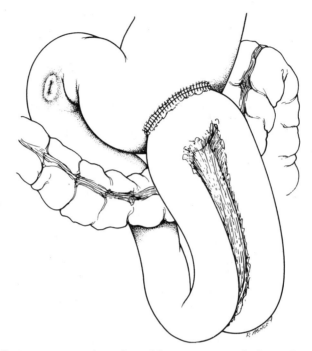

Figure 9–4. Gastroenterostomy is performed by anastomosis of a loop of jejunum side-to-side to the stomach. This form of drainage procedure can be performed in conjunction with vagotomy, although it is not ideal, as stomal ulcer can occur, especially over time. Its main application is for cases in which a duodenal ulcer causes so much scarring in the area of the duodenum that dissection in this area, which would be required for antrectomy or pyloroplasty, is unsafe.

gastric motility by denervating the antral pump and thus require a concomitant drainage procedure. A *highly selective vagotomy* (Fig. 9–7), also called *superselective vagotomy, parietal cell vagotomy,* or *proximal gastric vagotomy,* preserves the nerves of Laterjet to the "crow's foot." This maintains innervation of the antral pump, obviating the need for a drainage procedure. Because the celiac branch is preserved in both selective and highly selective vagotomy, postvagotomy diarrhea should not result, whereas it can be a serious complication of truncal vagotomy.

Surgery for duodenal ulcer seems to be a tradeoff between the more extensive operations such as vagotomy and antrectomy, which have lower recurrence rates but slightly higher morbidity and mortality, and the less extensive procedures such as vagotomy and pyloroplasty or highly selective vagotomy, which have lower morbidity and mortality but somewhat higher recurrence rates.

Indications for Gastric Surgery

Intractability. As medical therapy has become more effective, the need for surgery for intractable disease has decreased. Moreover,

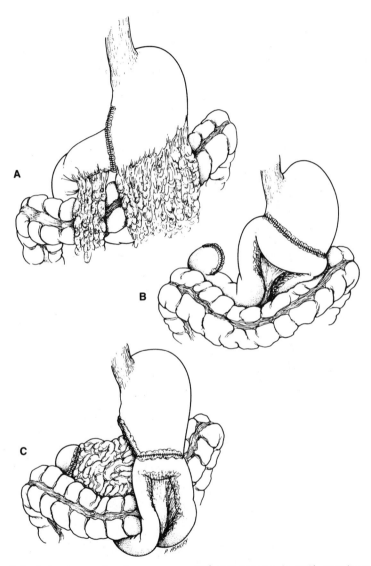

Figure 9–5. Antrectomy, also known as *partial gastrectomy,* is 50% gastric resection. Gastrointestinal continuity can be restored by Billroth I gastroenterostomy *(A),* in which the stomach is anastomosed to the duodenum, or by Billroth II gastrojejunostomy in the fashion of Polya *(B)* or according to Hofmeister *(C).*

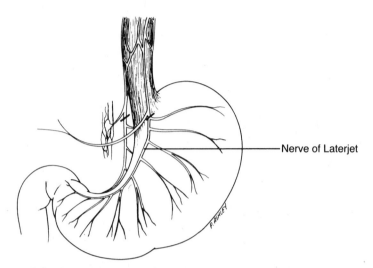

Figure 9–6. Selective vagotomy entails cutting the anterior and posterior vagus nerves below the takeoff of the hepatic and celiac branches, respectively. This has the advantage of preserving these branches and avoiding gallbladder stasis and postvagotomy diarrhea. The nerves of Laterjet are still interrupted, however, so that drainage must be performed.

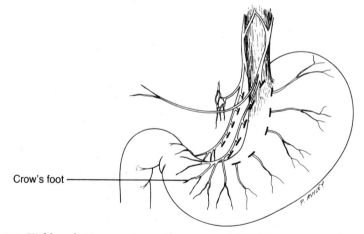

Figure 9–7. Highly selective vagotomy. The nerves of Laterjet are preserved so that the prepyloric pump is still innervated by the "crow's foot." The nerves of Laterjet are, however, isolated from the parietal cell mass; thus the other names, *parietal cell vagotomy* and *proximal gastric vagotomy*. It is important to continue the dissection 7 cm into the lower esophagus if the parietal cell mass is to be adequately denervated.

as medical management has become more effective and aggressive, patients refractory to maximal medical therapy such as H2 blockers, proton pump inhibitors, eradication of *H. pylori,* cessation of smoking, aspirin, and NSAIDS may have a more virulent form of disease for which the lesser operation, highly selective vagotomy, may not be effective. However, the tradeoff just outlined is certainly apparent here, since vagotomy plus antrectomy probably has the lowest recurrence rate, but vagotomy plus pyloroplasty and highly selective vagotomy have lower mortality rates and lower incidences of side effects such as the dumping syndrome (discussed later). Even though highly selective vagotomy may be less likely to control today's intractable ulcers, medical therapy can be added to it. It has lower morbidity and mortality rates than more extensive procedures, and more extensive surgery such as antrectomy can still be done later if highly selective vagotomy fails to cure the ulcer diathesis.

Obstruction. Duodenal ulcers can cause *gastric outlet obstruction.* In some cases the obstruction resolves with nasogastric tube drainage, fluid resuscitation, and medical therapy, including nutritional support as edema resolves. Endoscopic dilatation of the stricture may help postpone or even eliminate the need for surgery; however, obstructing duodenal ulcers may require operation. A procedure consisting of vagotomy and hemigastrectomy (antrectomy) would be reasonable in this setting, although many complications of ulcer surgery are caused in attempts to close a scarred duodenum after gastrectomy. If scarring in this area makes gastrectomy hazardous, a vagotomy may be done and drainage can be provided by gastroenterostomy, the scarred duodenum being avoided entirely. Similarly, pyloroplasty may be problematic in the face of a scarred duodenum. Some authors have advocated highly selective vagotomy combined with gastrotomy and dilatation of the narrowed duodenal bulb with dilators. Experience with this technique is limited, and its merit has not yet been determined. It should be remembered that copious nasogastric drainage in the preoperative period in a patient with an obstructing duodenal ulcer can cause hypokalemic, hypochloremic metabolic alkalosis. This is due to loss of sodium, chloride, and hydrogen ions from the stomach and to the loss of hydrogen ions and potassium ions in the renal tubules because of increased aldosterone secretion. Preoperative correction with sodium chloride and potassium chloride is necessary.

Perforation. A *perforated duodenal ulcer* presents as an acute surgical emergency. The first priority is, of course, resuscitation, and resuscitation is predicated on the *ABC*s (establish an *a*irway, make sure the patient is *b*reathing adequately, and then maintain the *c*irculation).

The admonition to establish an airway if necessary and to make sure the patient is ventilating adequately is more than theoretical in this setting, as intraabdominal sepsis from a perforated ulcer or from any other cause can result in respiratory insufficiency, which can evolve into circulatory collapse. It is important that the circulation be maintained, as it is jeopardized by several phenomena associated with perforated ulcer.

First, gastroduodenal contents free in the peritoneal cavity produce peritonitis, with sequestration of fluid in the peritoneal cavity (so-called third-space loss). This fluid is lost to the vascular compartment, and the resulting hypovolemia can cause inadequate cardiac output and inadequate tissue perfusion, obvious manifestations of which include tachycardia, hypotension, oliguria, and decreased central venous and wedge pressures if such measurements are available.

In addition, the acute insult can cause a vasovagal response, resulting in vasodilatation and hypotension. If there is a delay between perforation and operation, the bacteria in the gastroduodenal contents can set up bacterial peritonitis, manifested by sepsis, and possibly septic shock. In addition to vasodilatation and shunting at the periphery resulting in decreased oxygen consumption, a myocardial depressant factor may be liberated.

The treatment of choice for perforated duodenal ulcer is rapid resuscitation followed by prompt operation. Although series of nonoperative management have been reported, expeditious surgery is the safe, conservative approach. Resuscitation consists of volume replacement with a balanced salt solution such as normal saline or Ringer's lactate. Although use of 5% albumin is controversial, it can be added to the regimen. An inotropic agent such as dopamine can be added if cardiac output is down in the face of adequate wedge pressure.

Although omentum or contiguous organs sometimes seal off the perforation, one cannot rely on this and prompt operation is necessary to stop continued contamination of the peritoneal cavity. The conservative management is to oversew the perforation, buttressing it with an omental patch (Fig. 9–8). The gross contamination is removed, and the peritoneal cavity is irrigated with copious amounts of saline in the hope of minimizing the inoculum with which the body's immune system must cope.

In selected cases, a definitive ulcer operation such as highly selective vagotomy plus omental patch, vagotomy and pyloroplasty with the pyloroplasty incision made through the perforation, or vagotomy and antrectomy (in which the perforation is included in the resection) can be done in the hope of minimizing the possibility of recurrence. These definitive antiulcer operations might be appropriate when the interval between perforation and surgery is short (and thus bacterial peritonitis is unlikely to have developed), when the patient is a good surgical risk whose condition was hemodynamically stable with no major associated illnesses, and when the patient has a long history of peptic ulcer disease, including previous complications refractory to maximal medical treatment (making it unlikely that he would remain asymptomatic were definitive surgery not done). It must be emphasized that, when the perforated ulcer is gastric in origin biopsy or resection *must* be done to rule out gastric cancer.

Bleeding. Treatment of a bleeding duodenal ulcer requires rapid resuscitation. After initial resuscitation with a balanced salt solution (crystalloid) such as normal saline or Ringer's lactate solution, blood may be required if the bleeding was profuse. Replacement usually consists of packed red blood cells. Fresh-frozen plasma may be added if there is copious blood loss and large-volume transfusion in order to replace clotting factors and prevent a "washout coagulopathy." Platelet administration may be required with massive transfusion.

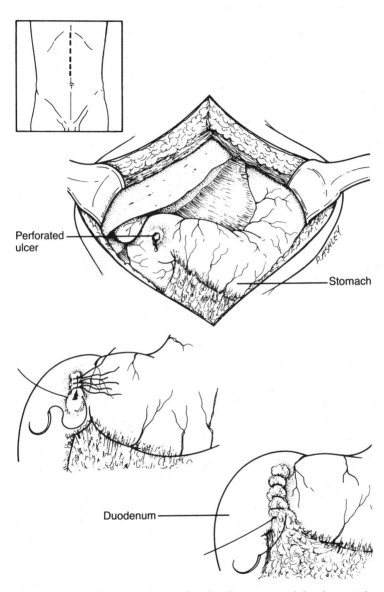

Figure 9–8. A perforated duodenal ulcer is closed with sutures, and the closure is buttressed with a patch of omentum. When the anterior duodenal wall is too edematous and friable to be approximated directly by sutures, an omental patch can be employed without first suturing the hole closed. Notice that the sutures used in duodenal closure can be left long, so that they can be used to tie the patch of omentum in place.

Prevention of hypothermia with a rapid infuser-warmer is important, as hypothermia can cause peripheral vasoconstriction, push the oxyhemoglobin dissociation curve to the left (making it more difficult to deliver oxygen to the tissues), depress the myocardium, and cause coagulopathy with diffuse bleeding. Early endoscopy is important with upper GI bleeding of any sort. Endoscopic therapy with the heater probe or with injection of epinepherine may stop the bleeding. If a bleeding duodenal ulcer is identified, surgery must be considered. A visible vessel in the ulcer bed suggests that nonoperative endoscopic therapy is unlikely to be successful and that surgery will be necessary. Blood loss of approximately 30% of the patient's blood volume or recurrent bleeding after initial stabilization indicates the need for surgery. The older the patient and the greater the magnitude of associated disease are, the earlier one needs to consider operation. These very sick people can ill afford to cope with the hemodynamic shifts that occur with repeated bleeding and transfusion.

Gastroduodenotomy with ligation of the bleeding point (often the gastroduodenal artery in a posterior duodenal ulcer) and closure of the gastroduodenotomy as a pyloroplasty, in association with truncal vagotomy, is an effective and mainstream treatment for bleeding duodenal ulcer (Fig. 9–9). In exceptional low-risk patients whose aggressive duodenal ulcer disease is refractory to maximal medical therapy, vagotomy plus antrectomy may be considered. This procedure has a lower recurrence rate but a slightly higher mortality rate. When there is bleeding from a gastric ulcer, surgery should be undertaken earlier, as patients tend to be older, bleeding is less likely to stop, and the specter of gastric carcinoma is ever present. The treatment of choice in bleeding gastric ulcer would be to excise the ulcer or include it as part of a distal gastrectomy, as malignancy must be considered.

Complications of Gastric Surgery

Acute Complications. Complications of ulcer surgery need to be considered. Obviously, complications associated with general anesthesia and major surgery in general, with its attendant hemodynamic shifts, can occur—myocardial infarction, atelectasis, postoperative pneumonia, deep vein thrombosis, and renal failure. Postoperative hemorrhage from a suture line can occur, and, because of the stomach's abundant blood supply, may be more common after gastric surgery than in some other types of intraabdominal procedures. Rebleeding from the ulcer itself can occur after vagotomy and pyloroplasty. After partial gastrectomy and Billroth II gastrojejunostomy, leakage from the oversewn duodenal stump is a particularly treacherous complication. This tends to occur approximately 1 week postoperatively and can lead to peritonitis or subphrenic abscess. Emergency reoperation may be required. If the effluent finds its way out through a drain, a duodenal fistula may occur instead of the complications mentioned previously. In the latter situation, the patient may be kept NPO and placed on total parenteral nutrition (TPN), in the hope that the fistula will close in approximately 6 to 12 weeks without needing reoperation.

There are several long-term complications of ulcer surgery, and the

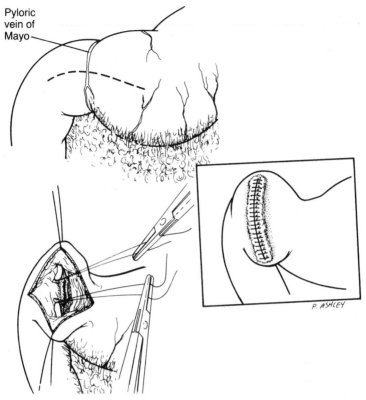

Pyloric
vein of
Mayo

P. ASHLEY

Figure 9–9. If a bleeding duodenal ulcer has first been identified by endoscopy, gastroduodenotomy can be performed, extending 3.5 cm onto the stomach and 2.5 cm onto the duodenum. After the bleeding gastroduodenal artery at the base of the ulcer has been ligated, the longitudinal gastroduodenotomy can be closed transversely, as in a Heineke-Mikulicz pyloroplasty.

surgical trainee should be familiar with their frequency and the degree of discomfort they cause patients so that he can make intelligent judgments about the benefits and risks of surgery for peptic ulcer disease.

Postvagotomy Diarrhea. Even though postvagotomy diarrhea is disabling in only a small percentage of patients after truncal vagotomy, in this relatively small number it can detract significantly from the quality of life. Avoidance of this complication is an argument for selective or highly selective vagotomy rather than truncal vagotomy, since section of the celiac branch of the vagus nerve is thought to play a causal role in postvagotomy diarrhea. Antidiarrheal agents such as loperamide or the somatostatin analogue octreotide may prove useful. As a last resort, postvagotomy diarrhea is sometimes treated by interposing an antiperistaltic 7- to 10-cm segment of jejunum 80 to 100 cm from the ligament of Treitz. This slows intestinal transit, reducing the diarrhea.

The Dumping Syndrome. Dumping is a classic postgastrectomy syndrome caused by rapid influx of hyperosmolar gastric contents into the small bowel, resulting from the absence of pyloric competence and the inability after vagotomy of the stomach to relax in order to accommodate a bolus of food. Since simple sugars have high osmotic pressure, liquids containing them, such as soft drinks, are especially likely to cause the problem. Symptoms of the dumping syndrome include cramps, diaphoresis, palpitations, and flushing. They are believed to be precipitated by fluid volume leaving the intravascular compartment in favor of the intestinal tract because of its high osmotic pressure. Hypovolemia or intestinal distention or stimulation of release of intestinal hormones such as serotonin, and vasoactive bradykinin VIP, or GIP can cause the symptoms, and administration of the somatostatin analogue octreotide may mitigate the symptoms. A 10-cm antiperistaltic loop of jejunum can be interposed between the remaining sections of the stomach and duodenum to treat dumping syndrome (Fig. 9–10A). Another surgical approach is conversion of the partial gastrectomy to a Roux-en-Y reconstruction,

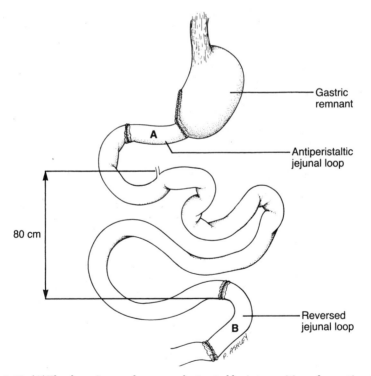

Gastric
remnant

Antiperistaltic
jejunal loop

80 cm

Reversed
jejunal loop

Figure 9–10. *(A)* The dumping syndrome can be treated by interposition of an antiperistaltic jejunal loop between stomach and duodenum after antrectomy and Billroth I gastroenterostomy. *(B)* A reversed jejunal loop placed 80 to 100 cm from the ligament of Treitz may be useful in treating postvagotomy diarrhea. Although the two operations are depicted in the same diagram, they are used to treat two different conditions.

which may slow down peristalsis by transecting neural pathways. Both operations are very significant, have highly unpredictable results, and should be considered only in the most disabling cases, when dumping is well-documented, other causes of the symptom complex have been excluded, and medical therapy has been exhausted.

Afferent Loop Syndrome. Afferent loop syndrome is caused by the buildup of bile under pressure, presumably resulting from kinking of a long afferent limb after gastrectomy and Billroth II gastrojejunostomy. This presents as bloating and pain relieved by projectile vomiting. Complete obstruction of the afferent loop can lead to gangrene. Remedial surgery for afferent loop syndrome may consist of resection of the previous anastomosis with shortening of the afferent limb, or it may consist of enteroenterostomy (Fig. 9–11).

Bile Reflux Gastritis. Bile reflux gastritis occurs as a result of bile reflux into the gastric remnant. Because after gastrectomy bile usually refluxes into the stomach, it is not clear why some patients get bile reflux gastritis and others do not. In any event, the treatment is to divert the bile away from the stomach by constructing a Roux-en-Y gastrojejunostomy (Fig. 9–12). This would be very ulcerogenic if complete vagotomy and adequate gastric resection had not been performed previously, because the alkalinizing bile is diverted away from the gastroenterostomy stoma. Before considering surgery for bile reflux gastritis, one must be comfortable that the symptoms are severe enough to warrant it and that other potential causes of the symptoms have been ruled out.

Rebound Hypoglycemia ("Delayed Dumping"). So-called delayed dumping that occurs several hours after meals is thought to be rebound hypoglycemia caused by a high level of endogenous insulin secretion caused by rapid influx of simple sugars into the gut. When conservative measures (such as avoidance of glucose-rich drinks) and administration of octreotide fail to relieve symptoms of dumping, interposition of an antiperistaltic loop of jejunum (see Fig. 9–10) has been used.

Recurrent Ulcers. As mentioned earlier, surgery for peptic ulcer seems to provide a choice between (1) procedures such as truncal vagotomy and antrectomy (hemigastrectomy), which have the lowest recurrence rates but somewhat higher rates of mortality, and of postgastrectomy syndromes such as dumping, and (2) procedures such as truncal vagotomy and pyloroplasty, or highly selective vagotomy without a drainage procedure, which have lower mortality rates and incidences of dumping. Recurrence after vagotomy and gastroenterostomy or vagotomy, antrectomy, and Billroth II gastrojejunostomy takes the form of marginal (otherwise known as *stomal* or *jejunal*) ulcer (Fig. 9–13). This is an ulcer on the jejunal side of the anastomosis, and it can cause recurrent symptoms, bleed, or perforate. The perforation may be into the colon—a gastrojejunocolic fistula (Fig. 9–14). The classic causes of recurrent ulcer after vagotomy and antrectomy are (1) incomplete vagotomy, (2) retained and excluded antrum, (3) Zollinger-Ellison syndrome, and (4) inadequate antrectomy.

Incomplete vagotomy is the most common cause of recurrence. It can be treated by completing the vagotomy. This is sometimes performed transthoracically. The pathophysiology of marginal ulcer after

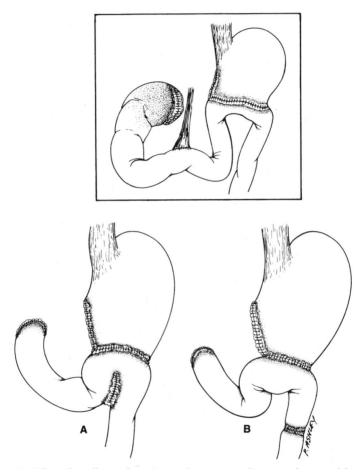

Figure 9–11. When the afferent loop is too long, it can become obstructed by kinking. Chronic manifestations of this include bloating relieved by bilious vomiting; gangrene of the afferent loop may be an acute manifestation. Operative treatment may consist of *(A)* enteroenterostomy, in which the afferent limb is decompressed into the efferent limb, or *(B)* resection of the gastrojejunostomy and shortening of the afferent limb.

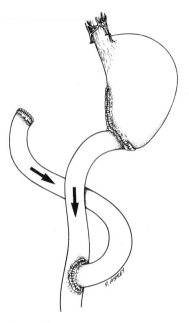

Figure 9–12. Bile reflux gastritis can be treated by Roux-en-Y conversion of the gastroenterostomy. This diverts bile away from the stomach and may be curative. A *caveat:* This operation is ulcerogenic when the vagotomy is not complete or the extent of antrectomy is insufficient.

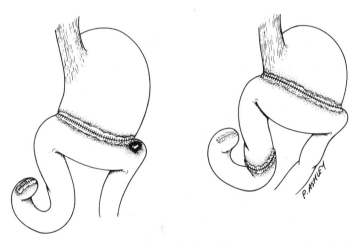

Figure 9–13. A recurrent ulcer on the jejunal side of the anastomosis (marginal or stomal ulcer) can occur if the vagotomy has been incomplete or the extent of gastrectomy insufficient. This may present as recurrent pain, upper gastrointestinal bleeding, a perforation, or a gastrojejunocolic fistula. The anastomosis is resected along with additional stomach. A jejunojejunal anastomosis and a new gastrojejunostomy are fashioned, and the vagotomy is completed if it was inadvertently left incomplete.

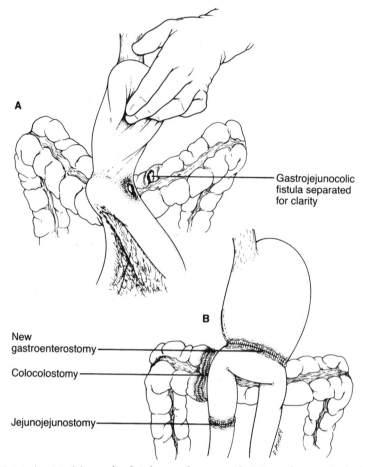

Gastrojejunocolic
fistula separated
for clarity

New
gastroenterostomy

Colocolostomy

Jejunojejunostomy

Figure 9–14. A gastrojejunocolic fistula may be a manifestation of a marginal ulcer *(A)*. This is treated surgically by resection of the anastomosis along with additional stomach and the involved segment of colon, and gastrointestinal continuity is restored by jejunojejunostomy, gastrojejunostomy, and colocolonic anastomosis *(B)*. Repeat vagotomy is performed when indicated.

retained and excluded antrum is a lesson in gastric physiology. There is ordinarily a negative feedback mechanism: acid bathing the antrum lowers its pH, shutting off gastrin release and thus decreasing acid production. If a bit of antrum is included mistakenly in the duodenal stump—that is, if the pylorus is left behind (Fig. 9–15)—the excluded antrum is no longer bathed in stomach acid. The antrum secretes large amounts of gastrin, unopposed by the usual negative feedback mechanism, and the excess acid leads to recurrent ulceration. Zollinger-Ellison syndrome occurs when a gastrin-secreting tumor (gastrinoma) develops in the islet cells of the pancreas. If this is not identified at the first operation and vagotomy plus partial gastrectomy

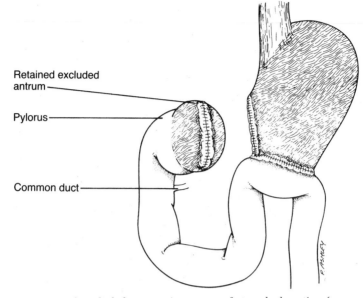

Retained excluded
antrum

Pylorus

Common duct

Figure 9–15. Retained excluded antrum is a cause of stomal ulceration (recurrent ulceration). The excluded antral segment, which is released from the inhibiting influence of gastric acid, secretes large amounts of gastrin. The gastrin stimulates copious acid secretion and resultant stomal ulceration.

is performed, the ulcer will recur. Zollinger-Ellison syndrome should be suspected when the peptic ulcers are multiple or atypical (e.g., beyond the first part of the duodenum). If the serum gastrin determination is greater than 1000 pg/mL in a patient with atypical ulcers, the diagnosis of Zollinger-Ellison syndrome is likely. Sometimes provocative tests—with secretin injection, calcium infusion, or a test meal—may be necessary to make the diagnosis if the serum gastrin level is borderline. Since gastrin-secreting tumors may be multifocal, hard to localize, and hard to resect, total gastrectomy may palliate by removing the end-organ. Maximal medical therapy directed at suppressing acid secretion can sometimes obviate the need for surgery.

GASTRIC CANCER

The incidence of gastric cancer is decreasing in the United States, but it still occurs frequently enough to command the surgeon's attention. Gastric cancer occurs so frequently in Japan that mass screening efforts are cost effective, and in that country screening with endoscopy and contrast studies may be responsible for the high prevalence of early, curable lesions. Foods that are converted to nitrites have been implicated in the causation of gastric cancer. Moreover, bacteria in the gastric remnant after previous gastric surgery are thought to increase the amount of nitrites in the stomach, predisposing to gastric cancer. Accordingly, some have advocated long-term screening of patients after gastric surgery. *H. pylori* may play an role.

Symptoms of gastric cancer include abdominal pain, melena, hematemesis, early satiety, anorexia, weight loss, nausea, and vomiting. Physical findings may include an epigastric mass. The presence of a left supraclavicular node (Virchow's node), Bloomer's shelf, Sister Joseph's nodule (metastatic implant in the umbilicus), an enlarged, nodular liver, or a fluid wave from ascites suggests that the gastric cancer is incurable. Iron deficiency anemia obligates the clinician to suspect carcinoma of the stomach and of the colon. Both organs need to be screened by endoscopy or barium studies, or both. Healing of a gastric ulcer on medical treatment, as demonstrated by upper GI series or endoscopy, does not rule out gastric carcinoma. One must perform esophagogastroduodenoscopy and multiple biopsies—and possibly brush cytology of the gastric ulcer—to confidently rule out cancer of the stomach.

The usual operation for carcinoma of the midstomach or antrum is subtotal gastrectomy (Fig. 9–16). Most patients have involvement of the regional lymph nodes at the time of surgery. Those with negative lymph nodes and no tumor involvement of the serosal surface of the stomach

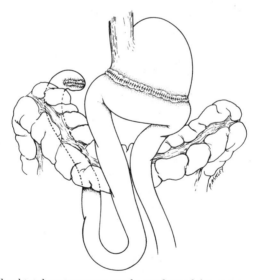

Figure 9–16. Distal subtotal gastrectomy can be performed for gastric carcinoma if a 5-cm margin of uninvolved stomach can be resected with the tumor. Gastrointestinal continuity is restored by gastrojejunostomy. Radical subtotal gastrectomy includes the spleen and distal pancreas in the resection, but this probably increases morbidity and mortality without increasing long-term survival. Radical lymph node dissection as practiced in Japan and some Western centers may improve survival or may merely stage the disease more accurately, placing many patients in a worse, albeit more accurate (higher-stage), prognostic category. This would improve survival stage for stage but not for the entire population, which would merely include more patients with more advanced-stage disease.

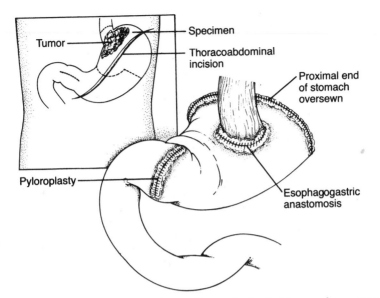

Figure 9–17. Gastric carcinoma near the cardia can be treated by esophagogastrectomy, which consists of resecting the distal esophagus and proximal stomach. This can be performed through a thoracoabdominal incision, left thoracotomy, or laparotomy combined with right thoracotomy. Continuity is restored by the anastomosing of the esophagus end-to-side to the stomach. Pyloroplasty is required because the vagus nerves are, of necessity, interrupted in the dissection required for the esophagogastrectomy. Some surgeons believe that distal esophagectomy and total gastrectomy plus esophagojejunostomy is a better cancer operation for proximal gastric cancer, although removing the entire stomach can increase morbidity and mortality.

have a much better prognosis than patients with lymph node or serosal involvement. Radical lymph node dissection, as practiced in Japan, may or may not increase survival. Resection en bloc of adjacent organs such as spleen and distal pancreas probably increases morbidity without prolonging survival. When the tumor is near the cardia (esophagogastric junction), an esophagogastrectomy (Fig. 9–17) may be required. Carcinoma of the cardia tends to have a diffuse histologic appearance, which has a worse prognosis, whereas carcinoma of the distal stomach tends to have "intestinal-type" histology, which has a better prognosis. The relative incidence of carcinoma of the cardia seems to be increasing as compared with distal gastric cancer. In the United States, a significant number of patients with symptomatic gastric cancer never undergo operation because the lesions are deemed incurable, and a significant percentage of patients explored for gastric cancer do not undergo resection because the operative findings demonstrate, that again, cure is not possible. Even those resected for cure have less than 50% 5-year survival, presumably owing to occult residual disease.

Recommended Reading

1. Zuidema GD, Ritchie WP Jr (eds): *Shackelford's Surgery of the Alimentary Tract,* ed 4, vol II. Philadelphia: W.B. Saunders, 1996.
2. Griffin SM, Raimes SA, (eds): *Upper Gastrointestinal Surgery.* Philadelphia: W.B. Saunders, 1997.
3. Sleisenger MH, Fordtran JS (eds): *Gastrointestinal Disease,* ed 5, vol 2. Philadelphia: W.B. Saunders, 1993.
4. Pappas TN: Historical aspects, anatomy, pathology, physiology, and peptic ulcer disease. In Sabiston DC, Lyerly HK (eds): *Textbook of Surgery: The Biological Basis of Modern Surgical Practice,* ed 15. Philadelphia: W.B. Saunders, 1997, pp 847–868.

10

Gastrointestinal Bleeding

Gastrointestinal bleeding can be a life-threatening event. Treatment may require resuscitation simultaneous with diagnosis. Accurate determination of the cause, along with precise localization, facilitates effective operative treatment.

For the purposes of our discussion, this subject is divided into upper and lower gastrointestinal bleeding. Common causes of upper gastrointestinal bleeding are duodenal ulcer, gastritis, gastric ulcer, and esophageal varices. Mallory-Weiss tear (from violent retching) can cause upper gastrointestinal bleeding but does not usually require surgery. Lower gastrointestinal bleeding can be caused by arteriovenous malformations (angiodysplasia), bleeding diverticula, colonic neoplasms, or inflammatory bowel disease.

The bleeding can be rapid, presenting as hematemesis and melena when from the upper tract or hematochezia (bright red blood per rectum) when from the lower gastrointestinal tract (that is, below the ligament of Treitz). Although bright red blood per rectum usually signifies lower gastrointestinal bleeding, it can be a sign of extremely rapid bleeding from the upper tract, as blood is a cathartic and the resulting shortened transit time prevents breakdown of the blood. Alternatively, the bleeding can be occult, from a carcinoma of the cecum or stomach, and no findings other than iron deficiency may be present. The following two case reports illustrate some important principles in the management of gastrointestinal bleeding.

CASE 10–1
Upper Gastrointestinal Bleeding

A 43-year-old man was admitted to the hospital with the chief complaint of tarry stools.

Seven years before admission, the patient underwent vagotomy and pyloroplasty and suture ligation of a bleeding duodenal ulcer. He was asymptomatic until 5 years before admission, when he developed epigastric pain in temporal relationship to business reversals. The symptoms were treated successfully with tranquilizers and antacids, and the patient remained well until 3 days before admission, when he developed some epigastric discomfort. On the day of admission he had several black, tarry stools, followed by a massive hematemesis and a syncope attack. He was brought to the hospital in an ambulance.

Past medical history was negative for heart disease, diabetes mellitus, hypertension, and other serious illnesses. The patient had not been taking ulcerogenic medications. There were no known allergies. The review of systems was unremarkable.

Physical examination on admission revealed a blood pressure of 100/60 mm Hg and pulse of 110 supine. Sitting, the blood pressure was 80 palpable and the pulse was 130. The patient was pale and diaphoretic. The sclerae were not icteric. There was no neck vein distention. The pulse was regular but thready; no murmurs, rubs, or gallops were heard. Examination of the abdomen revealed it to be soft and nontender, with no masses or organomegaly. There was a well-healed upper midline incision. Rectal examination revealed no masses or tenderness. There was black, tarry stool on the examining glove. No spider angiomas and no gynecomastia or testicular atrophy were noted.

The hematocrit was 44%, and the white blood cell count was 7500. The platelet count was normal, as were prothrombin and partial thromboplastin times.

Two large-bore peripheral intravenous catheters were inserted, 1500 cc of normal saline was infused, and supplemental oxygen was administered (40% by face mask). A Salem sump was inserted into the stomach, and 500 ml of "coffee-ground" material mixed with bright red blood was recovered. A Foley catheter inserted into the bladder yielded 60 ml of dark urine. At the time the intravenous lines were inserted, blood was drawn for type and cross-match of 4 units of packed red cells and for determination of CBC, electrolytes, BUN, blood sugar, prothrombin time, and partial thromboplastin time. ECG, chest x-ray, and definitive physical examination were done simultaneously with the resuscitation.

The patient's blood pressure increased to 140 mm Hg systolic, and his pulse decreased to 90 after the administration of 1500 ml of saline and 2 units of packed cells. Two more units of blood was ordered to be available. The gastroenterologist was asked to see the patient to perform early endoscopy, and the surgeon was informed of the patient's admission. The patient was transferred to the intensive care unit, where his urine output was found to have been 20 cc in the preceding hour.

Bright red blood was passing from the nasogastric tube. The tube was lavaged with room-temperature saline, and endoscopy revealed a large posterior ulcer in the duodenal bulb. An arterial "pumper" was identified at the base of the ulcer crater.

A third unit of packed cells and another liter of saline were given, and the repeat hematocrit was 31%. At that time blood pressure was 105/60 and pulse 105. Bright red blood was still coming from the nasogastric tube, and after 2 additional units of packed red cells and 2 units of fresh-frozen plasma, the hematocrit was 29% and the pulse 110. Urine output was 25 ml in the last hour. Another unit of blood was hung, the patient was brought to the operating room, and antrectomy was performed. No residual vagal fibers were found intact.

The patient had no further bleeding postoperatively. He tolerated a regular diet and had bowel movements. His incision healed per primum, and he was discharged to home on the 10th postoperative day.

DISCUSSION OF CASE 10–1

History. The chief complaint of tarry stools (melena) immediately suggests upper gastrointestinal bleeding. The history of present illness mentions that the patient had a vagotomy and pyloroplasty for a bleeding duodenal ulcer 7 years before admission and outlines a long-standing history of symptoms' being exacerbated by stress. Once again, the history provided a clue to the diagnosis, even before the physical examination and before any sophisticated tests were performed. That the patient had an episode of massive hematemesis and a syncopal attack signifies that the blood loss has been substantial and that resuscitation must be aggressive.

Significant negatives must also be mentioned in the past medical history. It is noted here that the patient had not been taking potentially ulcerogenic medications such as aspirin or NSAIDs. This information is important because, if the patient were taking any of these medications it would be reasonable to determine whether they might be discontinued.

Physical Examination. The patient was mildly hypotensive and tachycardic when supine. The blood pressure dropped, and the tachycardia increased considerably when the patient sat up; these orthostatic signs indicate hypovolemia. That the abdominal examination was unremarkable except for the surgical scar is not surprising in a patient with peptic ulcer disease with no perforation or gastric outlet obstruction. The absence of hepatomegaly, spider angiomas, gynecomastia, testicular atrophy, and caput medusae (enlarged veins of the abdominal wall near the umbilicus) argue against cirrhosis of the liver with portal hypertension and bleeding esophageal varices as a cause of the upper gastrointestinal bleeding.

Laboratory Examination. The initial hematocrit of 44% is normal. This is not surprising, as the patient lost whole blood and the hematocrit would not be expected to fall until interstitial fluid had time to enter the intravascular space as a homeostatic response aimed at maintaining circulating blood volume.

Hospital Course. It should be noted that administration of large amounts of fluid and of supplemental oxygen early in this patient's course is consistent with the principle that resuscitation and definitive diagnosis must occur simultaneously in seriously ill patients. This is analogous to the *ABCs* of emergency medical treatment, in which the *a*irway is established, adequate *b*reathing is ensured, and *c*irculation is supported. Only then is definitive diagnosis begun, as resuscitation efforts continue. The Foley catheter was inserted here because hourly monitoring of urine output is an excellent way to follow the patient's state of hydration, oliguria being one of the first signs of hypovolemia.

Some surgeons would insert either a central venous pressure

catheter or a Swan-Ganz catheter at this point. This was not done because this patient responded to volume expansion, because the central venous pressure does not accurately reflect what the left heart is doing, and because the patient was relatively young and without evidence of intercurrent cardiopulmonary disease. The two large-bore peripheral lines established were believed to afford superior forms of access in this patient.

The surgeon was asked to see the patient soon after he had arrived in the emergency department, so that he could have input into management and would be aware that the patient might need emergency surgical intervention. Lavage with saline may remove clots and facilitate endoscopy. Saline should be room temperature; iced saline is no longer used.

The nature of the lavage fluid returned may give insight into the rapidity of the bleeding. Early endoscopy is important in the treatment of rapid upper gastrointestinal bleeding. Knowledge of the source of the bleeding is especially helpful to the surgeon when operation is required, and this information may facilitate performance of the operative procedure.

In this case, early endoscopy affected the decision for prompt operation, since bleeding in a patient with an "arterial pumper" visible at the bottom of an ulcer crater is unlikely to stop. Also, there would be no reason to expose a patient with such a finding to the hemodynamic shifts of continued blood loss and transfusion or to the risk of hepatitis or other blood-borne infections and of "washout coagulopathy" that goes along with massive transfusion (see next paragraph). The bleeding point can be treated with the heater probe, bipolar cautery, epinephrine injection, or YAG laser through the endoscope. This may stop the bleeding, allowing the patient's medical status to be optimized before surgery. Some patients may not rebleed, in which case surgery is avoided. It is difficult to prove, however, that endoscopic treatment improves survival in upper gastrointestinal bleeding. In patients whose bleeding has stopped, significant rebleeding in hospital is an indication for surgery. Endoscopic treatment would not be indicated in a patient with a visible "arterial pumper." Such a patient should have prompt surgery.

Other factors that enter into the decision for early surgery in this case were the continued presence of bright red blood in the nasogastric tube, the drop in hematocrit in spite of transfusion, and persistent tachycardia and oliguria. Even more aggressive volume replacement with blood and physiologic saline would be required in this patient while preparations were being made to take him to the operating room. The fresh-frozen plasma was given to replace clotting factors (absent from banked blood), to prevent washout coagulopathy. Blood and fluids must be warmed in a rapid infuser-warmer to prevent hypothermia, which can cause coagulopathy in addition to decreasing oxygen delivery.

As was mentioned in Chapter 9, vagotomy, pyloroplasty, and oversewing of the ulcer is the operation commonly performed for bleeding duodenal ulcer. If there is a recurrence of bleeding later, a second vagotomy would be performed if any remaining vagal fibers were found, and antrectomy should be done with resection of the duodenal ulcer, if feasible. Successful treatment of this patient was predicated on rapid resuscitation, early endoscopy, and expeditious surgical intervention. There are, of course, many patients with bleeding of considerably less magnitude, and bleeding may stop spontaneously. The source should be documented with upper endoscopy. In the case of a duodenal ulcer, healing can be achieved with H_2 blockers, proton pump inhibitors, or Carafate (sucralfate). *Helicobacter pylori* should be eradicated, when possible. Alcohol, smoking, and potentially ulcerogenic medications should be avoided, when feasible. Bleeding gastric ulcers must at least be studied by multiple endoscopic biopsies to rule out gastric cancer, whose treatment is outlined in Chapter 9. If bleeding persists, the gastric ulcer must be treated with either wedge resection or partial gastrectomy. Esophageal varices are treated by endoscopic sclerotherapy or banding, portasystemic shunt, esophagogastric disconnection, transjugular intrahepatic portosystemic shunt (TIPS), or liver transplantation. The choice of treatment for bleeding esophageal varices is dependent on the patient's risk (Child's classification) as assessed by serum bilirubin, albumin, nutrition, and the presence or absence of ascites and encephalopathy.

CASE 10–2

Lower Gastrointestinal Bleeding

A 68-year-old man was admitted with bright red rectal bleeding. Two years before admission, the patient had been hospitalized with hematochezia. Sigmoidoscopy and barium enema at that time revealed only diverticulosis coli, and this was assumed to be the source of bleeding. The bleeding stopped and the patient was discharged. One year before admission the patient again had an episode of bleeding, this time mild. He had colonoscopy as an outpatient, but no bleeding point was found. The endoscopist saw blood up to the middle of the descending colon, and none above. The colonic mucosa appeared normal all the way to the cecum. The bleeding stopped again, and the patient experienced no further hematochezia until the day of admission, when he noticed bright red blood in the toilet bowl, called his physician, and was told to come to the emergency department.

Past medical history revealed angina pectoris treated with nitroglycerin paste.

Physical examination revealed blood pressure of 110/70 mm Hg and pulse of 90. There were no orthostatic changes. The conjunctivae were pink. Examination of the abdomen was unremarkable, and rectal examination revealed bright red blood on the examining glove, but no masses or tenderness.

The hematocrit was 42% and prothrombin time, partial thromboplastin time, and platelet counts were normal. Flat and upright abdominal films showed no abnormal results.

A nasogastric tube passed into the stomach yielded green bile, but no blood. This argued against rapid upper gastrointestinal bleeding as the cause of the bright red blood per rectum (which can reflect rapid transit from the laxative effect of the blood). It was thought that the patient was not bleeding rapidly enough for an angiogram or bleeding scan to be helpful, so colonoscopy was performed again but was not diagnostic. That night, the patient passed bright red blood with clots per rectum, and the blood pressure dropped to 80 systolic with a pulse of 120. One liter of Ringer's lactate solution and 3 units of packed red blood cells were infused, and emergency arteriography was performed. This revealed extravasation in the descending colon, with early filling of a large vein. The diagnosis of an arteriovenous malformation (AVM, angiodysplasia) was made; segmental resection of the left colon, including the bleeding site, was carried out, followed by end-to-end anastomosis. Postoperatively, the patient did well and had no further bleeding.

DISCUSSION OF CASE 10–2

History. This patient was admitted with a chief complaint of bright red blood per rectum; this suggests lower gastrointestinal bleeding. Brisk upper gastrointestinal bleeding might, however, be manifested by hematochezia instead of melena (the latter being the more common manifestation of upper gastrointestinal bleeding), since the rapid transit caused by the cathartic effect of blood might not allow enough time for the bright red blood to be changed to melena. From a structural point of view, it is important to note that the history of present illness begins at its temporal onset (that is, the first time the patient had any symptoms referable to the disease process in question).

Diagnostic Evaluation. It is not surprising that the findings on sigmoidoscopy were negative, as were those on colonoscopy later, as bleeding can obscure the lesion. Additionally, arteriovenous malformations may not be visible on endoscopy. In spite of its low yield, sigmoidoscopy is important to rule out bleeding sites in the anorectum that would not be addressed by abdominal colectomy and ileorectostomy. The use of colonoscopy in the diagnosis of lower gastrointestinal bleeding is controversial, because it is hard to visualize a bleeding point in the face of copious intraluminal blood. Because blood is a cathartic and can cause evacuation of stool, some endoscopists try to localize the bleeding point. It is of interest that the barium enema revealed only diverticulosis coli. The problem with doing a barium enema as part of the workup of lower gastrointestinal bleeding is that, if a lesion *is* demonstrated, there is still no direct evidence that the bleeding is coming from that lesion. Additionally, diverticulosis coli is so common that it might well be merely coincidental. Before the advent of angiography as part of the diagnostic evaluation of lower gastrointestinal bleeding, many instances of bleeding caused by angiodysplasia must have been attributed to diverticuli.

Hospital Course. The nasogastric tube was placed to rule out rapid upper gastrointestinal bleeding as the cause of hematochezia. Presumably, angiography was not planned initially because the bleeding was not considered heavy enough for arteriography to have a reasonable yield (0.5 ml per minute is considered the minimum rate of bleeding necessary for angiography to demonstrate the bleeding point). The episode of hypotension and tachycardia, however, convinced the radiologist that bleeding was, indeed, rapid enough. Angiography not only demonstrated the bleeding point but verified the diagnosis of an arteriovenous malformation on the basis of the classic finding of an early-filling vein. Two nuclear medicine (scintigraphy) techniques have been used: either radioactive technetium or isotope-tagged red cells are injected and the point of extravasation is detected with a scanner. They are sometimes used to identify bleeding too slow to be visualized by angiography. They must be interpreted with caution, however, especially with regard to the localization of bleeding since bowel contraction can propel the radiopharmaceutical cephalad or caudad.

The operative morbidity and mortality are markedly decreased when the bleeding point is known preoperatively. This is because the bleeding point is notoriously difficult to find intraoperatively, as the entire large bowel is usually filled with blood. If one is forced to operate when the source of bleeding is still obscure, subtotal colectomy may have to be done so that there is a reasonable expectation of including the bleeding point in the resected specimen.

GENERAL CONSIDERATIONS

Rapid upper gastrointestinal bleeding is usually manifested by melena and hematemesis. Orthostatic changes may be present if bleeding is brisk. Included in the differential diagnosis are duodenal ulcer, gastritis, gastric ulcer (or ulcerated gastric cancer), and bleeding esophageal varices. The Mallory-Weiss syndrome refers to bleeding from a tear near the gastro-esophageal junction caused by continued and violent retching. Resuscitation for upper gastrointestinal bleeding must be prompt, and early endoscopy appears to improve survival in patients whose bleeding is rapid. Operation is usually indicated when large amounts of blood are required to maintain stable vital signs.

Iron deficiency anemia can be caused by an occult gastrointestinal neoplasm such as gastric carcinoma or carcinoma of the cecum, and these should be ruled out either by endoscopy or barium studies early in the workup of anemia. Failure to do so can lead to delayed diagnosis and a poor prognosis.

Lower gastrointestinal bleeding can be caused by neoplasms, diverticulosis coli, angiodysplasia, or inflammatory bowel disease such as ulcerative colitis or Crohn's disease. In addition, anal lesions such as anal fissure and bleeding internal hemorrhoids must be considered. If bleeding is rapid, arteriography with injection of the inferior and superior mesenteric arteries may be extremely helpful in establishing a diagnosis. Establishment of the correct diagnosis preoperatively facilitates the operation.

Recommended Reading

1. Griffin SM, Raimes SA (eds): *Upper Gastrointestinal Surgery.* Philadelphia: W.B. Saunders, 1997.
2. Peterson WL, Laine L: Gastrointestinal bleeding. In Sleisenger MH, Fordtran JS (eds): *Gastrointestinal Disease: Pathophysiology/Diagnosis/Management,* ed 5. Philadelphia: W.B. Saunders, 1993, pp 162–192.
3. Murray JJ: Lower gastrointestinal bleeding. In Mazier WP, Levien DH, Luchtefeld MA, Senagore A (eds): *Surgery of The Colon, Rectum, and Anus.* Philadelphia: W.B. Saunders, 1995, pp 762–773.
4. Reeders JWAJ, Rosenbusch G: *Clinical Radiology and Endoscopy of the Colon.* New York: Thieme Medical 1994.

11

Surgery of the Colon, Rectum, and Anus

It is of utmost importance for surgical clerks and residents to be knowledgeable about surgery of the colon, rectum, and anus. Colorectal cancer afflicts one in 20 Americans. Benign anorectal disorders are pervasive. Complications of colon and rectal surgery such as anastomotic leak are responsible for prolonged hospitalizations, protracted stays in the intensive care unit, and significant mortality.

The principal functions of the colon are absorption of water and storage of fecal material. The colon also propels its contents in an aborad direction and secretes mucus. Pathologic lesions involving the colon can be classified as congenital, traumatic, neoplastic, inflammatory, and vascular. In this chapter, congenital lesions discussed are Hirschsprung's disease and malrotation of the midgut. The discussion of colon trauma emphasizes penetrating injury. Adenocarcinoma of the colon receives emphasis in the section on neoplastic diseases of the large bowel. The inflammatory lesions discussed are diverticulitis, Crohn's disease, and ulcerative colitis. Perianal disease is discussed in the section on inflammatory lesions.

CONGENITAL COLON LESIONS

Congenital lesions of the large bowel usually come within the domain of the pediatric surgeon, although some lesions, such as malrotation of the midgut, may not become evident until later in life and are thus encountered by the general surgeon. (Many excellent texts are devoted entirely to pediatric surgery.) Hirschsprung's disease and malrotation of the midgut are discussed here to introduce the reader to the subject, since some exposure to pediatric surgery is usually incorporated into general surgical training.

Hirschsprung's Disease

Hirschsprung's disease results from the absence of ganglion cells in the distal colon and rectum. This makes reflex relaxation of this segment

101

impossible and results in functional obstruction. Constipation is usually present early in life, and failure to pass meconium in the first 24 hours after birth forces consideration of this diagnosis. A contrast enema frequently demonstrates proximal dilatation of the colon. Rectal biopsy demonstrating an absence of ganglion cells confirms the diagnosis. Absence of the rectoanal inhibitory reflex on anal manometry (the usual response is a drop in anal pressure when a rectal balloon is inflated) may aid in the diagnosis. The initial treatment often consists of colostomy, allowing the return of bowel function so that the patient's general condition can be improved. A definitive procedure can be performed later. These procedures consist of resecting the aganglionic segment and anastomosing the proximal colon to very distal rectum, leaving as little aganglionic rectum as possible. Continuity is reestablished by operations identified by eponyms such as Soave's, Duhamel's, and Swenson's (Fig. 11–1).

Malrotation of the Midgut

Malrotation of the midgut occurs when normal rotation around the superior mesenteric artery fails to occur in embryonic life and bands extending from the malpositioned cecum to the right abdominal wall (Ladd's bands) obstruct the duodenum (Fig. 11–2). There may be associated twisting of the small bowel around the superior mesenteric artery (midgut volvulus) with vascular compromise and gangrene of the bowel (Fig. 11–3). Malrotation of the midgut with midgut volvulus may present

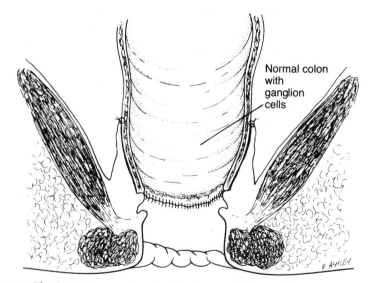

Normal colon with ganglion cells

Figure 11–1. The Swenson procedure for Hirschsprung's disease. The aganglionic segment is removed, and the proximal colon is anastomosed to distal rectum 1 cm above the anus.

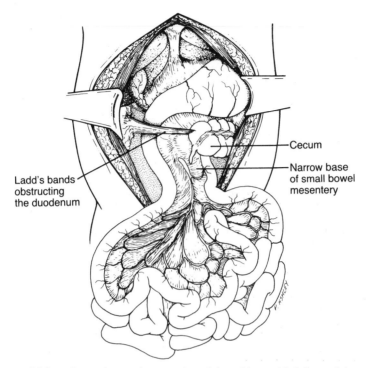

Figure 11–2. Malrotation or incomplete rotation of the midgut with failure of the cecum to achieve its normal position in the right lower quadrant. Ladd's bands, which connect the cecum to the abdominal wall, must be lysed to prevent duodenal obstruction. The narrow base of the mesentery predisposes to twisting of the small bowel (midgut volvulus).

with bilious vomiting and bloody stools. A barium enema may demonstrate malrotation of the cecum. Surgical treatment consists of untwisting the small bowel to restore perfusion, lysing Ladd's bands, placing the cecum in the left lower quadrant, and performing an appendectomy (see Fig. 11–3). If there is a question of intestinal viability, a second-look operation can be performed 24 hours later and remaining nonviable bowel resected.

TRAUMA TO THE COLON AND RECTUM

CASE 11–1

Colon Trauma

A 23-year-old man was wounded at close range by a shotgun blast directed at the right flank. He was brought to the hospital in profound shock, was resuscitated with 2 L of crystalloid and 3 units of packed

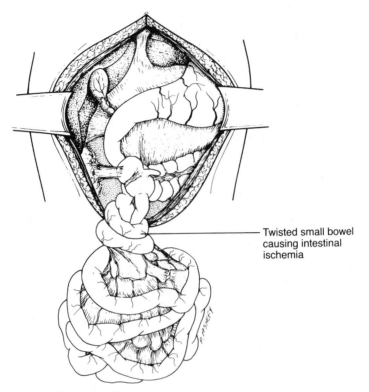

Twisted small bowel
causing intestinal
ischemia

Figure 11–3. Small bowel volvulus is corrected by counterclockwise rotation. Ladd's operation entails placing the cecum in a completely unrotated position in the left lower quadrant, with the small bowel on the right side of the abdomen. This is believed to widen the small bowel mesentery, lessening the possibility of recurrent midgut volvulus.

cells, and was taken to the operating room. Surgery revealed that the right kidney was shattered beyond repair and that the right renal artery was injured. A large hole in the cecum had permitted fecal soiling of the peritoneal cavity. Intraoperative intravenous pyelography demonstrated prompt functioning of the contralateral kidney, and accordingly right nephrectomy was performed in conjunction with a ileocolic resection, and ileostomy, and formation of a mucous fistula (see later discussion). The patient did well and was discharged from the hospital on the 10th postoperative day. Three weeks later he was readmitted, and intestinal continuity was restored by ileocolic anastomosis.

DISCUSSION OF CASE 11–1

Our knowledge of the best treatment of trauma to the colon and rectum derives largely from wartime experience. A basic tenet of war surgery is that, for penetrating injuries of the colon the injury should be either exteriorized or the organ defunctionalized by a completely diverting stoma (colostomy or ileostomy; Fig. 11–4). This principle is predicated on the fact that disruption of an anastomosis or leakage from a colonic closure is likely to result in peritonitis and sepsis and with the associated hazards of great morbidity and high mortality. The missiles used in warfare tend to be of high velocity and to cause massive tissue destruction. Moreover, in the pre-Vietnam era patients were sometimes lost to follow-up for significant periods during post-operative transport. This would seem to make use of primary anastomosis unwise for wartime injuries to the colon.

Although exteriorization or diversion is still often the safest approach, some surgeons advocate either primary repair or resection and primary anastomosis for certain low-velocity civilian injuries of the colon (Fig. 11–5). Primary repair or resection and anastomosis may be performed when shock is not present, when the interval between injury and treatment is not great, when contamination and tissue injury are minimal, and when there are no associated injuries. Because the patient in Case 11–1 had profound shock, fecal soilage was significant, and another organ was injured (shattered right kidney), it was felt that resection with ileostomy and mucous fistula was the safest course.

If the injury to the colon is caused by the colonoscope, primary repair without colostomy may be appropriate, since the patient has usually undergone bowel preparation with enemas and laxatives in anticipation of the procedure and peritoneal contamination may be minimal. When there is significant contamination, proximal diversion of feces with either repair or resection may be prudent.

Rectal Trauma

Rectal injury may be caused by missiles or sharp objects such as icepicks or by objects inserted during the course of anal eroticism. The injury may be iatrogenic, from instrumentation with a sigmoidoscope, colonoscope, thermometer, or enema tip. Injury above the peritoneal reflection usually requires laparotomy, as there is potential for peritoneal soiling. Rectal injuries below the peritoneal reflection may be treated by repair, presacral drainage, and temporary proximal colostomy (Fig. 11–6). Rectal washout to decrease contamination is sometimes indicated.

NEOPLASMS OF THE COLON, RECTUM, AND ANUS

CASE 11–2

Carcinoma of the Right Colon

A 58-year-old man was admitted to the hospital with a known carcinoma of the cecum and was scheduled for right hemicolectomy.

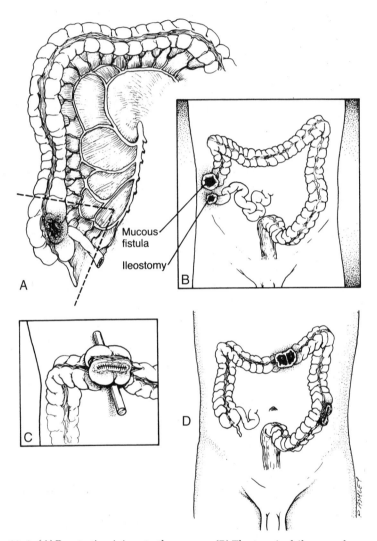

Figure 11–4. *(A)* Penetrating injury to the cecum. *(B)* The terminal ileum and cecum have been resected, an ileostomy has been performed, and a mucous fistula has been fashioned. This method of dealing with the injury leaves no intraabdominal anastomosis at risk of disruption. *(C)* A method for dealing with a penetrating injury to the transverse colon. The laceration has been sutured closed but exteriorized over a glass rod or bridge to prevent retraction. When leakage occurs, it is extraabdominal and cannot cause peritonitis. If after 10 days the closure remains secure, it can be dropped back into the abdomen in a relatively minor operation. *(D)* An injury to the descending colon or rectosigmoid can be sutured primarily and a completely diverting proximal colostomy performed at a convenient site in the mobile transverse colon. A colostomy closure can be performed later.

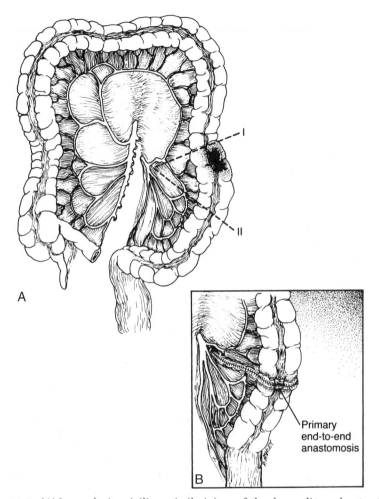

Figure 11–5. *(A)* Low-velocity civilian missile injury of the descending colon treated by resection of the involved segment and primary anastomosis. The arteries and veins in the mesentery supplying this segment are clamped, transected, and ligated, and the colon is transected at points I and II. *(B)* The ends are anastomosed (I to II). This may obviate a second operation, but it exposes the patient to the risk of anastomotic leak and possible sequelae of peritonitis and sepsis. This technique may be acceptable when (1) shock is not present, (2) there are no associated injuries, (3) contamination is minimal, and (4) only a short time has elapsed between injury and operation.

Three weeks before admission the patient had gone to his internist complaining of fatigue and malaise. There had been no history of weight loss, anorexia, hematochezia, or melena; nor had there been a change in bowel habits. Because the patient was found to have iron deficiency anemia, the internist performed sigmoidoscopy and barium enema examination. The latter revealed a large carcinoma of

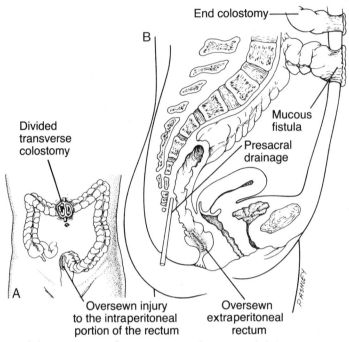

Figure 11–6. *(A)* An injury to the intraperitoneal portion of the rectum (i.e., above the peritoneal reflection) can be treated with primary closure and a proximal divided colostomy. An injury to the rectum below the peritoneal reflection *(B)* caused by a penetrating injury from below can be explored through the perineal wound, which is enlarged and débrided, sparing the sphincters when possible, to preserve continence. The rectum is repaired and presacral drainage is instituted. A completely diverting proximal colostomy is performed by laparotomy.

the cecum. The patient was referred to a surgeon, who prescribed bowel preparation at home and admitted him for colectomy.

Physical examination on admission revealed no supraclavicular lymphadenopathy and no abdominal masses or hepatosplenomegaly. Rectal examination revealed no masses and no rectal shelf. The alkaline phosphatase level was normal, and chest x-ray findings were negative. A carcinoembryonic antigen determination was ordered as a baseline measure.

The patient was admitted the morning of surgery, after receiving at home the night before mechanical and antibiotic bowel preparation. The former consisted of drinking 1 L of chilled polyethylene glycol solution, which cleared the colon of feces overnight. The latter consisted of taking neomycin (1 g) and erythromycin base (1 g) at 1:00 PM, 2:00 PM, and 11:00 PM the day before surgery.

The patient received prophylactic subcutaneous heparin 2 hours before surgery, and compression boots were placed preoperatively to decrease the risk of deep vein thrombosis or pulmonary embolus. On the morning of admission, the patient underwent right hemicolectomy. There was no evidence of liver metastases or intraperitoneal spread at surgery. The pathology report available several days later classified the surgical specimen as a stage II (Dukes B or B2) lesion. The patient had an unremarkable postoperative course and was discharged from the hospital on the 7th postoperative day.

Postoperative follow-up included serial physical examinations, hematocrit, carcinoembryonic antigen and alkaline phosphatase determinations, chest x-rays, and colonoscopy. Two years postoperatively there was no evidence of recurrence.

CASE 11–3
Obstructing Carcinoma of the Left Colon

A 43-year-old woman presented to the emergency department with a 1-week history of nausea, vomiting, and obstipation. On further questioning she reported a 3-month history of diarrhea alternating with constipation, decreased caliber of stools, and blood streaking on the outside of the feces; she attributed the latter finding to hemorrhoids.

Physical examination revealed the abdomen to be markedly distended, with moderate tenderness in the right lower quadrant. Bowel sounds were hyperactive. There was no generalized rebound tenderness or involuntary guarding. The findings on rectal examination were negative.

Flat and upright films revealed a markedly distended colon, the cecum being 10 cm in diameter. Sigmoidoscopy performed in the emergency department revealed a friable mass 18 cm from the anal verge. A biopsy and frozen section examination revealed the lesion to be an infiltrating adenocarcinoma of the sigmoid colon.

The patient was rehydrated and underwent emergency transverse colostomy. Ten days later, she underwent bowel preparation including three-way irrigations with neomycin solution (through the proximal and distal limbs of the colostomy and via the rectum); she received cathartics and oral doses of neomycin and erythromycin base. Resection of the sigmoid colon with end-to-end anastomosis was performed. The patient did well and was discharged on the 10th postoperative day after instruction in colostomy care. Supervision of colostomy care by an enterostomal therapy nurse had been arranged. Six weeks later the patient was readmitted, and closure of the transverse colostomy was performed without incident.

DISCUSSION OF CASES 11–2 AND 11–3

Neoplasms of the colon can be benign or malignant. There is a polyp-carcinoma sequence in which polyps of varying malignant potential can progress to carcinoma. Of the adenomatous polyps, the tubular adenoma has the least malignant potential (although it does have some); the villous adenoma has the greatest malignant potential (which increases with the size of the adenoma); and the villotubular adenoma is intermediate in malignant potential.

Many years ago, polyps were usually discovered during barium enema examination, and laparotomy and colotomy were required to remove them (Fig. 11–7). With the advent of colonoscopy, many pedunculated and some sessile polyps could be removed endoscopically with a snare. The hope is that this method will decrease the mortality from carcinoma of the colon. This would be an example of *secondary prevention. Primary prevention* would be to inhibit the development of polyps by strategies such as a high-fiber, low-fat diet and chemoprotection with agents such as the prostaglandin inhibitor sulindac (Clinoril).

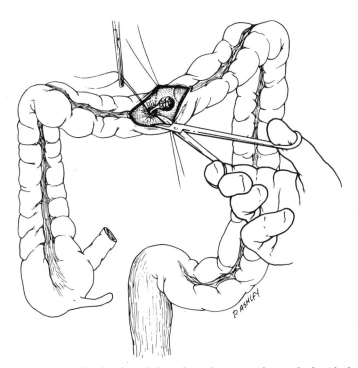

Figure 11–7. A pedunculated polyp of the colon, if it cannot be reached with the colonoscope because of redundancy or angulation of the colon, can be treated with colotomy, ligation of the stalk, excision of the polyp, and subsequent closure of the colotomy. More often, laparotomy is avoided by removing pedunculated polyps with a colonoscope. Although sessile polyps (polyps without a stalk or pedicle) may be removed through the colonoscope by fractionation techniques, they may require laparotomy and segmental colon resection if they are of substantial size and thus pose significant risk of harboring a carcinoma. Very small sessile polyps can be biopsied and destroyed through the colonoscope with the hot biopsy forceps.

Adenocarcinoma of the Colon and Rectum

Carcinoma of the colon is the neoplasm with which we are most concerned when we discuss tumors of the large bowel. One of 20 United States citizens gets colorectal cancer. In discussing the diagnosis of carcinoma of the colon, we will consider symptoms, signs, simple laboratory tests and imaging techniques, and invasive diagnostic methods such as endoscopy and biopsy. Then we will discuss the treatment, prognosis, and special considerations, such as the operative treatment of complicated colon cancer (e.g., with associated perforation or obstruction).

Symptoms

The most common *early* symptom of colorectal cancer is *none.* In other words, by the time colorectal cancer is symptomatic, it is already advanced, and although it may not be incurable, the chances for cure are diminished. This fact, coupled with the fact that colorectal cancers occur so frequently, explains why so much emphasis has been placed on screening for this disease. When symptoms do occur, they include change in bowel habits, transanal bleeding, and mucus per rectum. Abdominal, back, and rectal pain are late symptoms, as are nausea, vomiting, anorexia, and weight loss.

The symptoms in colorectal cancer depend on the location of the tumor in the large bowel. Because of the large caliber of the right colon and the liquid consistency of its fecal contents, a neoplasm there is less likely to obstruct than is a left colon lesion. Accordingly, carcinoma of the right colon may grow large without producing obstructive symptoms, and it may outgrow its blood supply, fungate, ulcerate, and bleed. The bleeding, however, usually is not clinically apparent, presenting as neither melena (tarry stools) nor hematochezia (passage of bright red blood per rectum). Slow, steady blood loss can result in anemia, which can be responsible for the weakness and malaise often associated with right-sided colon cancer. Because these carcinomas of the cecum and ascending colon often become large without obstructing, they may be the cause of vague right lower quadrant abdominal pain.

Cancers of the left colon are often signaled by bloody bowel movements. This symptom is often attributed by the patient to hemorrhoids, resulting in considerable delay in diagnosis. The physician must be careful not to contribute to this delay. It is often said that right-sided cancers bleed (slowly) and left-sided lesions obstruct, and obstruction can be responsible for the other symptoms of left-sided colon cancer. Constipation gets worse as the tumor begins to obstruct the flow of solid feces through the relatively narrow left colon. Diarrhea alternating with constipation must suggest the possibility of left colon cancer. As the obstruction progresses, nausea and vomiting may occur. Carcinoma of the colon can perforate, resulting in severe abdominal pain associated with nausea and vomiting. The perforation can be at the site of the tumor or at the cecum, which may dilate from an obstructing cancer of the left colon.

Signs

The signs of carcinoma of the colon and rectum can be related to the tumor mass itself. A large tumor of the right colon can present as a right lower quadrant abdominal mass. The astute examiner may even palpate a left lower quadrant abdominal mass in association with cancer of the sigmoid colon. An enlarged, nodular liver may be palpable when there are liver metastases. A fluid wave due to malignant ascites may be present in far advanced disease. Virchow's node is a palpable, hard, left supraclavicular node caused by metastases from a malignant tumor of the gastrointestinal tract. Blumer's shelf ("frozen pelvis") can be palpated on rectal examination when the rectovesical or rectouterine pouch contains tumor as a result of transcelomic spread of an intraabdominal malignant tumor. Krukenberg's tumor on occasion is palpable. This is a mass in the ovary metastatic from a gastrointestinal cancer, usually gastric but sometimes colorectal. Carcinoma of the rectum frequently is within reach of the examining finger.

When carcinoma of the colon becomes obstructing, abdominal distention and tympany are usually present. Laplace's law dictates that, when the colon becomes distended as a result of an obstructing malignant tumor of the rectosigmoid, the large-caliber cecum is most distended. Accordingly, an obstructing lesion of the left colon may result in significant right lower quadrant abdominal tenderness if the cecum is distended and perforation impending. Perforation of the colon, either at the site of the colon cancer or proximally at the site of the distended cecum, results in the physical signs of peritonitis: diffuse tenderness with generalized rebound, involuntary guarding, absence of bowel sounds, and a rigid, boardlike abdomen.

Relevant Lab Tests and Imaging

Laboratory Tests. Simple laboratory tests may prove useful in the diagnosis of colon cancer. The hemoglobin and hematocrit levels may indicate anemia. In fact, iron deficiency anemia should always alert the physician to the possibility of carcinoma of the cecum or stomach. It should lead to a thorough evaluation of the gastrointestinal tract in a search for malignant disease early in the course of the diagnostic workup for anemia. Leukocytosis may be found if perforation has occurred. A free perforation is usually apparent because of the symptoms and signs of peritonitis, but a sealed-off perforation with a pericolic abscess may present with few physical findings, and the presence of leukocytosis with fever may aid in the diagnosis. An elevated alkaline phosphatase level can indicate liver metastases. The carcinoembryonic antigen level may be elevated in colon cancer. Because of overlap in levels in patients with and without colon cancer, the carcinoembryonic antigen level is not a good screening measure for colon cancer. It is useful, however, if a patient with colon cancer has an elevated level that drops to normal after resection. A later rise in the carcinoembryonic antigen level often indicates a recurrence, and a "second look" operation may be indicated in this event. The presence of white blood cells and bacteria, along with fecal particles and air bubbles, in the urine may signal the presence of a colovesical fistula caused by colon cancer.

Imaging Techniques. Imaging techniques are helpful in evaluating for carcinoma of the colon. The flat and upright abdominal views can demonstrate a dilated colon in a case of large bowel obstruction secondary to obstructing carcinoma of the rectosigmoid colon. A cecum with a diameter of 8 cm or more signals impending perforation. The upright view may demonstrate free air under the diaphragm when there is a perforation. The chest x-ray detects pulmonary metastasis.

A barium enema may demonstrate the polypoid or constricting lesions of carcinoma or filling defects representing adenomatous polyps. Good preparation of the bowel to eliminate fecal material is necessary if the results of the barium enema are to be properly interpreted. A double-contrast barium enema (insertion of air plus barium) may be better at detecting small polyps than a single-contrast barium enema.

Although the cost effectiveness, and even reliability, of intravenous pyelography in the preoperative evaluation of patients with colon and rectal cancer has been questioned, it may help to evaluate the collecting system of the kidneys. This information may prove valuable at surgery, since, if the collecting system is involved by tumor, reconstruction of the collecting system will be necessary after tumor resection. If one kidney must be sacrificed, it is mandatory to demonstrate by preoperative intravenous pyelography (IVP) that the other kidney is functioning. If a double collecting system is present, preoperative IVP should have demonstrated it, making intraoperative injury less likely. CT is used to evaluate for liver metastasis and transcelomic spread, and it demonstrates the kidneys and collecting system, usually eliminating the need for IVP. The role of MRI in preoperative evaluation of patients with colorectal cancer is evolving. It may be helpful, in conjunction with gadolinium contrast, to distinguish between postoperative scar and pelvic recurrence. Even when liver metastases are present, it is often advisable to proceed with resection of the colon or rectum to prevent intestinal obstruction, necrosis, bleeding, or tenesmus, which can occur before widespread metastases cause the patient's demise.

Invasive Techniques. Rigid sigmoidoscopy to the 25-cm level has traditionally been the endoscopic procedure performed in conjunction with barium enema examination. The rationale is that the barium enema examination is not reliable in evaluating the rectum, and, therefore, sigmoidoscopy and the barium enema examination complement each other. The flexible 60-cm sigmoidoscope can also be used to complement barium enema. The colonoscope can replace both the sigmoidoscope and barium enema and has the advantage of identifying smaller polyps and allowing biopsy of other polyps or carcinomas anywhere in the colo-rectum.

Treatment

The treatment of carcinoma of the colon is essentially surgical. Only through surgical resection is there any hope of cure, and surgical extirpation in most instances also provides the best palliation. Until recently, adjuvant chemotherapy did not seem to offer much advantage in colon cancer that seemed resectable for cure. Recently, however, the National Institutes of Health convened a consensus conference that recommended that adjuvant therapy with 5-fluorouracil (5-FU) and levamisole (an anti-helminthic agent that stimulates the immune system) be used after resection for Stage III (Dukes C) colon cancer (i.e., cancers with involved mesenteric lymph nodes). Leucovorin is now often used instead of le-vamisole. In addition, The National Cancer Institute of The National Institutes of Health recommends 5-FU plus radiation therapy for adjuvant treatment after resection of Stage II (Dukes B—carcinoma through the bowel wall with negative lymph nodes) and Stage III (Dukes C) rectal cancers. Some surgeons prefer to give preoperative (neoadjuvant) chemo-irradiation for rectal cancer. Chemotherapy and immunotherapy have been used with variable success for Stage IV (Dukes D) colorectal cancer (metastasis present).

Surgical Treatment of Right Colon Carcinoma. One must resect the venous and lymphatic drainage (which runs in parallel with the arterial supply) en bloc with the colon to increase the chance of cure. Carcinoma of the cecum is treated by right hemicolectomy and ileotransverse colos-tomy, resection of the terminal ileum and right colon, and anastomosis of the cut end of the ileum to the remainder of the transverse colon (Fig. 11–8).

Surgical Treatment of Left Colon Carcinoma. Carcinoma of the recto-sigmoid colon is usually treated by sigmoid resection. A lesion that is more proximal in the descending colon may require left hemicolectomy if the draining lymphatics and veins are to be encompassed (Fig. 11–9).

Surgical Treatment of Rectal Carcinoma. The classic operation for carcinoma of the rectum has been *abdominoperineal resection* of the rectum, or Miles' procedure (Fig. 11–10). This operation consists of resecting the sigmoid colon, rectum, and anus, using both a laparotomy incision and an elliptical incision in the perineum, circumscribing the anus, and removing the specimen from below. The specimen is removed via the perineal incision, and the left colon is brought out through the abdominal wall as a permanent end colostomy. The perineum then can be dealt with—by (1) closing the perineal skin and the levator ani muscles, leaving the peritoneum unapproximated, or (2) by closing the peritoneum from the intraabdominal aspect ("reperitonealizing") and leaving the perineum open and packed with gauze, which is removed later. The abdominoperineal resection historically was the standard against which all other operations for carcinoma of the rectum were

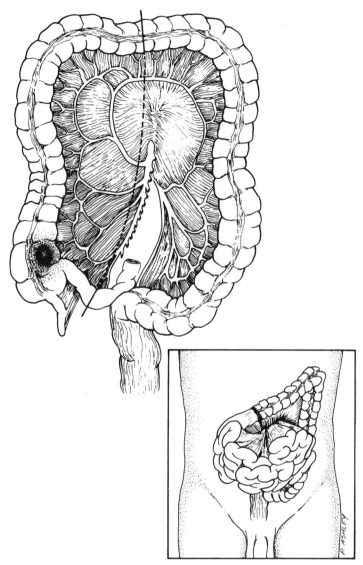

Figure 11–8. A right hemicolectomy and ileotransverse colostomy (anastomosis of the terminal ileum to the transverse colon) performed for carcinoma of the cecum. Resection of this extent is required for an adequate cancer operation, since the mesentery with its arterial and venous supply also contains draining lymphatics.

compared for operative morbidity and mortality, quality of life, and long-term survival.

In an effort to preserve the anal sphincter by performing a sphincter-sparing operation and to obviate a permanent colostomy, *anterior resection* was developed for the treatment of rectal cancer (Fig. 11–11). This

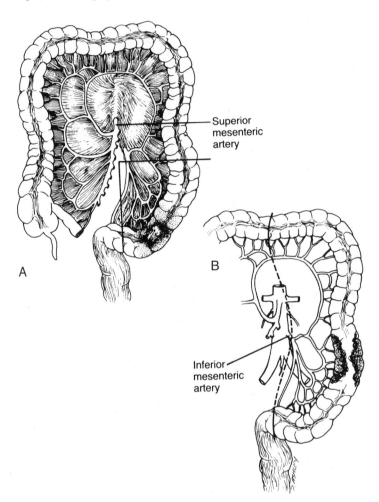

Figure 11–9. *(A)* A sigmoid resection or segmental resection of the sigmoid colon performed for carcinoma of the sigmoid colon. *(B)* A formal left hemicolectomy for carcinoma of the descending colon. Ligating the inferior mesenteric artery near its point of origin from the aorta allows inclusion of more lymph nodes.

operation consists of resecting the segment of rectum harboring the cancer along with a margin of rectum 2.0 to 2.5 cm distal to the tumor plus some sigmoid colon proximally. It was believed that a 5-cm distal margin was required because this seemed to be the limit of intramural spread of tumor and the lymphatic drainage was shown to be cephalad. It was originally believed that 7 cm of anorectum had to be preserved to retain fecal continence. The rationale was that continence required a reflex arc, the sensory receptors for which resided in the anal mucosa. Simple arithmetic dictates that a malignant tumor closer to the anal

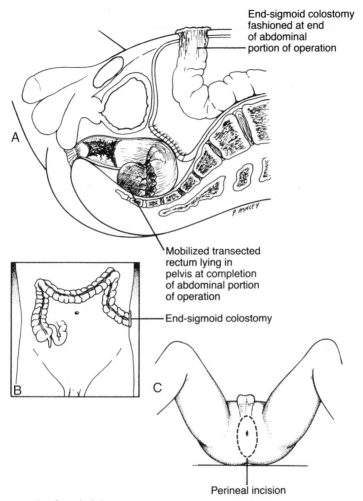

End-sigmoid colostomy
fashioned at end
of abdominal
portion of operation

Mobilized transected
rectum lying in
pelvis at completion
of abdominal portion
of operation

End-sigmoid colostomy

Perineal incision

Figure 11–10. Combined abdominoperineal resection of the rectum for a low-lying carcinoma of the rectum. *(A)* The rectum is mobilized from above at laparotomy. *(B)* The proximal end of the divided colon is brought out as a permanent end colostomy. *(C)* With the patient in lithotomy position an elliptical incision is made, circumscribing the anus. The dissection is continued cephalad to meet the dissection begun intraabdominally, and the rectum is removed from below. The perineal wound is then closed.

verge than 12 cm required treatment by abdominoperineal resection and permanent colostomy if these limits were to be respected (Fig. 11–12).

In recent years, however, there has been a tendency to believe that a distal margin of 2.0 or 2.5 cm is adequate and will not compromise survival unless the tumor is poorly differentiated. In addition, studies have suggested that the afferent limb of the reflex arc may reside in proprioceptive fibers in the levator ani muscles, through which the left

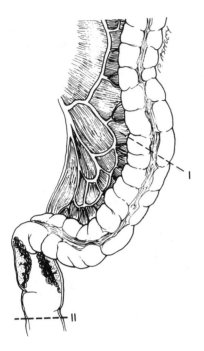

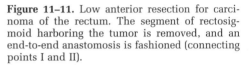

Figure 11–11. Low anterior resection for carcinoma of the rectum. The segment of rectosigmoid harboring the tumor is removed, and an end-to-end anastomosis is fashioned (connecting points I and II).

colon must pass after low anterior resection and anastomosis. Accordingly, in recent years low anterior resection and anastomosis have been performed for lesions much closer to the anal verge than 12 cm. This has never been much of a technical problem in women, with their wide, gynecoid pelvis, but the anastomosis can be technically demanding in a man with a narrow, android pelvis. Anastomosis of the proximal sigmoid colon to the distal rectum, or even to the anus, has been facilitated recently by the use of stapling techniques (Fig. 11–13) or by suturing the proximal colon to the dentate line per anus. Most cancers of the upper and middle thirds, and some cancers of the lower third, of the rectum can be treated by anterior resection. Anterior resection (and avoidance of a colostomy) can be performed with good long-term survival—equivalent to that for abdomo perineal resection—if the mesorectum that contains the draining lymph nodes is excised also.

Surgical Treatment of Carcinoma of the Anus. Carcinoma of the anus tends to be of the epidermoid variety. It is now often treated without abdominoperineal resection, owing to its dramatic response to the combination of chemotherapy and radiation therapy.

Surgical Treatment of Complicated Colon Cancer. Complications of colon cancer such as perforation and obstruction dictate a somewhat different approach. A carcinoma of the colon can perforate, or, if it is obstructing, can cause perforation of a grossly dilated cecum. In any event, the perforation leads to fecal soiling of the peritoneal cavity with

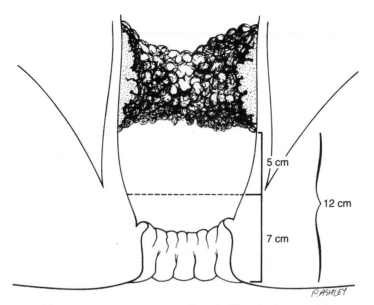

Figure 11–12. These measurements are used to decide whether a sphincter-preserving operation (anterior resection) can be performed or whether the patient must undergo abdominoperineal resection of the rectum with permanent colostomy. The old limit was approximately 12 cm. It is now deemed acceptable to use a distal margin of 2.0 to 2.5 cm. In addition, less than 7 cm of anorectum is required for fecal continence. Accordingly, low anterior resection of the rectum could technically be done for a carcinoma 5 or 6 cm from the anal verge. This would preserve the anal sphincter and avoid a colostomy. Because of the technical requirements of performing such a low anastomosis, one must guard against anastomotic leak and make sure that there is not too much compromise of the distal margin. The mesorectum should be excised to encompass draining lymph nodes.

resultant peritonitis, which markedly increased the operative mortality risk (Fig. 11–14). Although a perforated carcinoma of the right colon is often treated successfully by right hemicolectomy and primary anastomosis (ileotransverse colostomy), a perforated cancer of the left colon is believed to require resection and end colostomy. The distal colon either can be brought out as a defunctionalized limb that drains only mucus (called a mucous fistula) or can be oversewn and dropped back into the pelvis. The latter is called *Hartmann's procedure* (Fig. 11–15). The peritoneal inflammation resulting from perforation makes a primary anastomosis in the left colon too tenuous, and the risk of anastomosis disruption with resultant sepsis prohibitive.

Carcinoma is the most common cause of large bowel obstruction. Resection and primary anastomosis of an obstructing left-sided colon cancer is also considered unwise in such cases. The disparity in size between the dilated proximal bowel and the collapsed distal bowel, along with the edema of the bowel and the loading of the proximal colon with copious liquid and feces, would render the results of anastomosis

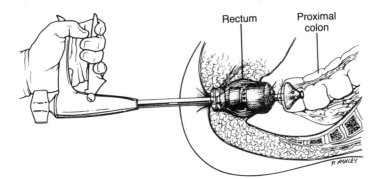

Rectum   Proximal colon

Figure 11–13. End-to-end stapling instrument used to perform a low anterior resection. The rectosigmoid was resected at laparotomy. The instrument is inserted through the anus, and the proximal and distal bowel are approximated over it. The instrument simultaneously fashions the connection (stoma) with a circular knife and connects the two ends with a double layer of staggered staples.

unpredictable, thus making resection with primary anastomosis hazardous. Therefore, large bowel obstruction secondary to colon carcinoma may be treated initially by transverse colostomy (Fig. 11–16). One to two weeks later, after the colon has been decompressed, mechanical and antibiotic preparation of the bowel can be done. An appropriate resection of bowel, tumor, and draining mesentery then can be performed along with anastomosis. The transverse colostomy can be closed in a third-stage operation. An alternative method of dealing with an obstructing carcinoma of the left colon is to perform primary resection with an end colostomy. The distal limb could be brought out as a mucous fistula or could be oversewn and dropped back into the pelvis (Hartmann's procedure). Gastrointestinal continuity can be reestablished at a second operation weeks later by means of an anastomosis. This is similar to the procedure performed for perforated left colon cancer, except that the second-stage operation to restore intestinal continuity need not be delayed as long as for the former procedure, as the surrounding inflammation would not be expected to be as great. The two-stage procedure has the advantage of resecting the tumor at the first operation, so that, should myocardial infarction or an other medical problem force delay of the next stage, at least the tumor will have been removed. The three-stage operation (diverting transverse loop colostomy as the first operation) has the advantage of being quicker and less extensive than resection plus colostomy but the disadvantages of leaving the cancer in place until the second stage and of requiring three operations instead of two. Nevertheless, the three-stage procedure may be indicated for patients who are too medically compromised on presentation to tolerate anything other than a transverse loop colostomy.

An obstructing lesion of the right colon is frequently treated by resection and primary anastomosis. Perhaps because the dilated ileum actually is closer in caliber to the transverse colon than it would nor-

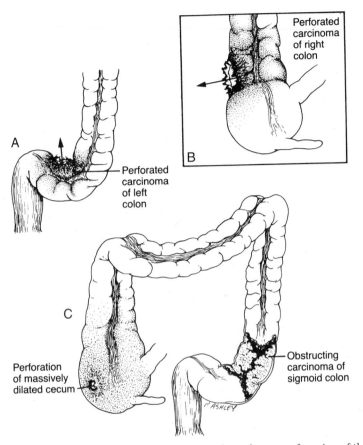

Figure 11–14. *(A)* Carcinoma of the left colon can perforate because of erosion of the tumor through the bowel wall, as can *(B)* carcinoma of the right colon. Alternatively, the cecum can perforate as a result of massive dilatation when a large bowel obstruction caused by left-sided colon cancer is present *(C)*.

mally be, a primary anastomosis can be performed with relative safety, even in the presence of obstruction.

Prognosis

The prognosis for colorectal cancer depends on the presence or absence of distant metastases, the presence or absence of involvement of the mesenteric lymph nodes, and the depth of invasion through the bowel wall. Carcinoma of the rectum historically has been staged according to Dukes ABC classification. Dukes A category refers to the stage at which the tumor is confined to the bowel wall; Dukes B is the stage when the tumor extends into the perirectal fat; and stage C denotes involvement of the mesenteric lymph nodes. Subsequently, this staging system was

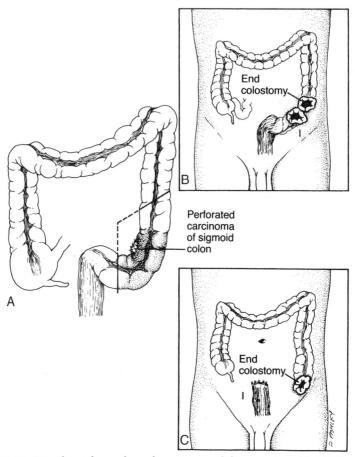

Figure 11–15. Procedures for perforated carcinoma of the rectosigmoid. *(A)* The segment of rectosigmoid harboring the tumor is resected. *(B)* When the tumor is high enough in the colon and there is enough distal limb, the distal limb can be brought out as a mucous fistula. *(C)* If the lesion is low lying, the distal limb may be too short to allow it to be brought to the abdominal wall. In that case, the rectal stump can be oversewn and dropped back into the pelvis.

applied to carcinoma of the colon, and stage D was added to denote the presence of distant metastases. Several refinements of the staging system have been suggested, but there is some feeling that we should continue to use Dukes original classification, since it has such prognostic significance.

Patients with Dukes A, B, and C tumors have approximately 70% to 90%, 60% and 30% 5-year survival rates, respectively. Stage D has a more dismal prognosis. Five-year survival approximates the cure rate for colorectal cancer, because most recurrences occur within the first 2 years. The 5-year survival rate is higher than the rate stated above when the

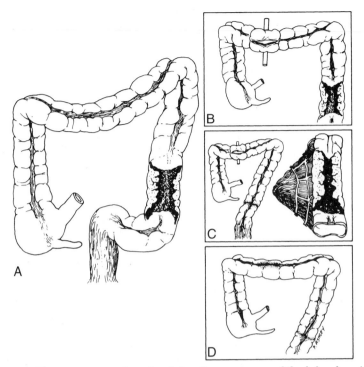

Figure 11–16. Three-stage procedure for obstructing carcinoma of the left colon. *(A)* Large bowel obstruction due to an annular (napkin-ring) carcinoma of the descending colon. *(B)* The obstruction has been relieved with a transverse colostomy. This can be performed through a small incision in the right upper abdominal quadrant. *(C)* At the second-stage operation, the segment of colon harboring the tumor has been resected. Since bowel preparation has been given through the stomas and the anus and per os, an end-to-end anastomosis can be performed safely. The presence of the proximal diverting colostomy adds another element of safety. *(D)* In the third stage, the colostomy is closed. A good alternative to the three-stage procedure for obstructing carcinoma is Hartmann's procedure, which is also done for perforated diverticulitis.

data are corrected actuarially (i.e., for patients who die of other causes). Chemotherapy has now been shown to improve survival for Dukes C cases of colon cancer, and a combination of chemotherapy and radiation therapy has improved survival in Dukes C carcinoma of the rectum. The TNM staging system has been officially sanctioned and is being used more frequently. Stages I, II, and III roughly correspond to Dukes A (confined to bowel wall), B (through bowel wall, no nodes), and C (positive lymph nodes). If there are metastases, the cancer is stage D (Stage IV), regardless of depth of invasion or node status.

INFLAMMATORY LESIONS OF THE COLON, RECTUM, AND ANUS

Inflammatory lesions of the colon, rectum, and anus include diverticulitis, ulcerative colitis, and Crohn's disease. Perianal problems such as anal fissure, fistula in ano, perianal abscess, and hemorrhoids are discussed in this section.

CASE 11–4

Perforated Sigmoid Diverticulitis

A 65-year-old woman was admitted via the accident room with severe abdominal pain associated with fever and shaking chills. She had been unable to eat or drink for 3 days and had last voided 18 hours before admission. She had undergone cholecystectomy 5 years before admission and had a history of hypertension treated with a low-salt diet.

Physical examination on admission revealed blood pressure of 100/60 mm Hg and a pulse rate of 120. The rectal temperature was 102°F. The abdomen was diffusely tender, with generalized rebound and involuntary guarding. Bowel sounds were absent. The rectal examination was unremarkable.

The white blood cell count was 16,400 with a shift to the left. The flat and upright abdominal films revealed a small amount of free air under the left hemidiaphragm.

A peripheral large-bore intravenous catheter and a central venous catheter were inserted, as was a Foley catheter. Fifteen milliliters of concentrated urine was drained. The central venous pressure was 0 cm H_2O. Fifteen hundred cubic centimeters of normal saline was administered over the next hour, blood for culture was drawn, and the patient was given gentamicin, clindamycin, and ampicillin. The central venous pressure increased to 10 cm H_2O, the pulse rate decreased to 96 beats per minute, the systolic blood pressure increased to 130 mm Hg, and 40 ml of urine was excreted over the course of 1 hour.

Laparotomy was performed, and feces and purulent material were found in the left lower abdominal quadrant, along with a perforated sigmoid diverticulum. Sigmoid resection with end colostomy and oversewing of the rectal stump (Hartmann's procedure) was performed. Postoperatively, the fever decreased and the colostomy began to function. The antibiotics and intravenous fluid administration were discontinued, and the patient tolerated a regular diet. She was discharged on the 14th postoperative day. Three months later she was readmitted, and intestinal continuity was reestablished with a colorectal anastomosis.

DISCUSSION OF CASE 11–4

Diverticulitis is a common form of inflammation as it relates to the large bowel. The majority of people over 60 years of age in Western countries are believed to have diverticulosis of the colon. A diet low in fiber—a result of the processed food consumed in Western countries—has been implicated in the pathogenesis of diverticulosis coli. According to Laplace's law, the colon must generate increased pressure to evacuate the small stools common to Westerners. This theoretically causes outpouching of the mucosa through defects in the muscular layers, where the mesenteric vessels penetrate the bowel wall (Fig. 11–17). Because these outpouchings do not contain all layers of the bowel wall, they are really pseudodiverticuli. Diverticuli have little significance unless they become inflamed (diverticulitis) or bleed. They do not usually do both. A high-fiber diet has been advocated to prevent both the development of diverticuli and the onset of acute inflammation in patients with diverticulosis coli.

Diagnosis

Symptoms and Signs. The sigmoid colon is a common site of diverticulitis. Sigmoid diverticulitis frequently presents with left lower quadrant abdominal pain, sometimes associated with reflex nausea and vomiting. Fever and chills may be present. A change in bowel habits with constipation, diarrhea, and decreased caliber of the stool may occur if there is an obstructive component to the diverticulitis. Urinary tract symptoms such as dysuria and frequency are common in patients with diverticulitis.

Physical examination may reveal left lower quadrant tenderness. A tender mass may be present if there is a peridiverticular abscess, and signs of peritonitis such as diffuse tenderness, generalized rebound, involuntary guarding, and a rigid, boardlike abdomen may be present if there is a free perforation. A tender mass may be discovered on rectal examination.

Laboratory Tests and Imaging Techniques. Leukocytosis is likely when diverticulitis is present, and the flat and upright abdominal films may reveal free air under the diaphragm (pneumoperitoneum) with perforated diverticulitis. The abdominal films may also show an ileus pattern (air-filled loops of small and large bowel) resulting from peritoneal irritation. Blunting of the psoas shadow may be noted when an intraab-

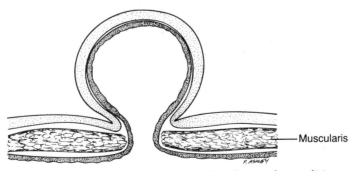

Figure 11–17. Section of the bowel wall showing that diverticulosis coli is composed of pseudodiverticuli. The mucosa pouts out through defects in the muscle coat.

dominal abscess is present. Barium enema examination is usually deferred until resolution of the acute episode, for fear of causing perforation of a previously intact inflamed diverticulum. The combination of barium and feces free in the peritoneal cavity causes particularly severe peritonitis and is thus to be avoided. A contrast enema with Gastrografin is safer and may expedite the diagnosis; however, if the acute episode subsides with nonoperative therapy, sigmoidoscopy and barium enema examination are often performed during a quiescent period to rule out carcinoma as a cause of the illness. Alternatively, colonoscopy can be performed on a nonemergency basis, but is avoided in the acute phase for fear of causing perforation. CT, now the gold standard in the diagnosis of sigmoid diverticulitis, can demonstrate diverticula and diverticulitis manifested by a thickened sigmoid colon and streaking of the surrounding fat due to inflammation. It may show a peridiverticular abscess, which can then be drained percutaneously under CT guidance, converting an emergency operation to an elective one in which a primary anastomosis can be performed and avoiding a temporary colostomy. An air-fluid level in the bladder on CT suggests a colovesical fistula, which can be due to diverticulitis.

Treatment

The treatment of diverticulitis without perforation usually involves "putting the bowel at rest" by withholding oral feedings, providing intravenous fluids, and perhaps decompressing the gut with a nasogastric tube if there is nausea, vomiting, and distention due to secondary ileus or to reflexes mediated by the autonomic nervous system. Intravenous doses of antibiotics are ordered. Many patients experience resolution of the acute attack on this regimen and can be discharged. If, however, the patient develops recurrent attacks, it may be prudent to perform definitive surgery such as sigmoid resection and primary anastomosis during a quiescent phase as prophylaxis against a serious complication such as a free perforation or a sealed-off perforation and abscess formation.

Diverticulosis can be a source of lower gastrointestinal bleeding (see Chapter 10). Diverticulitis can cause a host of complications—free perforation with peritonitis and sepsis, a sealed-off perforation with pericolic abscess, large bowel obstruction due to the inflammatory mass, and colovesical, colovaginal, and colocutaneous fistulas. Fistulas, of course, are not unique to diverticulitis: they also occur with Crohn's disease and carcinoma of the colon.

Historically in the treatment of perforated diverticulitis, a three-stage procedure was performed. The first stage was transverse colostomy and drainage of the perforation. The second stage, usually performed 6 to 12 weeks later, involved resecting the area of colon affected by diverticulitis (usually the sigmoid colon) and performing an anastomosis (connecting the proximal and distal parts of the colon by sutures). The third stage involved closure of the original transverse colostomy. The three-stage procedure is now of historical interest only.

Objections to the three-stage procedure were raised because the operation does not extirpate the inflamed segment of bowel, the transverse loop colostomy does not produce complete diversion, and, in any event, the distal colon is full of feces, which can subsequently bathe the area of perforation for days. These factors may be responsible for persistent sepsis after the first-stage operation (transverse loop colostomy and drainage of the pelvis). Moreover, the combined morbidity and mortality of all three stages is greater than that for either the one-stage or the two-stage procedure (described later), as is the duration of hospitalization.

Resection of the segment of bowel involved with diverticulitis and primary anastomosis of the remaining colon (Fig. 11–18) has been advocated by some investigators, even in cases of free perforation and perito-

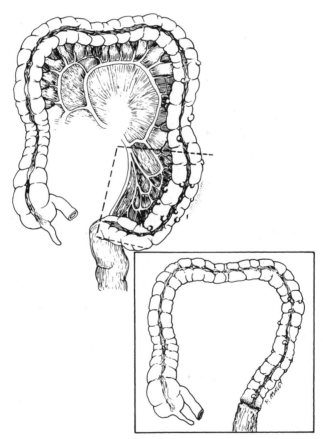

Figure 11–18. Resection of the segment of sigmoid colon that is most extensively involved down to the rectum followed by end-to-end anastomosis has been advocated for treatment of perforated sigmoid diverticulitis. Most surgeons believe that primary anastomosis in the face of perforation is too hazardous because acute inflammation increases the possibility of anastomotic leakage.

nitis or perforation with formation of a pericolic abscess. Those who object to this method believe that the likelihood of anastomotic disruption in the setting of acute inflammation is great, and the sequelae of persistent sepsis can be catastrophic. The one-stage operation is indicated mostly when one operates during a quiescent phase, after the acute inflammation has subsided.

A two-stage procedure (Hartmann's) has therefore been advocated in the presence of acute inflammation that does not resolve with medical treatment. This entails resecting the involved segment of colon and draining any pericolic abscess. The proximal segment of colon is brought out as an end colostomy, and the distal end is oversewn and dropped back into the pelvis. A second laparotomy can be performed later, when a colorectal anastomosis can be used to restore gastrointestinal continuity. Sigmoid resection with end colostomy and oversewing of the rectal stump has been illustrated in the discussion of perforating and obstructing carcinomas of the rectosigmoid colon and is also very useful when the surgeon must operate in the acute phase of diverticulitis. Colovesical and colovaginal fistulas can sometimes be repaired in one stage when the inflammation is of low grade. This is because any abscess present has typically drained itself through the bladder or vagina, respectively, allowing the acute inflammation to resolve.

It is not necessary to resect all proximal colon that contains diverticuli, but if complications such as postoperative colocutaneous fistula are to be avoided it is important to resect all of the sigmoid colon that harbors a thickened muscle layer and to anastomose uninflamed, nonthickened colon proximally to rectum distally. This is true whether a one- or a two-stage procedure is performed.

CASE 11–5

Ulcerative Colitis

A 35-year-old man was admitted because of an exacerbation of ulcerative colitis. Ulcerative colitis had been diagnosed at age 15, when a barium enema examination performed because of frequent bouts of bloody diarrhea revealed a foreshortened colon with loss of haustral markings and ulcerations. Multiple exacerbations and remissions had occurred until the month before admission, when the bouts became so frequent, in spite of use of steroids, sulfasalazine, and azathioprine, that the patient found the situation intolerable. He was also told by his gastroenterologist that the possibility of the colon's harboring a carcinoma was significant. Accordingly, he was hydrated and given a parenteral "prep" of corticosteroids to prevent an addisonian crisis, and underwent restorative proctocolectomy. A temporary ileostomy had been created at the time of this surgery, to allow the pouch to heal. He had an unremarkable postoperative course and was discharged on postoperative day 14. Three months later, the patient was readmitted and the ileostomy was closed. By 1 year after surgery, although the patient was still having six loose bowel movements per day, soiling of the underclothes during the day was rare. He was back at work by 7 months postoperatively.

DISCUSSION OF CASE 11–5

Inflammatory bowel disease is a fascinating subject that has received tremendous attention in the literature. Mastery of the terminology is an important first step in understanding inflammatory bowel disease, which can be categorized roughly as ulcerative colitis and Crohn's disease. A small group of lesions cannot be classified as one or the other of these, by virtue of either clinical manifestations or histologic appearance. This small group is said to be *indeterminate colitis.*

Ulcerative Colitis

Ulcerative colitis involves only the large intestine and is a mucosal and submucosal disease, not generally involving all the layers of the bowel wall. Bloody diarrhea and mucus per rectum are frequent findings, and fever may be present. Abdominal pain may occur with acute attacks. These patients may return to a baseline of rather good health between acute exacerbations. One extraintestinal manifestation is sclerosing cholangitis. Extraintestinal manifestations such as uveitis, ankylosing spondylitis, erythema nodosum, and pyoderma gangrenosum may can be associated with ulcerative colitis or with Crohn's disease. Chronic ulcerative colitis may be caused by the interaction of genetic and environmental factors. If one person in a family has ulcerative colitis, the risk for their family members increases. The immune system may play a role. It has been proposed—but not proven—that infection may also be implicated.

Diagnosis. The physical examination may reveal weight loss, but the findings on abdominal examination may be within normal limits if none of the complications of ulcerative colitis has occurred. Since ulcerative colitis almost never spares the rectum, sigmoidoscopy or colonoscopy and biopsy may confirm the diagnosis. Chronic ulcerative colitis may begin by affecting the rectosigmoid and progress in continuity to the ileocecal valve. Ulcers and pseudopolyps may be seen grossly, and crypt abscesses microscopically. Granulomas are not normally seen. Barium enema examination may demonstrate loss of haustrations and decreased caliber and foreshortening of the colon, but frank stricture in a case of ulcerative colitis should raise the suspicion of carcinoma of the colon, as strictures are a late finding in ulcerative colitis unless carcinoma of the colon has also developed. Colonoscopy may demonstrate ulcerative colitis much earlier in the course of the disease than does barium enema. There is a predisposition to colon cancer among patients with ulcerative colitis, and the incidence increases with duration of the disease. If colonoscopy and multiple biopsies show severe dysplasia, the risk of the colon's harboring carcinoma is significant and surgical extirpation of the colon and rectum must be considered. A small bowel series may show a "string sign" in the terminal ileum or involvement of other parts of the small bowel, suggesting the presence of granulomatous (Crohn's) rather than ulcerative colitis. Reflux of barium into the terminal ileum at the time of barium enema showing a diseased terminal ileum is also indicative of Crohn's disease with Crohn's colitis and ileitis (ileocolitis), rather than of ulcerative colitis.

Treatment. Exacerbations of ulcerative colitis are frequently managed with steroids, azathioprine, sulfasalazine, 5-ASA preparations, and sometimes cyclosporine. If the episode is severe, hospitalization may be required so that the patient can be given nothing by mouth, hydrated intravenously, and given intravenous steroids or ACTH and other medications. Total parenteral nutrition has proved useful in preventing malnutrition during periods when the patient is not eating. Active colonic bleeding may necessitate transfusion of packed red blood cells. The patient must be carefully monitored to ensure that toxic dilatation of the colon and perforation do not occur.

Surgery may be indicated for complications of ulcerative colitis such as *toxic megacolon.* This entity, also called *toxic dilatation of the colon,* presents with a markedly dilated colon that is filled with air and fluid and has the potential for perforation, with massive contamination of the peritoneal cavity and resultant peritonitis and sepsis.

Toxic megacolon may be precipitated by the use of antidiarrheal drugs such as diphenoxylate hydrochloride or by barium enema examination of patients with ulcerative colitis. A short period of "medical management," consisting of nasogastric decompression, intravenous hydration, antibiotics, and steroids, may be tried for toxic dilation of the colon, but patients must be monitored exceedingly closely with serial physical examinations, frequent abdominal x-ray examinations, and meticulous attention to the state of hydration. If there is any evidence of peritonitis on physical examination, or increasing colonic dilatation, or evidence of air in the bowel wall or free air under the diaphragm on flat and upright abdominal x-ray views, emergency laparotomy must be carried out. Surgery also should be undertaken if no evidence of improvement is seen within a reasonable time, since significant morbidity and mortality are associated with continued ineffective nonoperative treatment.

The operative treatment for toxic megacolon is usually *subtotal colectomy* (also called *total abdominal colectomy*), with either oversewing of the rectal stump (which is merely dropped back into the pelvis) or the bringing out of a mucous fistula (Fig. 11–19). In either case, ileostomy is performed. The additional time it would take to remove the rectum through a perineal incision is considered inappropriate for these critically ill patients. Moreover, preserving the rectum allows for restoration of continuity later by performing a mucosal proctectomy with pelvic pouch–anal anastomosis after the patient recovers from the acute illness. In some chronically ill patients without indications for emergency surgi-

Figure 11–19. Subtotal colectomy for toxic megacolon. The massively distended intraabdominal colon is resected, care being taken to avoid perforation of the paper-thin, fluid-filled bowel (I). The terminal ileum is brought out as an ileostomy (II), and the rectal stump is oversewn (III). Alternatively, the distal rectosigmoid colon may be brought out as a mucous fistula (so called because it obviously drains only mucus, not enteric contents).

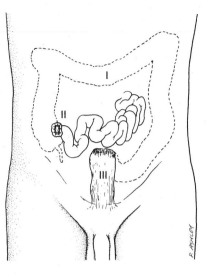

cal intervention, total proctocolectomy and permanent ileostomy are carried out to improve the quality of life and to prevent development of colon cancer, for which these patients are at increased risk. In contradistinction to Crohn's disease, these patients are not at risk for recurrence in the small intestine and are, therefore, cured after total proctocolectomy and permanent ileostomy.

Restorative proctocolectomy is now being performed for patients with ulcerative colitis undergoing elective surgery who are motivated to retain the normal route of defecation. The operation has a low mortality rate but high morbidity, and continence of feces may not be perfect thereafter. Moreover, it may take many months for patients to be able to return to work after the operation. Some patients may opt, therefore, for the simpler total proctocolectomy and permanent ileostomy, but most *patients* who have had both ileostomy and a restorative proctocolectomy (also known as a *pelvic pouch–anal anastomosis*) prefer life after the latter operation. The restorative proctocolectomy is performed by removing the entire colon and most of the rectum and stripping the mucosa from the remaining rectum. A "new rectum" is then formed in the shape of a J, an S, or a W by using a loop of small bowel, and the new rectum (neorectum) is brought through the sphincters and anastomosed to the dentate line. This is reasonable because there is only squamous epithelium below the dentate line, and it is only the columnar epithelium above the dentate line that is at risk for ulcerative colitis and adenocarcinoma. A temporary ileostomy protects against leaks. Small bowel obstruction (often requiring reoperation) and inflammation in the neorectum ("pouchitis") are common complications of this procedure. Enterovaginal fistula can also occur.

Crohn's Disease

Crohn's disease is a form of inflammatory bowel disease characterized by transmural involvement (that is, the entire thickness of the bowel wall is diseased). Granulomas may be present. Whereas ulcerative colitis is confined to the colon and rectum, Crohn's disease can involve any part of the gastrointestinal tract from mouth to anus. Ulcerative colitis tends to involve the left side of the colon, beginning at the rectum, whereas Crohn's disease tends to involve the right side of the colon when it involves that viscus at all. Crohn's disease tends to be characterized by multiple skip areas, whereas ulcerative colitis tends to involve one continuous area. When Crohn's disease involves the small bowel, it is often called *regional enteritis,* and since it frequently involves the terminal ileum, it may be called *terminal ileitis.* Crohn's disease of the large bowel is often called *granulomatous colitis.*

Diagnosis

Symptoms. Regional enteritis often presents with cramping abdominal pain, diarrhea, fever, and malaise. Patients are often chronically ill, never really returning to normal health. Extraintestinal manifestations such as ankylosing spondylitis, erythema nodosum, uveitis, and pyoderma gangrenosum can also occur with Crohn's disease. There are also increased incidences of associated gallstones, sclerosing cholangitis, and cholangiocarcinoma.

Physical Examination. The physical examination in Crohn's patients may reveal evidence of complications of the disease. There may be a tender mass if an intraabdominal abscess is present, and there may be abdominal distention if bowel obstruction has occurred. Free perforation is uncommon in this disease, but peritonitis can occur when an abscess ruptures into the free peritoneal cavity. The presence or absence of scars from previous abdominal surgery should be noted; drainage may indicate an enterocutaneous fistula.

Imaging Techniques. Plain abdominal films may show evidence of obstruction or a soft tissue density, the latter often displacing air-filled loops of bowel to one side of the abdominal cavity, suggesting an abscess. Barium examination, either an upper gastrointestinal series with small bowel follow-through or a barium enema with reflux into the terminal ileum, may show narrowing at the terminal ileum ("string sign") or elsewhere in the gut.

Endoscopy. Colonoscopy, in addition to barium enema, may demonstrate findings of Crohn's disease and help to define the anatomic pattern. Forty per cent of cases are ileocolic, 30% have small bowel involvement only, and 30% are only granulomatous colitis.

Treatment

Medical management of regional enteritis or granulomatous colitis usually consists of administration of steroids, sulfasalazine, 5-ASA; occasionally azathioprine, Flagyl, and antidiarrheal drugs; and sometimes bowel rest and total parenteral nutrition. It is the ASA moiety in sulfasalazine that is active and the sulfa moiety that is responsible for most of the side effects. Moreover, the two moieties are not cleaved until the colon, so sulfasalazine is useful only for colitis. Therefore, 5-ASA preparations are often used instead of sulfasalazine. Cyclosporine may aid in the closure of Crohn's fistulas. Surgery is indicated for the complications of Crohn's disease such as stricture causing partial or complete bowel obstruction, abscess formation in juxtaposition to diseased bowel, or the formation of fistulas with physiologic consequences. Surgery is also frequently performed for failure of medical therapy or failure to thrive. Repeated resections might put the patient at risk for the short-gut syndrome (malnutrition due to decreased absorptive surface), since the disease has a strong tendency to recur and may require many repeat resections over the years. Fear of short-gut syndrome is appropriate but should not cause the clinician to persist with nonoperative therapy when it has obviously become futile, for such a practice increases the risk of postoperative complications by allowing preoperative sepsis to supervene. Moreover, expeditious surgery allows for early rehabilitation and return to a state of well-being, even if recurrences throughout life are likely. Stricturoplasty—widening the stricture by opening it longitudinally and closing it transversely—applied to skip areas may further decrease the incidence of short-gut syndrome.

When Crohn's disease involves the terminal ileum and right colon (ileocolic Crohn's disease), it can cause obstruction or a sealed-off perforation with adjacent abscess requiring ileocolic resection with either a primary anastomosis or an ileostomy and mucous fistula to relieve the obstruction. A sealed-off perforation in the terminal ileum with an adjacent abscess probably requires resection of the involved segment of the small bowel along with drainage of the abscess. An entrectomy with end-to-end anastomosis can be performed for terminal ileitis with stricture, and skip areas can be treated by resection or by stricturoplasty. Enteroenteric and enterocolic fistulas do not always require surgical intervention. Enterovaginal and enterovesical fistulas are likely to be quite symptomatic.

Perianal disease—fistula in ano, anal fissure, or perianal abscess—often accompanies Crohn's disease. These entities can also occur in the absence of inflammatory bowel disease and are discussed separately. When they do occur with Crohn's disease, conservatism should be the rule, as the symptoms they cause can be mild in comparison with the appearance of the lesion, and wounds in the perianal region may not heal well after surgical intervention when Crohn's disease is present. Success has been achieved by treating the perianal manifestations of Crohn's disease with metronidazole (Flagyl). Anorectal abscesses still need to be drained, even in the presence of Crohn's disease, and carefully selected Crohn's patients with "garden-variety" fistula in ano may have a good result from fistulotomy, despite the risk of failure to heal.

Perianal Disease

Perianal disease frequently occurs in the absence of Crohn's disease, and although it is not usually life threatening, it can detract profoundly from the patient's quality of life. Entities to be discussed include hemorrhoids (piles), anal fissure (or anal ulcer), anal fistula, and perianal, ischiorectal, and pelvirectal abscesses.

Hemorrhoids

External hemorrhoids occur below the dentate line, where there is sensory innervation. They consist of dilated veins and overlying mucosa and skin. Thrombosis of external hemorrhoids is exceedingly painful, and incision with enucleation of the clot can afford dramatic relief (Fig. 11–20). Alternatively, a thrombosed hemorrhoid can be excised under local anesthesia.

Internal hemorrhoids can bleed, and even if the blood loss is small, rectal bleeding is usually alarming to the patient. One must be sure that the bleeding is not from an underlying carcinoma of the colon or rectum. It is a mistake to attribute rectal bleeding to hemorrhoids without per-

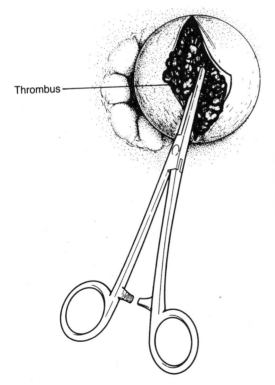

Thrombus

Figure 11–20. Enucleation of the clot from a thrombosed external hemorrhoid affords dramatic relief of pain. Local anesthetic is infiltrated, and the mucosa is incised. The clot is removed with a hemostat.

forming sigmoidoscopy and barium enema examination or colonoscopy. Internal hemorrhoids can also prolapse through the anus, and, since the mucosa secretes mucus, moist underclothes can cause pruritus ani.

Excision of the hemorrhoids by formal hemorrhoidectomy has been the treatment of choice (Fig. 11–21), but the postoperative discomfort experienced by the patient has led surgeons to search for less uncomfortable techniques. Internal hemorrhoids can be ligated with rubber bands in the expectation that they will slough (Fig. 11–22). This method can be employed on an outpatient basis but is suitable only for internal hemorrhoids, as it would cause extreme pain if used below the dentate line. There is good success with infrared coagulation for outpatient treatment of internal hemorrhoids to interrupt the blood supply and decrease bleeding and protrusion.

Anal Fissure

Anal fissures or ulcers are usually caused by trauma to the anal mucosa by hard stool. They often present with pain on defecation and blood on the toilet tissue. They result because a hard stool traumatizes the mucosa,

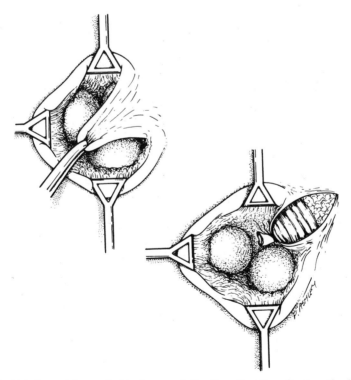

Figure 11–21. Formal hemorrhoidectomy entails dissecting free, ligating the base, and excising the right anterior and posterior and left lateral internal hemorrhoids.

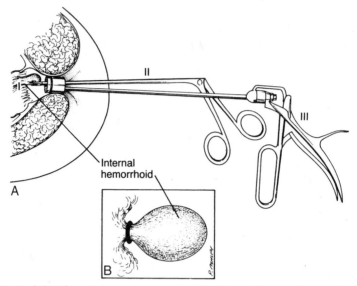

Internal
hemorrhoid

A

B

Figure 11–22. *(A)* Right anterior and posterior and left lateral internal hemorrhoids can be ligated without anesthesia as an outpatient procedure. Each hemorrhoid (I) is grasped with forceps (II) inserted through the hemorrhoid ligator (III). The trigger is pulled, and the band is placed tightly around the neck of the hemorrhoid. *(B)* Blood supply to the internal hemorrhoid is cut off, and it should slough and pass in 1 or 2 weeks.

causing spasm of the sphincter so that the next stool causes even more trauma. Because of the pain, the patient unconsciously avoids defecation, becoming more constipated and producing harder, more traumatizing stools. The increased pain causes more spasm, and the vicious cycle continues. Local ischemia can also play a role. Medical treatment consists of avoiding constipation by drinking more liquids, eating a high-fiber diet, taking a psyllium preparation, and exercising. Ointments are frequently prescribed. Anal fissure is not a listed indication for topical nitroglycerine ointment, but some clinicians find that it helps their patients with anal fissure, perhaps by relaxing the smooth muscle of the internal sphincter. Surgical treatment consists of sphincterotomy, the internal sphincter being incised to decrease its tone, leaving the external sphincter to preserve continence; this interrupts the vicious cycle of trauma, spasm, and more trauma.

Fistula in Ano

Fistula in ano arises in a crypt abscess. The tract then progresses in the intersphincteric plane, in the case of an intersphincteric fistula, often presenting as a perianal abscess. The fistula may not become apparent until after incision and drainage of a perianal abscess. Similarly, a transsphincteric fistula may lead to an ischiorectal abscess, and a suprasphincteric fistula to a pelvirectal abscess (Fig. 11–23).

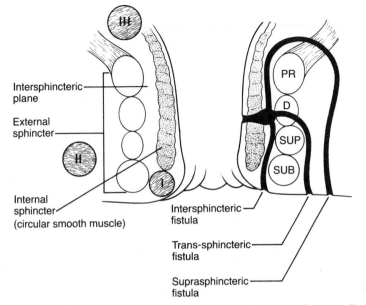

Figure 11–23. A fistula in ano begins as a crypt abscess. A plane exists between the circular internal sphincter (composed of smooth muscle) and the external anal sphincter (skeletal muscle). This is present because the outer longitudinal muscle coat of the bowel is attenuated down in this area. An intersphincteric fistula can develop after incision and drainage of a perianal abscess (I). A transphincteric fistula can develop after incision and drainage of an ischiorectal abscess (II). A pelvirectal abscess (III) can form above the levator muscles. Intersphincteric and transphincteric fistulas can be treated by unroofing, but because a suprasphincteric fistula lies above all the muscles of continence, unroofing or excision would result in incontinence. (Key: SUB, subcutaneous external sphincter; SUP, superficial external sphincter; D, deep external anal sphincter; PR, puborectalis muscle.)

Volvulus

Volvulus of the colon occurs when a loop of colon twists on redundant mesentery, causing compromise of the blood supply and creating potential for gangrene if the problem is not corrected soon enough. A sigmoid volvulus is a degenerative disease that tends to occur in chronically constipated, elderly, debilitated, and often institutionalized patients with redundant sigmoid colon. The colon often can be untwisted with a sigmoidoscope or colonoscope, and an emergency operation is thus avoided, but the recurrence rate is high. Therefore, elective sigmoid colectomy and end-to-end anastomosis is usually indicated to prevent recurrence, even though patients are often at increased operative risk because of associated medical problems.

Cecal volvulus is due to congenital failure of fixation of the right colon, so that it can twist on its mesentery. Under normal circumstances, the right colon is retroperitoneal and cannot twist. Because this lack of fixation is congenital in these patients, cecal volvulus tends to occur at an earlier age than does sigmoid volvulus. If surgery is performed before the onset of gangrene, the condition can be treated by tube cecostomy, which decompresses the colon before it perforates and also fixes the colon to the anterior abdominal wall, preventing recurrence of the volvulus. Two weeks later, the tube cecostomy can be removed and the colon remains fixed. The tract often closes without a second operation.

Mesenteric Infarction

Infarction of the colon, like that involving the small intestine, can be manifested by an acute surgical abdomen. It can be caused by arterial problems such as an embolus from a clot originating in the heart, by atherosclerotic narrowing of two or three visceral vessels such as the superior and inferior mesenteric arteries and celiac axis, by acute thrombosis of a narrowed visceral vessel, or by arteritis. An embolus is likely to lodge in the superior mesenteric artery, thus involving the small intestines and large bowel to the distal transverse colon. A mesenteric venous thrombosis may be caused by a hypercoagulable state such as polycythemia and can result in gangrene of the large or small bowel. Moreover, nonocclusive mesenteric infarction can occur when blood is shunted away from the splanchnic circulation as a homeostatic mechanism in low-flow states such as cardiogenic shock. This entity has a high mortality rate.

Ischemic colitis is often manifested by bloody diarrhea. It occurs when there is inadequate blood flow to the colon, owing, for example, to narrowing of the inferior mesenteric artery and disruption of collaterals from the marginal artery of Drummond. This can occur, albeit uncommonly, when the inferior mesenteric artery is sacrificed during resection of an abdominal aortic aneurysm. Ischemic colitis can heal without sequelae or can progress to gangrene or heal with stricture formation.

Recommended Reading

1. Mazier WP, Levien DH, Luchtefeld M, Senagore A (eds): *Surgery of the Colon, Rectum, and Anus*. Philadelphia: W.B. Saunders, 1995.
2. Levien DH (ed): Anorectal surgery. Surg Clin Am, 1994.
3. Cohen Z, McLeod RS: Inflammatory bowel disease. In Zuidema GD (ed): *Shackelford's Surgery of the Alimentary Tract*, ed 4, vol IV. Philadelphia: W.B. Saunders, 1996, pp 53–72.

12

Surgery of the Biliary Tract and Pancreas

Approximately 500,000 cholecystectomies are performed in the United States each year. Biliary tract disease is extremely common, and it is important for surgeons to master this fascinating subject.

CASE 12–1
Cholelithiasis and Chronic Cholecystitis

A 55-year-old woman presented to the surgeon's office with an 18-month history of intermittent right upper quadrant abdominal pain colicky in nature and precipitated by eating fatty foods. The pain often was severe, awakening her from sleep, and radiating to the right subscapular region. The attacks lasted approximately 2 hours, occurred three times per week, and were associated with nausea, and occasionaly vomiting. There was no history of dark, tea-colored urine or yellow stools. Her last attack was 2 days earlier.

Past medical history included hypertension but was negative for other illnesses. She had had no previous surgery or hospitalizations.

Physical examination revealed an obese female. There was no abdominal tenderness, mass, or organomegaly. Rectal examination was negative.

Laboratory reports obtained from the internist's office stated that the bilirubin, alkaline phosphatase, LDH, SGPT, amylase, and lipase values were within normal limits. An abdominal ultrasound study obtained by the internist revealed multiple echogenic foci in the gallbladder with beam blocking. The common bile duct did not appear dilated, and there were no dilated intrahepatic radicals. ECG and chest x-ray were normal.

The next week, the patient was admitted electively the morning of surgery and underwent laparoscopic cholecystectomy. She was able to eat the night of surgery, was discharged from the hospital the next morning, and returned to work the next week.

DISCUSSION OF CASE 12–1

Cholelithiasis (gallstones) is a common entity and its incidence increases with age. It is more common in women and in obese persons.

Multiparity and ingestion of birth control pills also increase the risk. There may be a genetic predisposition in some families and ethnic groups.

Diagnosis

Symptoms. The symptoms are often intermittent, and the patient frequently does not have the symptoms when she visits the surgeon. The pain typically is experienced in the right upper abdominal quadrant or epigastrium and often radiates to the right subscapular region. The pain is often accompanied by nausea and vomiting. The symptoms may be ill-defined and described as "heartburn" or dyspepsia. It is important to determine that there has been no dark, tea-colored urine or clay-colored stools, as these findings suggest a concomitant common bile duct stone (choledocholithiasis).

Physical Examination. Physical examination is often negative in a patient with cholelithiasis and chronic cholecystitis. This is in contradistinction to the findings in a patient with acute cholecystitis due to a stone obstructing the cystic duct, who may have a tender, palpable gallbladder.

Laboratory Findings. The complete blood count may reveal a normal white blood cell count, as acute inflammation is not present. The liver function tests (alkaline phosphatase, LDH, SGPT, and bilirubin) are likely to be normal unless there is also a common bile duct stone. The amylase value is normal unless there is associated gallstone pancreatitis.

Diagnostic Imaging. The diagnosis of cholelithiasis and chronic cholecystitis now is usually made by abdominal ultrasonography, which demonstrates the calculi as echogenic foci in the gallbladder with beam blocking. Thickening of the gallbladder wall and pericholecystic fluid can be identified on ultrasound, but they are indicative of *acute* rather than *chronic* cholecystitis. A dilated common bile duct or intrahepatic ducts can be appreciated by ultrasound and, if present, indicate concomitant common bile duct stones (choledocholithiasis). CT is less effective than ultrasound in diagnosing gallstones but is very effective in identifying dilated ducts (when IV contrast is given to distinguish portal veins and hepatic veins from ducts) and in identifying a thickened gallbladder wall and pericholecystic fluid.

Surgery

Cholecystectomy (removal of the gallbladder) is usually recommended for patients with symptomatic gallstones who are otherwise in reasonable health. This is done to relieve the symptoms of biliary colic and prevent the complications of gallstones—acute cholecystitis, common bile duct stones (choledocholithiasis) with obstructive jaundice, obstructive cholangitis, or both, cholecystoduodenal fistula with gallstone ileus, and gallstone pancreatitis. Whether completely asymptomatic gallstones identified as an incidental finding should be addressed surgically is a judgment call.

Laparoscopic Cholecystectomy

Although open cholecystectomy (by way of laparotomy) was historically the treatment for cholelithiasis and chronic cholecystitis, laparoscopic cholecystectomy has become the usual operation. This procedure entails placing four trocars through the abdominal wall, distending the abdomen with carbon dioxide, and visualizing the abdominal contents with a laparoscope inserted through the trocar placed through the lower end of the umbilicus. Instruments are then inserted through the other ports, and the procedure is visualized on a television screen as the surgical team removes the gallbladder, which can usually fit through the umbilical or upper abdominal puncture wound. The cystic duct and artery are doubly clipped and transected. Carefully identifying the junction of the gallbladder and cystic duct helps avoid common bile duct injury. The gallbladder is then dissected free from the liver bed and removed. To perform cholangiography at the time of laparoscopic cholecystectomy, a catheter is inserted through one of the ports or through a needle puncture in the abdominal wall into the cystic duct, dye is injected, and a radiograph is taken.

Laparoscopic cholecystectomy is becoming almost as safe (or as safe) as the traditional open method. This procedure is patient driven. Patients are demanding laparoscopic cholecystectomy because of the dramatic decrease in postoperative pain, the shorter hospital stay (1 or 2 days) or even outpatient surgery, and early return to work (approximately 1 week). Surgeons are striving to master this new procedure—so much in demand—and to monitor their results to make sure that it is at least as safe as the traditional operation. Patients must be informed that the surgeon will convert the operation to an open one if adhesions, bleeding, obscure anatomy, or other "surprises" are encountered that render laparoscopy unsafe.

Postoperative Course. Although a nasogastric tube and Foley catheter are often inserted preoperatively to prevent bladder or stomach injuries at the time of trocar insertion, they are taken out in the operating room or recovery room. Oral intake is usually resumed when the patient is fully awake, and the patient is encouraged to walk about. If there is no protracted nausea, vomiting, or unexpected fever or pain, the patient is usually discharged on the first postoperative day. Some surgeons are performing these operations as an outpatient procedure, although they must have a suitably "low threshold" for admitting a patient overnight when there is any question about the postoperative course.

Alternatives to Cholecystectomy for Chronic Cholecystitis

Dissolution of gallstones with chenodeoxycholic acid (chenotherapy) has fallen in disfavor. It was predicated on the premise that bile salts and phospholipids act in concert to keep cholesterol in solution and, when they are not present in adequate quantities, the cholesterol precipitates and gallstones form. Chenodeoxycholic acid tips the balance toward dissolution. For this technique to be effective, the gallbladder must be shown by oral cholecystography to function, so that the substance can be absorbed into it. The stones must be smaller than 1 cm, and they must not be radiopaque, as calcium interferes with dissolution. Symptoms must not be frequent, since it can take 2 years for chenotherapy to be effective. Because teratogenicity has not been ruled out, female patients must not be of childbearing age or must be using reliable birth control. Chenotherapy is thus appropriate for only a very small portion of those with cholelithiasis. Even when chenotherapy works, the gallstones can recur when therapy is discontinued. There has been some interest in breaking large stones nonoperatively with sound waves (extracorporeal shock-wave lithotripsy) and then dissolving the fragments with chenodeoxycholic acid. Enthusiasm for this has diminished since the advent of laparoscopic cholecystectomy.

CASE 12–2

Acute Cholecystitis

A 46-year-old woman presented to the emergency department with a 1-day history of severe right upper quadrant abdominal pain associated with nausea and vomiting.

Three years before admission, the patient had a similar, although milder, episode, at which time cholelithiasis was diagnosed on ultrasound. The decision was made to defer surgery at that time, and the patient had been asymptomatic until the present attack. On the evening before this admission, the patient also experienced a fever to 102°F and shaking chills. The symptoms persisted, and the patient came to the emergency department. No dark urine, clay-colored stools, or jaundice had been noted.

There was no history of diabetes mellitus or other serious medical problems.

Physical examination revealed an obese female in moderate distress. Temperature was 101.5°F, pulse 120 bpm, and blood pressure 150/90 mm Hg. Examination of the abdomen revealed marked right upper quadrant tenderness with Murphy's sign. There was a suggestion of a tender mass in the right upper quadrant. There was no generalized rebound or involuntary guarding. Bowel sounds were hypoactive. Rectal examination was normal.

The patient's white blood cell count was 17,500. The bilirubin, alkaline phosphatase, and LDH, amylase, and lipase values were within normal limits. Flat and upright abdominal films revealed no radiopaque gallstones, and repeat ultrasound confirmed the presence of gallstones but showed no dilatation of the common bile duct or intrahepatic radicals. A HIDA scan was performed, and after 4 hours dye was detected in the duodenum but not in the gallbladder. This suggested cystic duct obstruction.

The patient was given gentamicin and ampicillin intravenously. She was kept NPO, and a nasogastric tube was placed to suction. By the next day, however, the abdomen appeared even more tender; because the patient was still markedly febrile, cholecystectomy was scheduled. At surgery, the gallbladder was tense and acutely inflamed, with purulent exudate on its surface. A stone impacted at Hartmann's pouch obstructed the cystic duct. Laparoscopic cholecystectomy was attempted, but the gallbladder was too tense to be grasped. An attempt was made to decompress it with a large additional trocar placed through a separate stab wound under direct visualization, but this was unsuccessful because the gallbladder was completely filled with stones rather than bile. Thus, the surgeon converted the operation to open cholecystectomy. Because there were no indications for common bile duct exploration, it was not carried out.

Postoperatively, the patient's temperature returned to normal. Gastrointestinal function returned quickly; the nasogastric tube was removed, and the patient was allowed to eat. Liver function tests remained normal, and the white blood cell count returned to normal. Antibiotics and intravenous fluids were discontinued. The patient was discharged on the 7th postoperative day.

DISCUSSION OF CASE 12–2

Diagnosis

Symptoms. Acute cholecystitis usually presents as an emergency with severe symptoms early on. Typically the pain is in the right upper quadrant, radiating to the right subscapular region, although it may be experienced in the epigastrium. Nausea and vomiting are frequently present. Fever and chills can accompany acute cholecystitis in the same way that they accompany other abscesses, as the gallbladder can act like a collection of pus when the cystic duct is obstructed. Again, it is important to determine whether the patient has had dark urine or acholic stools, as these symptoms suggest concomitant common bile duct obstruction resulting from choledocholithiasis (common bile duct stones).

Physical Examination. In contradistinction to the patient with chronic cholecystitis, the patient with acute cholecystitis often has exquisite tenderness in the right upper quadrant. Murphy's sign is elicited when the examiner places his hand on the patient's right upper abdominal quadrant and asks the patient to take a deep breath. If an inflamed, tense gallbladder comes into contact with the examiner's hand as the gallbladder descends with downward movement of the diaphragm, the patient is likely to cease deep inspiration abruptly and to complain of pain; this suggests acute cholecystitis. The patient may even have diffuse abdominal tenderness and generalized rebound, making it difficult to exclude other intraabdominal disorders.

Laboratory Examination The white blood cell count is usually elevated because of acute inflammation. One would not ordinarily expect the bilirubin or alkaline phosphatase value to be elevated unless there is also a common bile duct stone, although, inexplicably, one can see mild elevations of these enzymes in acute cholecystitis, even without choledocholithiasis.

Imaging. Only 15% of gallstones are radiopaque enough to be seen on plain films of the abdomen. This is in contrast to the stones of urolithiasis, which are radiopaque in 85% of cases; however, plain abdominal films can document the presence of cholelithiasis in the 15% with radiopaque stones. Also, the plain films may demonstrate free air when the underlying problem turns out to be a perforated ulcer rather than acute cholecystitis. The abdominal films can also show air in the biliary tree when cholecystoduodenal fistula is present. Ultrasound is very useful to demonstrate gallstones and dilatation of the common bile duct and intrahepatic radicals in the event of concomitant choledocholithiasis. The presence of a thickened gallbladder wall or pericholecystic fluid suggests acute, rather than chronic, cholecystitis. The HIDA scan is an adjunct to history and physical examination in the diagnosis of acute cholecystitis. It requires that a radiopharmaceutic agent be injected into a vein and the right upper quadrant be imaged by scintigraphy. If dye appears in the duodenum after 4 hours but not in the gallbladder, the presumption is that the cystic duct is obstructed by a stone sitting in it or adjacent to it in Hartmann's pouch (Fig. 12–1). Cystic duct obstruction is the usual cause of acute cholecystitis.

Treatment

The patient must be kept NPO and rehydrated with intravenous fluids. The gastrointestinal tract may be put to rest with a nasogastric tube. Since the most common organisms in the biliary tract are *E. coli, Klebsiella* and *Enterococcus,* gentamicin and ampicillin would be an appropriate antibiotic combination.

If the patient's acute attack quickly subsides on this regimen, the patient can be allowed to go home, to return in 6 weeks for an interval cholecystectomy. This allows the surgeon to work in a field that is less edematous and inflamed, however the risk of a second attack during the interval is always present. It is often prudent to operate within a few days of admission, after the patient's condition has been optimized by rehydration, antibiotics, and bowel rest. One must sometimes operate even earlier if the patient fails to improve on the regimen described or in the rare case when free perforation of the gallbladder occurs. To proceed with cholecystectomy, the structures in the porta hepatis are carefully identified and the cystic artery is then ligated. The gallbladder is dissected free from the liver bed, the cystic duct is transected, and the gallbladder is removed (Fig. 12–2). A catheter can be inserted through the cystic duct stump into the common bile duct and cystic duct cholangiography can be performed (Fig. 12–3). If there are no filling defects in the common bile duct to suggest choledocholithiasis and there is free flow of dye into the duodenum, the catheter is removed and the cystic duct ligated. Many surgeons perform cystic duct cholangiography on all

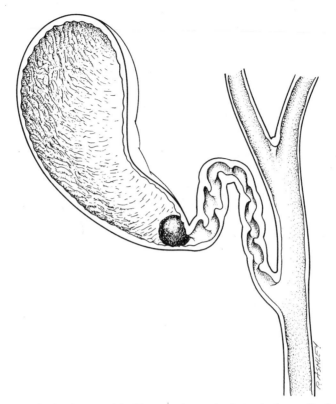

Figure 12–1. A calculus impacted in Hartmann's pouch obstructs the cystic duct. A stone obstructing the cystic duct by reason of its position in Hartmann's pouch or in the cystic duct itself is the mechanism of most cases of acute cholecystitis.

patients undergoing cholecystectomy, whereas others do only for a specific indication, such as a history of jaundice or cholangitis or pancreatitis; if there are multiple small stones in the gallbladder; or if the common bile duct is dilated.

The timing of surgery must be geared to the individual patient's clinical course. Although an acutely inflamed gallbladder was originally considered a contraindication to laparoscopic removal, many surgeons have now extended the indications for laparoscopic cholecystectomy to include acute cholecystitis. Since general anesthesia is still required for this procedure, it cannot be performed in patients who cannot tolerate such anesthesia.

Some patients are so elderly or critically ill, or both, that it seems unlikely they would survive cholecystectomy. In this desperate situation, cholecystostomy (Fig. 12–4) can be performed under local anesthesia through a small incision in the right upper quadrant. Cholecystectomy could be performed later, when the patient was in more a stable condi-

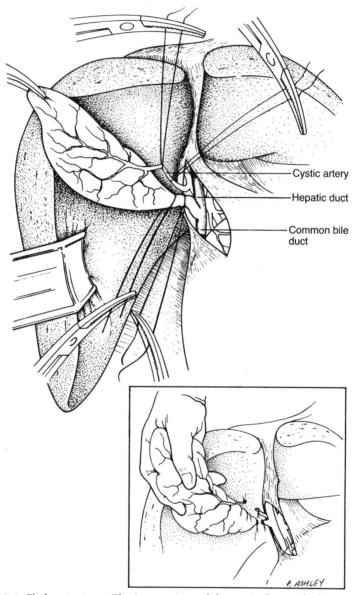

—Cystic artery

—Hepatic duct

—Common bile duct

Figure 12–2. Cholecystectomy. The intersections of the cystic duct with the common bile duct and of the cystic artery with the right hepatic artery are identified with care, and any anatomic variations are noted. The cystic artery is doubly ligated and transected. The gallbladder is dissected free from the liver bed. The cystic duct is transected and the gallbladder removed. Operative cholangiography may be performed via the cystic duct before it is ligated.

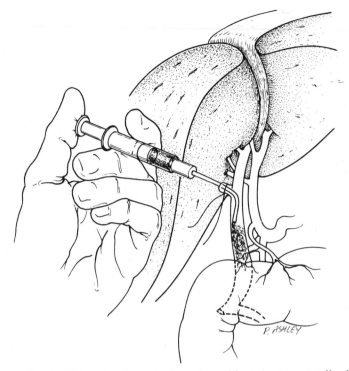

Figure 12–3. Cystic duct cholangiography is performed by inserting a small tube through the cystic duct into the common bile duct. Dye is injected with care, to avoid introducing air, as bubbles can mimic common duct stones. Findings are normal when no filling defects are noted in the hepatic ducts or common duct and there is free flow of dye into the duodenum.

tion, and in fact, some patients never go on to require definitive surgery (cholecystectomy). In a statistical quirk, the operation of lesser magnitude (cholecystostomy) has a higher mortality rate than the more extensive procedure (cholecystectomy). This reflects the fact that cholecystostomy is performed on "higher-risk" patients.

   Pathology. With chronic cholecystitis, gallstones are usually present, as are mononuclear cells. Rokitansky-Aschoff sinuses involve the mucosa, and acute inflammation is absent. With acute cholecystitis, there are usually gallstones; one of these may be obstructing the cystic duct. Polymorphonuclear leukocytes are present in acute cholecystitis, and the lumen of the gallbladder may be filled with pus (empyema of the gallbladder). The mucosa is usually ulcerated, and there may be black areas of necrosis in the wall. The omentum and surrounding organs usually prevent free perforation of the gallbladder; however, free perforation or sealed-off perforation with a pericholecystic abscess can occur, especially in diabetics. When the gallbladder is filled predominantly with mucus, the patient is said to have *hydrops of the gallbladder.*

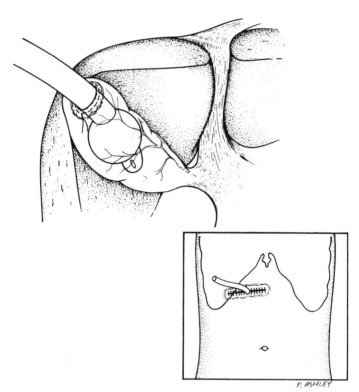

Figure 12–4. Cholecystostomy can be performed by (1) placement of a pursestring suture in the fundus of the gallbladder, (2) removal of the gallstones, and (3) tying down the pursestring suture around a catheter, which is brought out through the abdominal wall, effecting drainage. This can be done under local anesthesia through a small incision and is thus appropriate for selected critically ill patients whose condition is hemodynamically unstable. Cholecystectomy can be performed later, after the patient's condition has stabilized. Cholecystostomy has a high mortality rate because of the poor-risk group of candidates.

Complications of Cholecystectomy. The anatomy of the common bile duct, the cystic and hepatic ducts, and the hepatic and cystic arteries is variable. Injury to the right or left or common hepatic artery can cause necrosis of the liver, although not invariably, as most of the liver's blood supply is derived from the portal vein. Similarly, intraoperative injury to the common bile duct can result in a stricture that is exceedingly difficult to repair and can lead to cholangitis or obstructive jaundice later. These complications are more likely to occur when the anatomy is further obscured by the edema and inflammation of acute cholecystitis than when cholecystectomy is performed for chronic cholecystitis. Subhepatic abscess and wound infection are also more likely to occur after cholecystectomy for acute cholecystitis than for chronic cholecystitis. This provides a cogent argument for performing cholecystectomy when the diagnosis of cholelithiasis is made, rather than waiting for a complication such as acute cholecystitis, cholangitis, or cholecystoduodenal fistula to occur, since these complications of gallstones increase the likelihood of postoperative complications.

If the common bile duct is injured, the results are best if the injury is recognized promptly and treated. If, after laparoscopic cholecystectomy, a leak from the common bile duct or cystic duct stump is suspected because of fever, abdominal pain, nausea, vomiting, or distention, the leak can sometimes be demonstrated by HIDA scan. When a collection is recognized by ultrasound or CT, it may be drained percutaneously. The leak can sometimes be addressed by placing a stent across it, using endoscopic retrograde cholangio pancreatography (ERCP Fig. 12–5).

CASE 12–3

Cholelithiasis and Choledocholithiasis with Jaundice

A 70-year-old woman was referred to the surgeon's office with a 3-week history of dark, tea-colored urine, clay-colored stools, and itching. Her family thought that her skin was becoming yellow. She had experienced one or two episodes of abdominal pain, nausea, and vomiting over the past 5 years.

Physical examination revealed scleral icterus. The liver was not enlarged, and the gallbladder was not palpable. There were no spider angiomas, no palmar erythema, and no caput medusae. Abdominal masses, tenderness, and distention were not present. Bowel sounds were normoactive. Rectal examination was negative.

Laboratory examination revealed an alkaline phosphatase value of 300 and a total bilirubin of 19.5 mg/dL. The SGPT was normal. Ultrasound revealed multiple stones within the gallbladder with beam blocking. The common bile duct measured 12 mm in diameter, and dilated intrahepatic lakes were present. ERCP and papillotomy were performed (Fig. 12–6), and the stone impacted in the ampulla was extruded. Two smaller calculi were removed with a stone basket. The jaundice resolved; the liver function tests returned to normal; and elective laparoscopic cholecystectomy was performed 6 weeks later to prevent recurrent choledocholithiasis or another complication of cholelithiasis and chronic cholecystitis such as acute cholecystitis, cholangitis, or cholecystoenteric fistula.

Had the ERCP proved unsuccessful, the patient would have been taken to surgery and cholecystectomy performed. A cystic duct cholangiogram would likely reveal stones in the common bile duct or ampulla of Vater. The duct would be opened and the stone might be removed with Desjardin stone forceps or a biliary Fogarty catheter and the common bile duct closed over a T tube. If a T-tube cholangiogram made just before the termination of operation revealed no retained stone, the operation could be terminated. Seven days postoperatively, T-tube cholangiography would be repeated, and if it showed no retained stones and free flow of dye into the duodenum, the tube

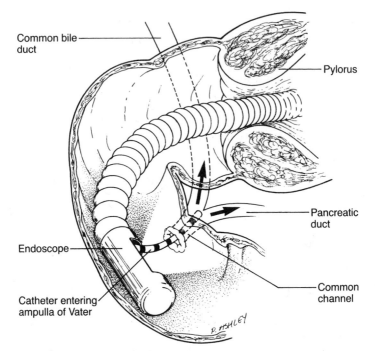

Figure 12–5. Endoscopic retrograde cholangiopancreatography (ERCP). Esophagogastroduodenoscopy is performed, and the ampulla of Vater is cannulated from within the duodenum. Dye is injected into the common bile duct and main pancreatic duct (duct of Wirsung) from within the duodenum. A common duct obstruction from neoplasm or stone can be identified, and irregularities of the pancreatic duct may suggest carcinoma of the pancreas. Effluent from the pancreatic duct can be sent for cytology, to test for malignant cells. A stent can be used to correct a stenosis, defunctionalize a leak due to operative injury, or bypass a neoplasm.

could be removed. Drainage of bile from the T-tube tract would be expected to be self-limited, allowing early discharge to home.

DISCUSSION OF CASE 12–3

Diagnosis

History. A patient presented with obstructive jaundice. The dark urine was caused by excretion of conjugated bilirubin into the urine and the clay-colored stool by the absence of bile pigment.

Physical Examination. The gallbladder was not palpable in this case. A tender, palpable gallbladder suggests acute cholecystitis, usually with cystic duct obstruction caused by a stone impacted in the cystic duct or in Hartmann's pouch. A palpable, nontender gallbladder in the face of jaundice (Courvoisier's sign) suggests carcinoma of the head of the pancreas or periampullary cancer obstructing the

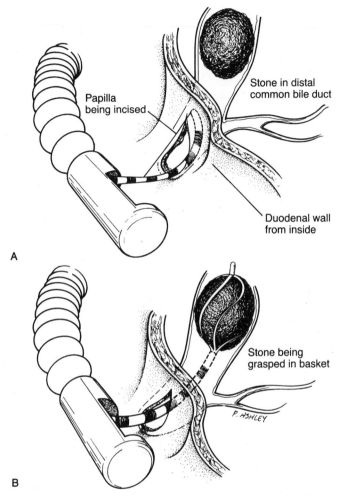

Figure 12–6. Endoscopic papillotomy. *(A)* Papilla of Vater is incised with cautery during the course of ERCP. Any common bile duct stones should then be able to pass into the duodenum and out through the gut. They can be removed with a stone basket *(B)* or can be allowed to pass spontaneously through the now patulous sphincter.

common bile duct. The absence of tenderness is due to the fact that the cancer obstructs the common bile duct slowly and there is no acute inflammation to cause tenderness. Spider angiomas and caput medusae (dilated veins near the umbilicus) and palmar erythema are signs of cirrhosis of the liver. They were not present in this case.

  Laboratory Examination. An alkaline phosphatase reading elevated out of proportion of the SGPT and LDH suggests obstructive jaundice rather than hepatocellular disease, as does a large direct component of the elevated bilirubin value.

Diagnostic Imaging. Ultrasonography demonstrated gallstones in addition to the dilated intrahepatic lakes, suggesting that the patient had obstructive jaundice rather than hepatocellular disease and that the obstructive jaundice was due to choledocholithiasis (common bile duct stones) rather than to a neoplasm. This interpretation does not apply in all cases, however, since it is not uncommon to have gallstones *and* pancreatic or periampullary cancer, the neoplasm being responsible for the obstructive jaundice. The extrahepatic biliary tree was imaged by ERCP (see Fig. 12–5), in this case, allowing definitive treatment at the time of ERCP using papillotomy and stone extraction. Percutaneous transhepatic cholangiography (Fig. 12–7) can also image the extrahepatic biliary tree and allow decompression when a catheter is left in situ, but it would not have provided the definitive treatment provided in this case by ERCP and papillotomy.

Surgical Treatment

As described under imaging, ERCP and papillotomy may allow stone extraction from the common bile duct, allowing definitive treatment of choledocolithiasis. If they are unsuccessful, however, operative treatment may be necessary. Common bile duct exploration is performed by first "kocherizing" the duodenum—incising its peritoneal cover and reflecting it anteromedially like a page of a book (Fig. 12–8). This allows the distal

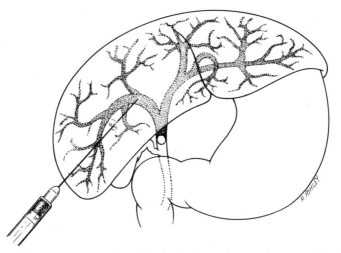

Figure 12–7. Percutaneous transhepatic cholangiography. A skinny needle is placed through the abdominal wall into the parenchyma of the liver under fluoroscopic guidance. Dye is injected under fluoroscopy until the needle is found to be within a bile lake. Further injection of dye should visualize the extrahepatic biliary tree. A dilated duct with a meniscus at the lower end suggests that common bile duct stones are responsible for the obstructive jaundice. This test can be performed in jaundiced patients.

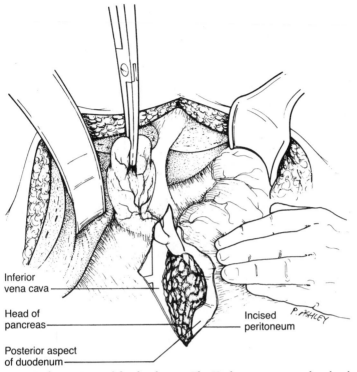

Figure 12–8. "Kocherization" of the duodenum. The Kocher maneuver, whereby the perito-neal covering of the duodenum is incised and the duodenum reflected anteromedially, like a page of a book, allows inspection of the posterior duodenum and pancreas and palpation of the distal common bile duct.

common bile duct to be more easily palpated for stones. Two traction sutures are then placed on the common bile duct, and it is incised (choledochotomy). Stone forceps are passed proximally into the right and left hepatic ducts and distally to the ampulla of Vater, and any stones encountered are grasped and removed (Fig. 12–9). (We no longer force stone forceps or Bakes dilators through the papilla of Vater, as we now know that this trauma can cause spasm.)

If the common duct stone cannot be removed with these maneuvers, a biliary Fogarty catheter (Fig. 12–10) can be passed around the stone. The balloon is then inflated and the catheter pulled back, bringing the stone with it. In addition, forceful irrigation of the bile duct with saline may float some common duct stones out of the duct. A fiberoptic choled-ochoscope may be inserted into the duct to search for residual stones, which can be removed with a basket passed through the scope.

When the surgeon is sure that there are no residual common bile duct stones, the duct is closed over a T tube (Fig. 12–11). An operative cholangiogram is made at the completion of the procedure, and the

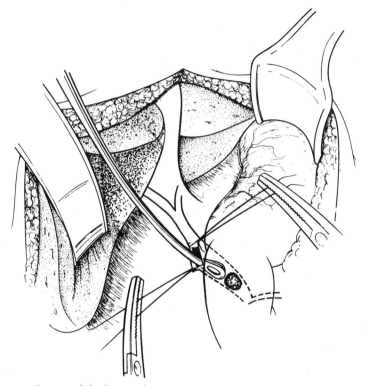

Figure 12–9. Common bile duct exploration. Two traction sutures are placed in the distal common duct, and an incision (choledochotomy) is made. Stone forceps are passed proximally into the common, right, and left hepatic ducts and distally into the common bile duct. Any stones encountered are removed. Irrigation of the ducts may cause other calculi to flow out via the choledochotomy incision. A fiberoptic choledochoscope can be passed into the common bile duct and hepatic ducts. Any stones that are found can be removed via a basket passed through the choledochoscope.

operation is terminated if no filling defects are seen on the cholangiogram and if dye passes into the duodenum.

The T-tube cholangiogram is repeated 1 week later, to make absolutely sure that there are no retained stones before the T tube is removed. If, indeed, there are none, the tube is removed with the expectation that drainage of bile through the tract will cease in a day or two because the bile will take the path of least resistance (i.e., through the papilla and into the duodenum). If the T tube were mistakenly removed in the presence of distal obstruction, bile leakage through the T-tube tract would not stop.

Some centers are now using intraoperative ultrasonography to check for stones in the bile duct before or after common bile duct exploration. This approach may detect stones that are not apparent when ultrasonography is done through the abdominal wall.

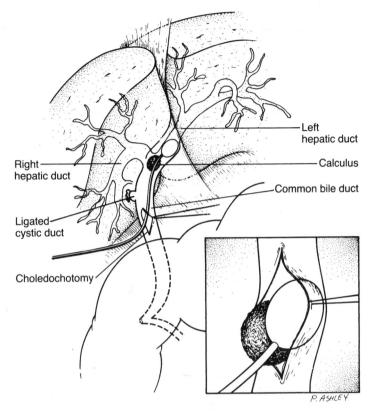

Left
hepatic duct

Right
hepatic duct

Calculus

Common bile duct

Ligated
cystic duct

Choledochotomy

P. ASHLEY

Figure 12–10. A biliary Fogarty catheter has a balloon at its tip and can be guided past a common bile duct stone with the balloon deflated during common duct exploration. It can then be pulled back with the balloon inflated, bringing the stone out with it.

Treatment of Retained Common Bile Duct Stones

The most common reason for finding a retained stone on T-tube cholangiography done 1 week postoperatively is that the stone was apparent on the operative cholangiogram but was not found by the surgeon. If this occurs, the patient can be sent home with the T tube in place and can return to the hospital after 6 weeks. T-tube cholangiography is repeated, and if the retained stone is still there, it can be retrieved with a ureteral stone basket placed through the now well-formed T-tube tract under fluoroscopic control.

The situation is worse when the patient presents with obstructive jaundice after a previous cholecystectomy at which no common bile duct exploration was performed and thus, no T tube was inserted. In this situation, the diagnosis of a retained common bile duct stone could be made by endoscopic retrograde cholangiopancreatography, and the pa-

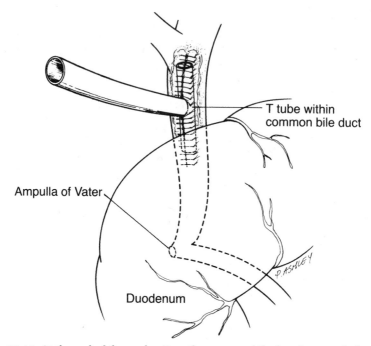

Figure 12–11. At the end of the exploration, the common bile duct is sutured closed over a T tube, whose end is brought out through a separate stab wound in the abdominal wall. T-tube cholangiography is performed before the abdomen is closed, to make sure that no stones are retained in the common bile duct. Seven days postoperatively, the T-tube cholangiogram is repeated to make absolutely sure that no stones were retained. If this study is negative, the tube is removed.

pilla could be incised during endoscopic papillotomy (see Fig. 12–6), allowing the stone to pass. If this is not successful, reoperation and common bile duct exploration might be necessary.

Common Bile Duct Stones in the Context of Laparoscopic Cholecystectomy

Exploring the common bile duct when choledocholithiasis is encountered at the time of open cholecystectomy (approximately 10% of cases) has long been standard procedure. When laparoscopic cholecystectomy became the most frequent approach to gallstones, new methods of addressing the possibility of concomitant common bile duct stones had to be devised. One way of dealing with the problem is to perform preoperative ERCP in patients who are more likely to have choledocholithiasis (i.e., those with a history of jaundice, cholangitis, pancreatitis, elevated alkaline phosphatase, or dilated common bile duct on ultrasound). Another way of addressing the possibility of intercurrent choledocholithiasis is to make an operative cholangiogram at the time of laparoscopic cholecystectomy by inserting a catheter into the cystic duct through one of the ports or through a separate puncture wound, injecting dye, and taking a radiograph. Instruments have been developed to dilate the cystic duct so that a choledochoscope can be passed into the common bile duct and stones can be retrieved. Advanced laparoscopic intracorporeal suturing techniques have even allowed laparoscopic common bile duct explorations through an incision in the common bile duct (choledochotomy) to be performed in some settings. At the time of laparoscopic common bile duct stone retrieval during laparoscopic cholecystectomy, it has proved possible in some settings to perform papillotomy (incision of the papilla of Vater) to prevent further retained common bile duct stones. Since these techniques are not always feasible, another approach is to perform the laparoscopic cholecystectomy and postoperative ERCP if retained common bile duct stones later become manifest.

CASE 12–4

Obstructive Cholangitis

A 68-year-old man presented to the emergency department with fever and chills, jaundice, and abdominal pain.

Three years before admission, the patient had undergone cholecystectomy and had had an unremarkable postoperative course. One week before admission he began to pass dark, tea-colored urine and yellow stools. On the day of admission, he had abdominal pain that was greatest in the right upper quadrant and he experienced a shaking chill. His wife noticed that he had become jaundiced and insisted he come to the hospital.

Past medical history included hypertension treated by diet and the previous cholecystectomy.

His temperature was 101.6°F, pulse 110, and blood pressure 160/100 mm Hg on admission. His sclerae were icteric. His abdomen was mildly tender in the right upper quadrant, with no rebound or guarding. The liver and spleen were not palpable, and there were no masses. Bowel sounds were normal, and rectal examination was negative.

The white blood cell count was 17,000 and the bilirubin was 6 mg/dL. The alkaline phosphatase value was 650. Flat and upright abdominal x-rays were negative. Blood cultures were drawn.

A large-bore catheter was inserted into the antecubital vein, and the patient was resuscitated with a liter of Ringer's lactated solution. Gentamicin, 1.7 mg/kg, and ampicillin, 2 g, was administered intravenously. A Foley catheter was inserted to monitor urine output.

Ultrasonography of the biliary tree revealed the common bile duct to be 22 mm in diameter; dilated intrahepatic radicles were present. ERCP was attempted but was unsuccessful. Percutaneous transhepatic cholangiography (PTC) was performed, and multiple stones were demonstrated within a dilated common bile duct. No dye could be seen in the duodenum. A catheter was passed into the common bile duct over a guidewire at the time of PTC. This was left in situ to decompress the common bile duct. Sepsis persisted, however.

Therefore, the patient was taken to surgery, and common bile duct exploration was performed. After performance of the choledochotomy, 12 small stones were removed from the common bile duct and several from the right and left hepatic ducts. A stone was impacted tightly in the ampulla, and this, presumably, was why ERCP was unsuccessful. The stone was pushed into the duodenum by a dilator passed through the choledochotomy. (The stone would be expected to pass harmlessly in the stool.) The choledochoscope was passed proximally into both hepatic ducts and distally through the ampulla of Vater into the duodenum. In light of the large number of small common bile duct stones, the surgeon could not be sure that all had been removed. Therefore he anastomosed the common bile duct to the duodenum (performed a choledochoduodenostomy) so that the ampulla of Vater was bypassed. Thus, any remaining stones could pass into the duodenum without causing repeat obstruction.

The patient had an unremarkable postoperative course. The antibiotics were stopped on the 7th postoperative day. The patient was eating well and having bowel movements with formed, brown stool. He was afebrile and his bilirubin and alkaline phosphatase levels were returning toward normal; he was discharged on the 10th postoperative day.

DISCUSSION OF CASE 12-4

Diagnosis

History. Fever and chills, jaundice, and abdominal pain compose *Charcot's triad,* which is indicative of obstructive cholangitis, formerly known as *ascending cholangitis.* Since this entity can be caused by choledocholithiasis (common bile duct stones), by neoplasm obstructing the common bile duct, or by iatrogenic stricture, historical details suggesting the presence of one of these causes should also be sought. For instance, a common bile duct injury leading to stricture may have occurred during previous gastric surgery. A stone may have been left in the common bile duct at previous cholecystectomy.

Physical Examination. Jaundice and scleral icterus may be apparent on physical examination. The patient may have few physical findings referable to the abdomen. Tachycardia, hypotension, and a thin, thready pulse may be present when obstructive cholangitis has led to septicemia.

Laboratory Examination. The bilirubin value is elevated—as is the alkaline phosphatase—out of proportion to the LDH and SGPT, as with obstructive jaundice in general. In hepatocellular diseases such as hepatitis and cirrhosis of the liver, the LDH and SGPT are likely to be elevated out of proportion to the alkaline phosphatase value. The white cell count is elevated because obstructive cholangitis is an acute infectious process, similar to an abscess with pus under pressure. The blood cultures are likely to be positive, although these results are not available until several days after blood is collected. The most frequent organisms isolated are *E. coli, Klebsiella,* and *Enterococcus.* The BUN, hematocrit, and serum sodium values may be elevated, reflecting intravascular depletion due to sepsis, increased insensible loss from fever, or, usually, decreased fluid intake. Vomiting can also contribute to the dehydration.

Diagnostic Imaging. Ultrasonography is the diagnostic tool *par excellence* in this setting. Although it is difficult to demonstrate stones in the common bile duct on ultrasonography (in contradistinction, stones in the gallbladder are easy to see), the abdominal sonogram can demonstrate a dilated common bile duct, whose internal diameter should normally measure not more than 6 to 7 mm on ultrasonography. This dilatation may indicate stones. In addition, dilated intrahepatic radicles can easily be demonstrated.

Treatment

Obstructive cholangitis is a grave emergency, since the infected bile is under pressure and predisposes to bacteremia and endotoxemia. Mental obtundation is an especially grave sign. Resuscitation and diagnosis must be conducted concurrently. Aggressive fluid administration is imperative. A Foley catheter may be helpful, since restoration of adequate urine output is an indication of successful volume repletion. Patients with a diseased left ventricle may require insertion of a Swan-Ganz catheter for physiologic monitoring. Antibiotic therapy must be instituted empirically, targeted against *E. coli* and *Klebsiella* and *Enterococcus* species.

The common bile duct must be decompressed. ERCP with papillotomy allows destruction of the competence of the sphincter of Oddi via esophagogastroduodenoscopy. This may prove to be the definitive treatment for choledocholithiasis (common bile duct stones), with or without obstructive cholangitis, *if* the stones pass after the papilla has been incised. A stone basket can be passed through the ampulla to facilitate stone retrieval and obviate surgical intervention. When ERCP and papillotomy proved unsuccessful in this case, PTC was performed. When this study demonstrates the obstruction, a catheter may be inserted into the common bile duct and left there for drainage. When the sepsis resolves with fluid resuscitation, antibiotics, and percutaneous drainage, surgery can be undertaken on a less emergent basis. Otherwise, emergency common bile duct exploration is performed with choledocholithotomy (removal of stones from the duct). If the surgeon can be sure that all the stones have been removed, he can close the common bile duct over a T tube (Fig. 12–11). If not, a choledochoduodenostomy can be performed (Fig. 12–12) to ensure that any retained stones can pass harmlessly into the duodenum. Choledochojejunostomy, with (Fig. 12–13) or without (Fig. 12–14) a Roux-en-Y or a transduodenal sphincteroplasty (Fig. 12–15), accomplishes the same goal.

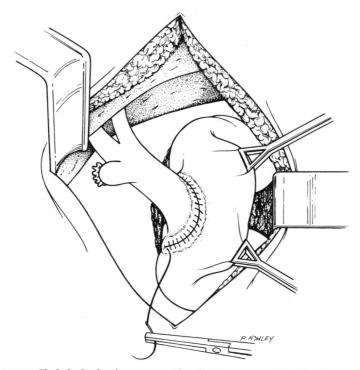

Figure 12–12. Choledochoduodenostomy. The distal common bile duct is anastomosed side-to-side to the duodenum, bypassing the papilla of Vater. This can be performed for palliation of carcinoma of the distal bile duct or to bypass a calculus that is impacted in the ampulla and cannot be removed. It is sometimes wise to perform choledochoduodenostomy if one cannot be sure that all stones have been removed from the common bile duct at the time of exploration. The bypass prevents a retained stone from causing obstructive jaundice and facilitates its harmless passage into the duodenum.

CASE 12–5

Pancreatitis

A 47-year-old man presented to the emergency department complaining of a 1-day history of severe epigastric pain radiating to the back and associated with nausea and vomiting. He admitted to drinking seven beers a day for the last 3 years but much more alcohol during the last week. He had had three loose bowel movements the day before admission.

Past medical history included a seizure disorder (treated with Dilantin) since evacuation of a subdural hematoma after a fall down stairs 3 years earlier.

On admission, the pulse was 130 and the blood pressure was 100/50. The pulse was thin and thready. The respiratory rate was 30

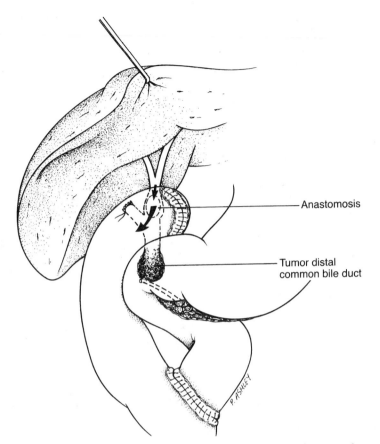

Anastomosis

Tumor distal
common bile duct

Figure 12–13. Roux-en-Y choledochojejunostomy. The anastomosis between the common bile duct and jejunum can be performed for the same indications as for choledochoduodenostomy. In the case of tumor, the choledochojejunostomy has the advantage of being less likely to be obstructed by advancing neoplasm than is choledochoduodenostomy, as the anastomosis is farther removed from the primary tumor in the former procedure. The Roux-en-Y configuration is designed to prevent jejunal contents from refluxing into the common duct. The fear that jejunal contents in the common bile duct might cause cholangitis is unfounded, however, as long as the anastomosis is ample.

breaths per minute. The patient was in marked distress. Abdominal examination revealed diffuse tenderness, greatest in the epigastrium, with generalized rebound and involuntary guarding. Bowel sounds were hypoactive. There was ecchymosis in both flanks. Rectal examination was negative.

Laboratory examination revealed a hematocrit of 40% and a white blood cell count of 13,500. The electrolytes included bicarbonate of 18, and the BUN was 34. Serum amylase was 2000 Somogyi units. Serum calcium was 8.2, and the arterial blood gases revealed a PaO_2 of 56 mm Hg.

The chest x-ray revealed a left pleural effusion and fluffy infil-

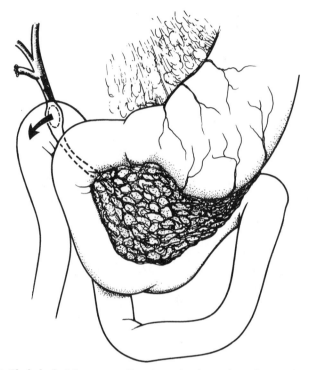

Figure 12–14. Choledochojejunostomy (loop)—a simpler and quicker method of bypassing the ampulla of Vater than the Roux-en-Y choledochojejunostomy. A loop choledochojejunostomy is a good operation for palliation of a neoplastic obstruction of the common bile duct and should not cause cholangitis if an ample anastomosis is created.

trates over both lung fields. The flat and upright abdominal films revealed multiple loops of air-filled small bowel with multiple air-fluid levels but with air in the colon consistent with ileus. Ultrasonography of the extrahepatic biliary tree revealed no gallstones and no dilated duct.

The patient was admitted to the hospital and kept NPO. A nasogastric tube was inserted and placed to suction. A large-bore intravenous line was inserted, and the patient received 2 L of Ringer's lactated solution over the next hour and a total of 5 L over the next 24 hours. A Foley catheter was inserted and the urine output, which was originally scanty, increased to 50 ml per hour after the first 3.5 L of intravenous fluid had been infused. Because the hematocrit dropped to 25%, 3 units of packed red cells were transfused. The partial pressure of oxygen increased to 70 mm Hg with a 40% face mask. The serum amylase returned to normal over the next 5 days, but attempts at refeeding resulted in a return of abdominal pain and an increase in serum amylase.

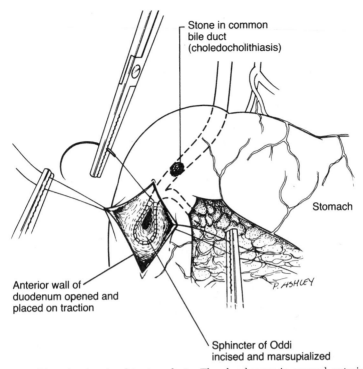

Figure 12–15. Transduodenal sphincteroplasty. The duodenum is opened anteriorly, and the ampulla of Vater identified and cannulated with a groove director. The sphincter of Oddi is incised, and care is taken to avoid injury to the pancreatic duct, which can be instrumented with a lacrimal probe. The mucosa of the distal common bile duct is marsupialized (that is, sutured to the duodenal mucosa) to prevent it from narrowing down later by fibrosis. This is an excellent method for removing a stone impacted at the ampulla. In addition, the sphincteroplasty allows any residual stones to pass harmlessly into the duodenum.

Accordingly, the patient was kept NPO and placed on total parenteral nutrition, which he received for the next 3 weeks. After he had been asymptomatic with normal serum amylase and 2-hour urinary amylase values for approximately a week, the patient was fed again, this time without recrudescence. Intravenous feeding was discontinued, and the patient was discharged.

DISCUSSION OF CASE 12–5

The most common causes of pancreatitis are alcohol abuse and gallstones; less common causes include hypercalcemia, hyperlipidemia, trauma, ischemia, bulimia, and drugs such as steroids and azathioprine. The relative proportion of the two—alcoholic pancreatitis and gallstone pancreatitis—seen in a given hospital depends on the magnitude of the alcoholism problem in the population the hospital serves. Although the treatment of alcoholic pancreatitis is usually nonoperative, these patients are frequently admitted to the surgical service because it is often difficult to be sure that they do not have some other acute abdominal condition that would require emergency surgery and because their fluid and electrolyte problems require aggressive resuscitation, which the surgeon is best able to provide. Patients with gallstone pancreatitis usually require cholecystectomy—and sometimes common duct exploration—to eradicate the underlying cause. Alcoholic pancreatitis is a serious entity with an appreciable mortality if close monitoring and aggressive treatment are not instituted.

Diagnosis

Symptoms. The symptoms of acute pancreatitis include severe abdominal pain, often located in the epigastrium and often radiating to the back. The pain may be precipitated by an alcoholic binge. The pain is usually associated with nausea and vomiting. Steatorrhea may be present if exocrine insufficiency has occurred. If the pancreatitis in caused by gallstones, the patient may have an antecedent history of biliary colic–right upper quadrant abdominal pain radiating to the right subscapular region and precipitated by fatty foods and associated with nausea and vomiting. Dark urine and clay-colored stools may be described if choledocholithiasis is also present.

Physical Examination. Physical findings in acute pancreatitis include severe epigastric tenderness, sometimes associated with diffuse tenderness over the entire abdomen, with generalized rebound and involuntary guarding. The abdomen may be rigid and boardlike. These findings could easily make it impossible to avoid exploratory laparotomy for a patient with pancreatitis: the patient might have a perforated ulcer or another intraabdominal lesion, masquerading as pancreatitis, that requires laparotomy. If the patient has hemorrhagic pancreatitis, he may have ecchymoses on the flanks (Grey Turner's sign) caused by hemorrhage into the retroperitoneum. Because pancreatitis causes tremendous loss of fluid into the peritoneal cavity, the signs of dehydration—tachycardia, thin, thready pulse, and hypotension—may also be present.

Laboratory Examination. The chemistry laboratory plays an important part in the diagnosis of acute pancreatitis. Typically, if the upper limit of normal for serum amylase in a given laboratory is 200 Somogyi units, a patient with acute pancreatitis would be expected to have an amylase value of at least 300—and up to 2000—Somogyi units. A 2-hour urine amylase reading can pick up pancreatitis when the patient has normal serum amylase, presumably because the blood was drawn at an instant when the serum amylase was not elevated. Since the 2-hour urine amylase is related to the serum amylase over time, it overcomes this problem. The other side of the coin is that elevated serum amylase does not ensure that the patient's findings are the result of pancreatitis, as a perforated peptic ulcer, strangulated hernia, or mesenteric infarction can also elevate the serum amylase value. The distinction is critical because these other conditions can be fatal if laparotomy is not carried out promptly whereas pancreatitis is often best managed nonoperatively.

To determine whether an elevation of serum amylase is due to pancreatitis or to another disease, the concept of the ratio of amylase to creatinine clearance has been formulated. The reader will remember that the formula for clearance of a substance from the blood by the kidney is $U \times V/P$, where U is the concentration of the given substance in the urine, V is the urine volume, and P is the concentration of the substance in the plasma. It can easily be seen that, if one divides the clearance of amylase by the clearance of creatinine to determine the amylase–creatinine clearance ratio, the urine volume cancels out. The advantage of this fact is that a spot urine specimen can be used for testing, rather than a timed collection, making the test logistically easier. It has been stated that, when the ratio is greater than 1:5 pancreatitis is likely to be the cause of the amylase elevation. In reality, however, this ratio is not more selective or specific than the simple serum amylase. An elevated serum lipase may aid in the diagnosis of pancreatitis, because results of this test can remain elevated longer than those of serum amylase. Thus, a certain percentage of patients with acute pancreatitis will still require laparotomy because another intraabdominal process presenting as acute surgical abdomen cannot be ruled out.

The hematocrit and blood urea nitrogen values may be elevated if the patient is dehydrated, because of the massive shift of fluid from the intravascular space into the peritoneal cavity and the bowel lumen. Conversely, the hematocrit may drop if the patient bleeds into the retroperitoneum as a result of hemorrhagic pancreatitis. A low serum calcium level correlates with poor prognosis in pancreatitis. The arterial blood gases may indicate hypoxia caused by a right-to-left shunt, since phospholipase A liberated in pancreatitis interferes with surfactant and causes microatelectasis with resultant perfusion of underventilated alveoli. In fact, pancreatitis is an example of a clinical entity that can lead to the systemic inflammatory response syndrome (SIRS) and release of cytokines, with resultant multi-system organ failure in the absence of infection.

Ranson has described 11 prognostic factors for patients with acute pancreatitis. On admission, age over 55 years, blood sugar greater than 200 mg/100 ml, and a leukocyte count above 16,000 are associated with a poor outlook. In the first 48 hours after admission, a serum calcium value below 8 mg/100 ml, a drop in hematocrit of 10 points or more, a base deficit greater than 4 mEq/l, a rise in blood urea nitrogen of 5 mg/100 ml, an LDH level above 700 IU per cent, an SGPT level over 250 Sigma Frankel units per 100 ml, a PaO_2 under 60 mm Hg, and fluid retention calculated to be more than 6 liters all correlated with poor prognosis. Patients with three or more of these serious findings were much more likely to die or to be extremely ill than those with one or two signs.

Diagnostic Imaging. Imaging techniques are helpful, but not always diagnostic, when acute pancreatitis is suspected. The chest film may show pleural effusion, which is often associated with pancreatitis. It may also show the fluffy infiltrates of adult respiratory distress syndrome that can occur with acute pancreatitis. The flat and upright abdominal x-rays may show a nonobstructive ileus pattern (air-filled loops of small and large bowel with air-fluid levels) or may show a "sentinel loop," which is an air-filled loop of small bowel near the pancreas presumably formed by localized ileus secondary to inflammation in the area. Another radiographic sign that may be present in pancreatitis is the "colon cutoff sign," an abrupt disappearance of the column of air in the transverse colon caused by edema (phlegmon) surrounding the pancreas, which lies in the leaves of the transverse mesocolon.

Either ultrasonography or CT may demonstrate the edematous, enlarged pancreas or the presence or absence of gallstones, with a high degree of accuracy. The physician can then deduce whether the patient has gallstone or alcoholic pancreatitis, since the other causes of pancreatitis are much less common.

Treatment

Treatment consists of fluid resuscitation and of "placing the pancreas at rest." The former is of prime importance, because massive amounts of fluid can be lost through extravasation of serum into the peritoneal cavity as a result of inflammation. This dehydration is compounded by the fact that fluid intake has often been voluntarily restricted by the patient because of nausea and pain. Vomiting also promotes abnormal loss of fluid, and fever increases insensible losses. The intravascular compartment must thus be expanded to prevent hypovolemic shock. The pancreas is "put at rest" by keeping the patient NPO and by decompressing the stomach with nasogastric suction. While nasogastric suction has not been proven to reduce mortality in patients with pancreatitis, it certainly makes some patients more comfortable, particularly when the pancreatitis has resulted in ileus or gastric atony. Pharmacologic manipulation with anticholinergic agents such as Pro-Banthine or with agents such as glucagon or Trasylol has largely been abandoned. Somatostatin analogues such as octreotide decrease exocrine secretion. Their efficacy in the treatment of pancreatitis remains uncertain. H2 blockers or sucralfate can be used to prevent stress ulcer and gastrointestinal bleeding. The efficacy of antibiotics in preventing the development of pancreatic abscess is open to question. Since many affected patients must be kept NPO for prolonged periods of time, nutritional support is often provided by total parenteral nutrition.

There is a continuum of severity of pancreatitis: in increasing order, edematous, hemorrhagic, and necrotizing. A low serum calcium value is a poor prognostic indicator, being lowest in the most severe cases. It may be due to the low albumin concentration often seen after fluid resuscitation, compounded by calcium accretion in areas of fat necrosis, and resistence to parathormone. Hypoxia usually is demonstrated by arterial blood gases in severe cases caused by ventilation-perfusion abnormalities.

Peritoneal dialysis has been proposed but has not been proven to reduce mortality in the severest cases. To the extent that it works, it may do so by removing noxious substances such as trypsin, chymotrypsin, phospholipase A, and histamine from the peritoneal cavity. Total pancreatectomy has been performed as a last-ditch effort to salvage patients with necrotizing pancreatitis. Physiologic monitoring with a Swan-Ganz catheter may be indicated to facilitate fluid management when cardiac function is compromised by either preexisting cardiac disease or the insult of severe pancreatitis. Ventilatory support may be required in the most severe cases.

Initially gallstone pancreatitis is treated in the same fashion. The presumed cause is the migration of gallstones from the gallbladder through the cystic and common ducts, past the papilla of Vater, and into the duodenum, transiently obstructing the pancreatic duct as the stones pass through the common channel. In fact, in studies of patients with gallstone pancreatitis many gallstones have been recovered from the stool. Accordingly, cholecystectomy to prevent subsequent attacks is thought to be indicated within several days after the acute attack subsides. By waiting until the acute attack has ended, one can often avoid common duct exploration. If cholecystectomy is delayed too long, however, the risk of a repeat attack of gallstone pancreatitis becomes greater.

Pancreatic pseudocyst, a complication of pancreatitis, often presents as early satiety, nausea, vomiting, and abdominal pain shortly after subsidence of an attack of acute pancreatitis. The serum or 2-hour urinary amylase level may also rise again. A mass may be palpable. It is called a *pseudocyst* instead of a true cyst, because it has no epithelial lining and results from edema and fibrinous exudate that pushes adjacent viscera in front of it. This phlegmon cavitates and ultimately becomes organized.

The emergence of ultrasonography as a widely available diagnostic modality has much enhanced the diagnosis of pancreatic pseudocyst, as it is very accurate for identifying hollow structures. CT is also very valuable in the diagnosis of pancreatic pseudocyst. Percutaneous drainage of pancreatic pseudocysts under CT or ultrasonographic guidance may prove helpful as a temporizing measure, but it is not usually a permanent solution, and operative intervention often is required.

It is certainly true that pancreatic pseudocysts can resolve without surgical intervention, but they can also cause symptoms from compression of adjacent organs or rupture and spillage of their contents into the abdominal cavity, causing peritonitis. They may leak slowly into the peritoneal cavity, causing pancreatic ascites, or they may erode into adjacent vessels such as the gastroduodenal or splenic arteries, causing exsanguinating hemorrhage. Six weeks is usually allowed to elapse before surgical decompression is undertaken, as the wall of the pseudocyst

must be allowed to mature before it is firm enough to allow safe anastomosis to a nearby organ. Cystogastrostomy (Fig. 12–16)—suturing of an
opening made in the cyst to an opening made in the posterior wall of
the stomach—is thought to be technically easiest, because the two structures are often already densely adherent. Some surgeons believe that a

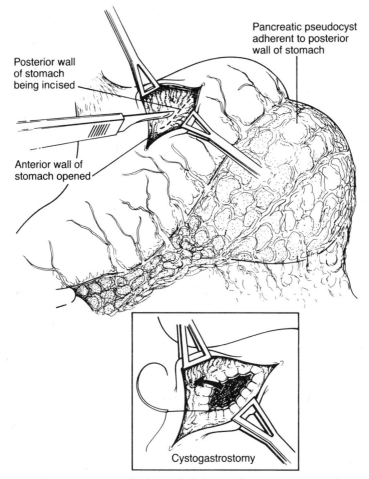

Figure 12–16. Cystogastrostomy for internal drainage of a pancreatic pseudocyst. This is
an excellent procedure in the usual case when the pancreatic pseudocyst is densely
adherent to the posterior wall of the stomach. Approximately 6 weeks must elapse before
the wall of the pseudocyst is mature enough to allow safe suturing. The anterior gastric
wall is incised, and the position of the pseudocyst is documented by aspiration through
the posterior gastric wall, which is then incised. After the pseudocyst is entered, it is
anastomosed to the posterior gastric wall from within the stomach using running, locking,
nonabsorbable sutures. This is more for hemostasis than for mechanical strength, as the
two structures are already densely adherent. The anterior wall of the stomach is then
sutured closed.

Roux-en-Y cystojejunostomy (Fig. 12–17) produces more efficient dependent drainage. In either case, draining the cyst to an adjacent organ causes obliteration of the cyst over time.

CASE 12–6

Carcinoma of the Head of the Pancreas

A 50-year-old man was referred to the surgeon with a 3-week history of increasing pruritus (itching).

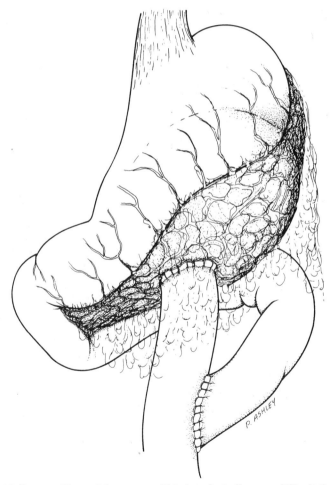

Figure 12–17. Roux-en-Y cystojejunostomy. This is technically more difficult than cystogastrostomy but may allow greater dependent drainage. Moreover, it may be necessary when the pseudocyst and the stomach are not contiguous.

For a year before admission, the patient had experienced vague pain in the lower back that was treated with intermittent bed rest, a heating pad, and muscle relaxants. Three weeks before admission, the patient began to experience generalized pruritus, and his wife began to notice his eyes turning yellow. The patient had dark, tea-colored urine and clay-colored stools. His total bilirubin and alkaline phosphatase values, obtained during a visit to his doctor, were found to be 6 mg/dL and 850, respectively. Outpatient ultrasonography revealed a dilated common bile duct and dilated intrahepatic ducts. A dilated gallbladder was shown to be devoid of stones. The pancreas was obscured by overlying bowel gas. CT revealed a mass in the head of the pancreas with no apparent involvement of surrounding structures such as the portal vein and no evidence of hepatic metastasis. Percutaneous needle biopsy of the pancreatic tumor under CT or ultrasound guidance was felt to be unnecessary, if surgical resection for cure was contemplated. ERCP showed distal common bile duct obstruction and encasement of the pancreatic duct. Brush cytology specimens collected through the ampulla demonstrated malignant cells. The diagnosis of pancreatic cancer was made, and the patient was referred for definitive surgery.

On admission, the chief complaint and history of present illness were as outlined. The past medical history was entirely negative. Physical examination on admission revealed scleral icterus. The abdomen was soft and not tender, and a nontender gallbladder was palpable in the right upper quadrant. There were no other masses, and the liver was 8 cm to percussion. Rectal examination revealed no Bloomer's shelf.

Laboratory examination on admission included a total bilirubin value that had increased to 13 mg/dL and alkaline phosphatase that had increased to 900. The prothrombin and partial thromboplastin times were normal. Chest x-ray revealed no evidence of metastasis.

The patient underwent laparotomy with the plan that, if the tumor could be resectable for cure, pancreaticoduodenectomy (Whipple's procedure) would be carried out. Unfortunately, at surgery there was invasion of the portal vein that was not appreciated on preoperative CT. Accordingly, a double bypass (cholecystojejunostomy and gastrojejunostomy) was carried out (Fig. 12–18). Postoperatively, the jaundice continued to resolve, with concomitant resolution of the itching. The patient was able to tolerate a regular diet, was producing brown stool, and was discharged. Four months later, the patient entered a hospice program.

DISCUSSION OF CASE 12–6

Diagnosis

Symptoms. Carcinoma of the pancreas has a very poor prognosis, at least in part because of the typically late diagnosis. Delay occurs because the symptoms—weight loss, anorexia, and epigastric pain radiating to the back—are rather nonspecific. Jaundice may occur relatively early in carcinoma of the head of the pancreas if the lesion

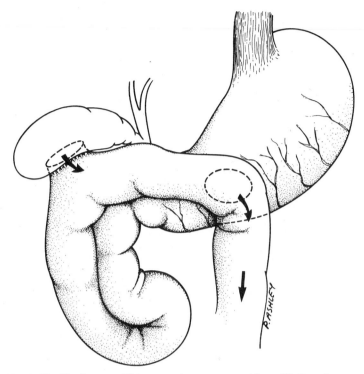

Figure 12–18. Double bypass. This operation may provide palliation for a pancreatic carcinoma that is not resectable for cure. The extrahepatic biliary tree is bypassed by anastomosis of the jejunum to the gallbladder (cholecystojejunostomy). The gastric outlet obstruction caused by the tumor in the C loop of the duodenum is bypassed by anastomosis of the stomach to the jejunum (gastroenterostomy).

obstructs the common bile duct. Pruritus can occur in any case of obstructive jaundice. Nausea and vomiting occur if the pancreatic cancer causes gastric outlet obstruction by reason of its position in the duodenal C loop.

Physical Findings. The classic physical finding in malignant obstruction of the common duct is a nontender, palpable gallbladder in the presence of jaundice (Courvoisier's sign). An epigastric mass, the pancreatic cancer, may also be present. Migratory thrombophlebitis can be seen in association with pancreatic cancer.

Simple Laboratory Tests. Simple laboratory tests are helpful in the diagnosis of pancreatic cancer. One expects to find an elevated direct (conjugated) bilirubin value with obstructive jaundice. An alkaline phosphatase level elevated out of proportion to the LDH and SGPT also suggests obstruction rather than hepatocellular disease as the cause of jaundice. The prothrombin and partial thromboplastin times may be elevated, as bile, which is required to absorb fat, cannot reach the small intestines. Since vitamin K is a fat-soluble vitamin and is required for synthesis of factors II, VII, IX, and X by the liver, obstructive jaundice is often associated with prolonged prothrombin and partial thromboplastin times. This derangement can be corrected with parenteral vitamin K.

Imaging Ultrasound is the simplest and least invasive diagnostic imaging study for pancreatic cancer. It can diagnose common bile duct obstruction and often can visualize a pancreatic mass, unless the pancreas is obscured by overlying bowel gas. When ultrasound demonstrates liver metastasis or ascites, percutaneous needle biopsy or aspiration of peritoneal fluid for cytology can be performed under ultrasound guidance. If widespread dissemination is demonstrated, no other diagnostic imaging may be required. CT can demonstrate the presence (or absence) of liver metastases, a dilated common bile duct, and the pancreatic mass. It may confirm unresectability owing to invasion of the portal vein. Because pancreatic cancer is so often unresectable, CT is more accurate for predicting unresectability than resectability. Angiography may demonstrate invasion of the portal, superior mesenteric, and inferior mesenteric veins, celiac axis, and superior mesenteric artery, indicating unresectability even when one would have thought otherwise from the CT. Thus, performing angiography in addition to CT may save some patients a futile laparotomy; however, as outlined below, operative palliation of obstructive jaundice may be more durable than lesser procedures. Percutaneous needle biopsy or aspiration cytology under CT or ultrasound guidance is performed to get a tissue diagnosis when it has been shown that the pancreatic cancer is wide-spread and laparotomy is not contemplated. It is usually avoided when resection for cure is planned, for fear of seeding the needle track with malignant cells. ERCP may aid in the diagnosis of pancreatic cancer when the mass is not visible on CT. It may show a distorted pancreatic duct in addition to a dilated common bile duct, and cells can be aspirated for cytology.

Treatment

The only potentially curative modalities for carcinoma of the pancreas entail formidable surgery. A pancreaticoduodenectomy (Whipple's procedure) is resection of the head of the pancreas along with the antrum of the stomach and the duodenum (Fig. 12–19). (This is necessary because the pancreas and duodenum share their blood supply.) Some surgeons advocate pylorus-preserving pancreaticoduodenectomy (in which the pylorus and gastric antrum are spared), in the hope of minimizing postoperative digestive problems. This may or may not decrease morbidity as compared with Whipple's procedure.

Once the head of the pancreas and duodenum have been resected for Whipple's procedure, gastrointestinal continuity is restored by anastomosing the common bile duct, the distal remaining pancreas, and the gastric remnant to the jejunum. The pancreatic anastomosis is treacherous because it tends to leak, causing sepsis, and it is associated with appreciable morbidity and mortality. Accordingly, total pancreatectomy (Fig. 12–20) is sometimes performed. It has the advantage of avoiding a

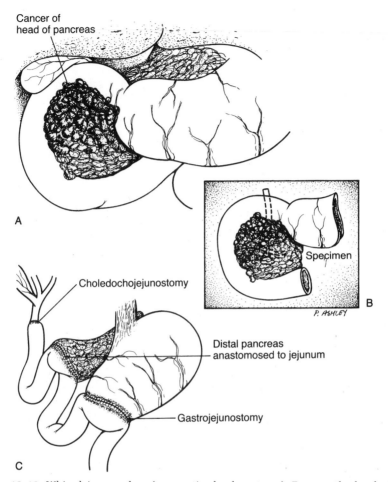

Figure 12–19. Whipple's procedure (pancreaticoduodenectomy). Because the head of the pancreas shares its blood supply with the duodenum, the head of the pancreas and duodenum must be resected en bloc for cure. The pylorus and gastric antrum are usually resected to remove the G cells and part of the parietal cell mass, to prevent stoma ulceration. The dilated common bile duct, the gastric remnant, and the remaining pancreas with its duct must then be anastomosed to the jejunum to reestablish gastrointestinal continuity. *(A)* Pancreatic carcinoma located in the head of the pancreas. *(B)* Specimen consisting of proximal pancreas, duodenum, gastric antrum, and distal common bile duct removed. *(C)* Gastric remnant, dilated common bile duct, and pancreas with its main pancreatic duct, all anastomosed to the jejunum.

difficult and dangerous anastomosis and removing the entire pancreas, which may be potentially helpful because pancreatic cancer can be multifocal. Total pancreatectomy has three disadvantages: it causes diabetes; it causes pancreatic exocrine insufficiency that requires replacement therapy; and it necessitates splenectomy.

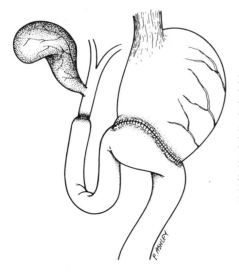

Figure 12–20. Total pancreatectomy, an alternative to Whipple's procedure for attempted cure of carcinoma of the head of the pancreas. The entire pancreas and spleen are removed. This obviates the treacherous pancreaticojejunal anastomosis, but it results in diabetes and exocrine insufficiency. The distal common bile duct and gastric remnant are anastomosed to the jejunum to reestablish gastrointestinal continuity.

Pancreatectomy has a high mortality rate (10%) in some centers, although in other institutions the mortality is extremely low. Because of the extent of the operation and the fact that the 5-year survival, even after potentially curative resection, is less than 15%, some surgeons might develop a defeatist approach and not even offer pancreaticoduodenectomy. One must remember, however, that there are *no* 5-year survivors after palliative surgery for carcinoma of the pancreas. In addition, periampullary cancers such as carcinoma of the papilla of Vater, of the duodenum, and of the distal common bile duct may be difficult to distinguish from carcinoma of the head of the pancreas at surgery, and these other conditions have a much more favorable prognosis after pancreaticoduodenectomy.

Palliative procedures for carcinoma of the pancreas are aimed at bypassing the obstruction of the common bile duct to relieve jaundice, with its associated severe pruritus and the potential for cholangitis, and at bypassing the gastric outlet obstruction caused by the tumor, alleviating persistent nausea and vomiting. The former goal is often accomplished by performing choledochojejunostomy or cholecystojejunostomy; the latter, by gastroenterostomy. The jaundice can sometimes be treated by a stent placed across the tumor at the time of ERCP, which temporarily relieves the jaundice and pruritus. Alternatively, placement of a catheter over a guidewire inserted during percutaneous transhepatic cholangiography can be used to relieve the jaundice and itching temporarily. Such a catheter can have side holes proximal and distal to the tumor, effecting internal drainage. The tube traverses the skin and may be connected to a drainage system for external drainage. This method can be used to improve the patient's medical status in preparation for definitive surgery or as the sole measure for a patient with limited life expectancy. The former use has become uncommon, because it can introduce bacteria into the duct and increase septic complications after the definitive pancreaticoduodenectomy.

Although the long-term outlook for carcinoma of the pancreas is extremely poor, in a small number of cases extensive surgery such as pancreaticoduodenectomy can be curative. If cure is not possible in a given case, bypass of the obstructed common bile duct or of the obstructed gastric outlet can effect significant palliation. Chemotherapy and radiation therapy before (neoadjuvant) or after (adjuvant) potentially curative surgery are under investigation, as is intraoperative radiation therapy (IORT).

Recommended Reading

1. Nahrwold, DL: The biliary system. In Sabiston DC, Jr., Lyerly HK (eds): *Textbook of Surgery, The Biological Basis of Modern Surgical Practice,* ed 15. Philadelphia: W.B. Saunders, 1997, pp 1117–1151.
2. Yeo CJ, Cameron JL: The pancreas. In Sabiston DC Jr., Lyerly HK (eds): *Textbook of Surgery, The Biological Basis of Modern Surgical Practice,* ed. 15. Philadelphia: W.B. Saunders, 1997, pp 1152–1186.
3. Garden OJ: *Hepatobiliary and Pancreatic Surgery.* Philadelphia: W.B. Saunders, 1997.
4. Zuidema GD (ed): *Shackelford's Surgery of the Alimentary Tract,* ed 4, vol III. Philadelphia: W.B. Saunders, 1996.

13

Trauma

Trauma is a frequent killer of young people. Prompt and appropriate intervention can salvage young people who have many productive years left to live. The situation tends to evolve quickly, and the surgeon must act almost reflexively, at least initially. However, mature judgment and a wide range of knowledge are required to make the important decisions about definitive therapy. Time spent in the study of trauma is rewarded by confidence in the management of these sometimes difficult situations.

CASE 13–1

Blunt Abdominal Trauma

A 21-year-old man was a passenger in the front seat of a car that ran off the road, hitting a tree. The ambulance drivers stated that he was unconscious at the scene, with blood pressure of 90/60 mm Hg and pulse of 120. There was deformity of the right leg with the tibia protruding through the skin. While in-line traction was maintained on the cervical spine, an airway was established by chin lift and an oral airway was placed. Oxygen was instituted by face mask, and a large-bore intravenous catheter was inserted into a forearm vein by the emergency medical technician (EMT). Ringer's lactated solution— "wide open"—was begun. The right leg was splinted. The patient was transported to the hospital.

Past medical history, family history, and review of systems were not available.

On arrival at the emergency department, the patient's airway was found to be compromised by blood, saliva, and loose teeth. His breathing was rapid and shallow. His circulation was judged to be marginal because blood pressure was 80 palpable, pulse was 130, and the lower extremities were cold and mottled.

The patient's neck was kept immobilized with the cervical collar, and an attempt was made to establish an airway by chin lift and by suctioning the contents from the mouth, at all times maintaining in-line immobilization of the cervical spine. When these efforts to establish an adequate airway and adequate breathing were not completely successful, an orotracheal tube was inserted with continued in-line immobilization of the cervical spine. A second large-bore peripheral intravenous catheter was inserted in the contralateral forearm. Blood specimens were taken for CBC, electrolytes, BUN, glucose, amylase, and toxicology, and the patient's blood was typed and cross-matched for 4 units of packed red blood cells. Two liters of Ringer's lactated solution was infused over 15 minutes with a rapid infuser–warmer.

After the initial quick assessment of airway, breathing, and circulation and after initial resuscitation, the patient was found to be responsive only to pain. He was undressed further to search for other injuries, and a more definitive examination was undertaken. A cross-table lateral x-ray of the cervical spine demonstrating C7 and the top of T1 showed no abnormality. He was "log-rolled" with in-line traction of the cervical spine, so that the examination could be completed. There was alcohol on his breath. He opened his eyes to pain, his best verbal response was to utter inappropriate words, and his best motor response was to localize pain, giving him a Glasgow Coma Scale score of 10. He moved all four extremities with normal deep tendon reflexes and no pathologic reflexes. Proprioception and pin prick could not be assessed. There was no Battle's sign. Pupils were equal, round, and reactive to light and accommodation.

There were good breath sounds over both lung fields, and the paradoxical motion of the left chest wall that had been present before intubation resolved after positive-pressure ventilation was instituted. There was no jugular vein distention, and no Kussmaul's sign. Pulsus paradoxus was absent. Heart sounds were strong, and there were no murmurs.

Examination of the abdomen revealed it to be not distended; involuntary guarding and moderate right upper quadrant tenderness were believed to be present. Bowel sounds were present. There was ecchymosis in the left flank. Rectal examination revealed the prostate to be in normal position, and there was normal sphincter tone.

Examination of the right lower extremity revealed a gross deformity, with a fragment of the tibia protruding through the skin. The posterior tibial and dorsalis pedis pulses were palpable bilaterally. The other three extremities appeared normal.

Because the cross-table lateral view of the cervical spine revealed no fracture or dislocation, it was believed that the patient could be moved for other studies, if indicated. The blood pressure had increased to 110/60 and the pulse had decreased to 96. The initial hematocrit came back at 40 and the white count was 13,600. The amylase value was 360. Formal cervical spine films were negative, and the chest x-ray revealed fractures in two places on the sixth through eighth ribs on the left. There was no widened mediastinum or evidence of pneumohemothorax.

Although there were no focal neurologic signs, it was thought that CT of the head was indicated because of the patient's diminished level of consciousness and because he would need to undergo surgery for the open fracture of the tibia—and probably for intraabdominal bleeding. Because the blood pressure and pulse had improved with the initial resuscitation, it appeared that the patient could be transported to the radiology department for CT.

CT of the head revealed no mass lesion. The blood pressure fell again to 90 mm Hg systolic, in spite of the fact that the patient had received 3 L of crystalloid. A repeat hematocrit sample was drawn, and a unit of packed red cells was transfused. CT of the abdomen revealed an estimated 1 L of free fluid and suggested a ruptured spleen and a liver laceration. A fracture of the left superior pubic ramus was identified, as was a retroperitoneal hematoma. Both kidneys functioned promptly with the injection of contrast medium.

The repeat hematocrit was 26. The blood pressure increased to 120/90, and the pulse decreased to 84 after 3 units of packed cells had been transfused. The patient was brought to surgery.

At surgery, 1.5 L of blood was found in the peritoneal cavity. Meticulous exploration of the peritoneal cavity was carried out. The injuries were believed to include a superficial laceration to the right lobe of the liver, which was no longer bleeding. The spleen was found to have an extensive network of intersecting ruptures. There was a large hematoma surrounding the left kidney, and a large pelvic hematoma. Both hemidiaphragms were intact. Three additional units of packed red blood cells was transfused.

The spleen was thought to be unsalvageable, especially in light of the associated injuries; thus splenectomy was performed. Because the liver laceration was no longer bleeding, a closed drainage system was placed in the area of injury and brought out through a separate stab wound. Hematomas in the left perinephric region and in the pelvis were left undisturbed. The orthopedic team debrided and irrigated the leg wound and then treated the tibial fracture with an intramedullary nail.

The patient was brought first to the recovery room and then to the intensive care unit. A central venous pressure line was inserted, and total parenteral nutrition was begun on postoperative day 1. The patient initially demonstrated a large right-to-left shunt with arterial oxygen desaturation. Chest x-rays demonstrated fluffy infiltrates thought to represent adult respiratory distress syndrome (ARDS), and an infiltrate on the left was thought to represent a lung contusion. The initial postoperative serum amylase value was 2000 Somogyi units.

Over the course of the next week, amylase returned to normal, the infiltrates resolved, and paradoxical motion of the chest wall resolved. The patient was successfully extubated, and gastrointestinal function returned so that he was able to tolerate a regular diet and have bowel movements. Parenteral nutrition was discontinued. Neurologic function returned toward normal. The patient was discharged from the hospital on the 14th postoperative day. The tibial fracture healed without sequelae.

DISCUSSION OF CASE 13–1

Chief Complaint and History of Present Illness

In the case of trauma, the chief complaint and history of present illness are often obtained from the ambulance drivers or police. The nature of the injury often gives important clues to the possible injuries sustained. A history of unconsciousness suggests that at the very least the patient has sustained a cerebral concussion. A steering wheel injury to the chest (deceleration injury) makes one think of traumatic rupture of the thoracic aorta at the ligamentum arteriosum, as it is at this fixed point that the shear forces could be expected to be greatest. Traumatic rupture of the thoracic aorta from blunt chest injury is usually lethal, and only the minority whose rupture is contained by the adventitia of the aorta or by pleura and other mediastinal structures survive transport to the ER. History of deceleration injury (e.g., steering wheel to the chest) and chest x-ray findings of widened mediastinum, apical cap, loss of the contour of the aorta, shift of the trachea to the right, and left pleural fluid (hemothorax) all suggest traumatic rupture of the thoracic aorta. Aortography confirms the injury. CT and trans-esophageal echocardiography findings may contribute to the diagnosis. Surgery must be expeditious, as exanguination can occur at any time. Cardiopulmonary bypass or a shunt is usually employed to decrease the likelihood of spinal cord ischemia.

Management by EMTs at the Scene

The cervical collar was applied to prevent injury to the spinal cord, should fracture-dislocation of the cervical spine be present. If the EMTs thought that the airway was severely compromised or that ventilation was inadequate, they might have been forced to intubate the patient, but there is a tradeoff that requires a judgment call: The more they do in the field, the longer it takes to get the patient to a hospital where definitive therapy can be instituted by the responsible surgeon. In this case, they settled for instituting supplemental oxygen via face mask.

Because the patient was hypotensive and tachycardic, the EMTs inserted a large-bore intravenous catheter and infused "physiologic saline" as fast as possible. Either Ringer's lactate or normal saline could have been chosen, because the electrolyte concentrations grossly approximate that of plasma and because the solutions are distributed in the extracellular space, maximizing expansion of the intravascular space. While a "plasma expander" such as 5% albumin might be expected to be even more efficient because it is distributed initially in the intravascular compartment, it is not routinely used early in this situation because of the belief that, in shock, the capillaries are more permeable to albumin, which will therefore leak into the interstitium, bringing fluid with it. Aggressive fluid resuscitation to restore normal intravascular volume (as manifested by normalization of blood pressure and pulse) is a time-honored practice that has been recently challenged on the grounds that normal blood pressure may actually exacerbate hemorrhage. Certainly, mechanical control of bleeding sites must take priority over fluid administration, and, of course, they are not mutually exclusive. The extent to which blood loss (volume) should be restored before operation in a patient with hemorrhage is a subject of active study.

The technicians follow the *ABCs* of establishing an *a*irway, making sure the patient is *b*reathing adequately, and supporting the *c*irculation, just as the surgeon will on the patient's arrival at the emergency department.

Other Aspects of the History

When the patient arrives, an effort is made to contact the family, as they must, of course, be notified of the injury. Informed consent should be obtained if possible from patient or a family member for any invasive procedures. A member of the team should be assigned to obtain the past medical history, to the extent possible. Knowledge of associated illnesses, allergies, or medications the patient is taking enhance proper care.

Initial Resuscitation in the Emergency Department

Resuscitation and diagnosis often must be carried out simultaneously, as one cannot afford to wait to institute treatment until a definitive determination of all the injuries has been made. An initial assessment of the airway was made in this patient. Blood, teeth, and other débris can obstruct the airway, producing anoxia. In an unconscious patient or one with facial fractures, the tongue can obstruct the airway. The jaw should be lifted with the fingers behind the angle of the mandible or under the chin, in an attempt to dislodge the tongue from the airway. In-line immobilization of the cervical spine must be maintained during this and all maneuvers. Suctioning and administration of high-flow oxygen via a nonrebreathing mask may then be adequate. If not, intubation and positive-pressure ventilation may be necessary. The key to intubation is to maintain immobilization of the cervical spine to prevent a spinal cord injury, should a cervical spine fracture or dislocation be present. Some surgeons recommend nasotracheal intubation to obviate hyperextension of the neck, which is sometimes required for orotracheal intubation. The theoretical disadvantage of this approach is that the nasotracheal tube could be pushed into the brain if the cribriform bone were fractured. Thus, this approach is relatively contraindicated when fracture of the facial bones is suspected. Orotracheal intubation can often be performed without hyperextending the neck, even in patients with facial fractures. When intubation cannot be accomplished, other options include needle cricothyroidotomy (performed by inserting a large-bore sheath over needle through the cricothyroid membrane), formal cricothyroidotomy, or emergency tracheostomy (Fig. 13–1).

Even though the airway is patent, the patient may not be breathing adequately, for a number of reasons. He may have depression of the respiratory center because of central nervous system injury or drug taking. The patient in Case 13–1 had inadequate breathing because of *flail chest*. This occurs when three or more ribs are fractured in at least two places (Fig. 13–2). It allows paradoxical motion of a segment of chest wall, decreasing the patient's effective tidal volume and increasing the work of breathing. Pain, splinting, and decreased tidal volume can lead to ineffective cough and sigh, with carbon dioxide retention and hypoxia

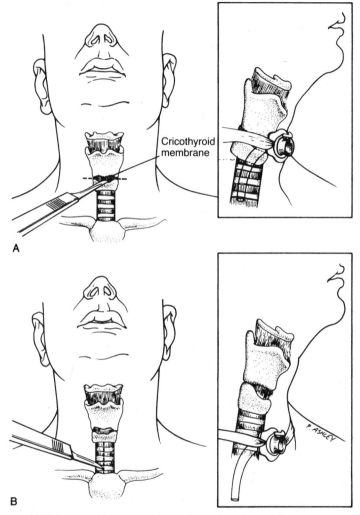

Figure 13–1. *(A)* Cricothyroidotomy can be performed rapidly under emergency conditions when there is upper airway obstruction. A transverse incision is made in the neck over the cricothyroid space, and the cricothyroid membrane is punctured with a scalpel and then dilated. A tracheostomy tube is inserted. This procedure is facilitated because the cricothyroid membrane is superficial. *(B)* Tracheostomy is performed by means of an incision (dotted lines) in the neck, separating the strap muscles and incising the trachea through the second and third rings. A tracheostomy tube is then inserted. Both procedures are more easily performed when an endotracheal tube is in place and when the patient can be brought to the operating room.

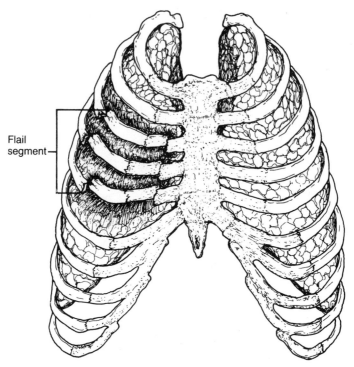

Flail
segment—

Figure 13–2. Three ribs are fractured in two places, resulting in flail chest. The flail segment moves paradoxically, diminishing the effective tidal volume. An underlying lung contusion may be contributing to respiratory failure. Modern treatment involves "internal splinting" with intubation and positive-pressure ventilation for more severe injuries.

due to retained secretions and atelectasis. Concurrent underlying lung contusion can be an even more significant cause of respiratory failure with flail chest. In times past, flail chest was stabilized with sandbags or with towel clips, but modern treatment entails "internal splinting," with endotracheal intubation and positive-pressure ventilation.

The circulation must be supported. Initially this is done by infusing approximately 2 L of crystalloid such as Ringer's lactate solution. If time allows, blood can be formally typed and cross-matched for safe transfusion. If blood is required sooner than formal cross-matching will allow type O blood or type-specific blood can be transfused, though the risk of transfusion reaction is somewhat greater. The benefits and the risks of using un–cross-matched blood must be weighed. If there is no evidence of trauma to the urethra, a Foley catheter can be inserted to monitor urine output, which is a good reflection of the adequacy of resuscitation. Pulse and blood pressure should be determined frequently. Restoration of premorbid intravascular volume and blood pressure may not be possible in a profusely hemorrhaging patient and may actually increase blood loss from an area of injury. Contrariwise, the heart needs adequate left ventricular end-diastolic volumes to perfuse the tissues, and without such volume myocardial infarction, stroke, mesenteric infarction, or acute renal failure, among other disasters, might be precipitated. At present, insertion of a Swan-Ganz catheter in the emergency department is rarely indicated.

Definitive Diagnosis

After the initial quick assessment (primary survey) of the *ABCs* (airway, breathing, circulation) and after resuscitation, *disability* is briefly assessed. That is, it is determined whether the patient is alert, responsive to verbal stimuli, responsive only to painful stimuli, or unresponsive. The patient is undressed completely and examined for other injuries, which may not have been immediately apparent. This completes the *ABCDE,* the *quick* neurologic examination for the disability and the undressing for exposure, in the *ABCDE* of resuscitation. Then, a head-to-toe physical examination is performed. This constitutes the secondary survey.

Central Nervous System. Evaluation of the patient's central nervous system requires that his mental status be described according to the Glasgow Coma Scale. Eye opening, best motor response, and best verbal response are evaluated to determine the score. Four points are given if the patient opens his eyes spontaneously, and one point if he does not open them at all. Two or three points are given, respectively, when he opens his eyes to pain only or to voice. Best motor response is quantified by an award of 6 points if the patient follows commands and 1 point if he is flaccid, intermediate points being given for responses that require less advanced brain function. Best verbal response is assessed by an award of 5 points if the patient is oriented and 1 point if there is no verbal response. Intermediate points are given for less organized verbal responses.

Basilar skull fractures may cause Battle's sign, manifested by ecchymosis behind the ear, or they may cause blood to be visible behind the tympanic membrane (*hemotympanum*) on otoscopic examination. *Raccoon's eyes* (ecchymosis in the periorbital area) may indicate an orbital fracture. Leakage of cerebrospinal fluid from the nose or ear indicates that the meninges have been torn.

A good neurologic examination can be performed quickly. It entails assessment of the cranial nerves, motor strength, and deep tendon reflexes, and determination of the presence or absence of pathologic reflexes such as Babinski's sign. A dilated pupil can signify brain stem compression from herniation caused by a subdural or epidural hematoma. Emergency *bur holes* may be life saving, as they relieve compression. In less desperate circumstances CT may be used to localize the space-occupying lesion. It should be recognized that head injury alone is rarely a cause of shock and that, when shock is present, another source, such as intraabdominal or intrathoracic injury, must be sought.

Cardiovascular System. Pulse, blood pressure, and urine output are valuable parameters to monitor. A patient who complains of being cold, who says he wants to sleep, and who is cold and clammy with mottled extremities is in shock.

A drop in blood pressure may be a relatively late manifestation of hypovolemia. The sympathetic response to blood loss causes peripheral vasoconstriction with an increase in total peripheral resistance, helping to support the blood pressure, and it causes constriction of the renal arterioles with decreased urine output (to conserve intravascular volume). It also causes reflex tachycardia; all these processes occur well before systemic pressure drops. Mental confusion may be caused by decreased cardiac output. The neck veins are collapsed in the patient with hemorrhagic shock, and elevated neck veins suggest cardiac tamponade or tension pneumothorax.

The pneumatic antishock garment (PASG), also known as military antishock trousers (MAST), is sometimes used to increase blood pressure in hemorrhagic shock patients by increasing peripheral vascular resistance. The hope was, that when the garment was inflated around the legs and abdomen it would increase flow to the heart, brain, and lungs. However, applying it before direct control of bleeding is achieved can actually increase blood loss, and even if it is accompanied by massive fluid resuscitation in the field or emergency department, it can result in severe hemodilution and decreased oxygen delivery. Concern about the PASG parallels concern about aggressive fluid resuscitation to restore blood pressure before operative or nonoperative direct control of bleeding: it might actually increase blood loss. This may be true especially if the injury is outside the area covered by the PASG, as to the heart or another intrathoracic structure. Cardiogenic shock, diaphragmatic injury, and pregnancy are contraindications to PASG. PASGs may have a role in stabilizing unstable pelvic fractures and tamponading retroperitoneal hematomas caused by pelvic fracture. Other measures in the treatment of pelvic fractures include external fixators, angiography with embolization, and open reduction and internal fixation.

Traumatic rupture of the thoracic aorta can occur at the ligamentum arteriosum, just distal to the left subclavian artery. The fact that the vessel is fixed there maximizes the effect of the shearing forces caused by deceleration injury. Most patients with traumatic rupture of the thoracic aorta do not arrive alive in the emergency department. Those who do may undergo operative repair with cardiopulmonary bypass or with a heparin-bonded shunt. Alternatively, one can clamp the thoracic aorta and merely work quickly in the absence of bypass, although this carries the risk of compromising the blood supply to the spinal cord and causing quadriplegia.

Respiratory System. The respiratory status of the patient must also be evaluated more thoroughly after the initial resuscitation. The patient may have flail chest, which requires positive-pressure ventilation. Before institution of positive-pressure ventilation, the flail segment moves paradoxically every time the patient breathes, decreasing the tidal volume and predisposing to respiratory failure. The underlying lung contusion may be an even more important cause of pulmonary dysfunction. Gastric atony and dilatation frequently accompany trauma. A nasogastric tube should be inserted to prevent aspiration of gastric contents, which can add considerably to morbidity. Contusion of the lung parenchyma can add to the right-to-left shunt. An air leak from a bronchus can result in a bronchopleural fistula with tension pneumothorax. This can cause a shift of the mediastinum, decreasing return of blood to the right side of the heart and leading to cardiac arrest.

Massive bleeding into the chest is usually apparent on chest x-ray. In this setting a chest tube must be inserted, and if the bleeding continues thoracotomy may be required to stop it. Hemorrhage may originate from an intercostal or internal mammary artery or from a branch of the pulmonary artery. Bleeding from the latter is more likely to stop spontaneously when the lung is reexpanded with a tube thoracostomy, since the pulmonary circulation is under low pressure. When significant hemothorax is present, blood should be removed by tube thoracostomy. Otherwise it will organize and result in restrictive lung disease from fibrothorax, which requires decortication for treatment.

Genitourinary System and Renal System. Blood at the meatus of the penis or inability to micturate suggests an injury to the urethra. A bulge in the penis, perineum, or scrotum suggests extravasation of urine from an injured urethra. In this case, catheterization of the bladder should be avoided, as it could exacerbate the urethral damage. Rectal examination can demonstrate a "floating prostate," which also indicates urethral damage. A retrograde cystourethrogram, obtained by injecting dye through the urethra, can help to evaluate this possibility. If intravenous pyelography shows prompt function of both kidneys, a major injury to the renal arteries is ruled out, obviating angiography. One would ordinarily try to avoid operating for a renal fracture because, if the tamponade is relieved by surgery, nephrectomy may be required for hemostasis. Conversely, if one or both kidneys do not function on intravenous pyelography, angiography is necessary, as injury to the renal pedicle may require renal artery repair.

If there is no apparent injury to the urethra, Foley catheterization may be helpful. Urine output can then be carefully monitored, reflecting the patient's state of hydration.

Gastrointestinal System: Abdominal Examination. Early diagnosis of intraabdominal injury has a salutary effect on outcome. If the patient has developed hemorrhagic shock, substantial blood loss must have occurred; the number of body cavities in which this blood can collect is limited. There is not enough room in the cranial vault to accommodate a large quantity of blood, and the patient would first develop neurologic findings. Massive hemorrhage can occur into the chest, but this should be readily apparent on chest x-ray.

A patient can lose a large quantity of blood into the thigh after a fracture of the femur, but this should be manifested as swelling or pain in the thigh, or as deformity or fracture on radiographs. Accordingly, if the patient is hypotensive and the chest x-ray shows no hemothorax, hemoperitoneum, or retroperitoneal hemorrhage is likely, and if the patient has a tender abdomen, laparotomy is indicated. If no symptoms or signs are referable to the abdomen, if the patient has a decreased level of consciousness that makes physical examination of the abdomen difficult to interpret, or if the patient will require general anesthesia for craniotomy or repair of an orthopedic injury, further testing may be needed to rule out intraabdominal bleeding caused by a ruptured solid viscus or a major vascular injury.

Peritoneal lavage is a good procedure for confirming hemoperitoneum. It is performed through a peritoneal dialysis catheter inserted through the linea alba into the peritoneal cavity. It can be inserted by percutaneous puncture or through a small incision made in the midline while the patient is still in the accident room. A syringe is used to aspirate. If unclotted blood is aspirated, laparotomy is required. Otherwise, 1000 ml of normal saline is instilled and then allowed to drain out. When there are more than 100,000 red blood cells or more than 500 white blood cells per mm^3, or food particles or bacteria are identified on Gram's stain, laparotomy is necessary. An elevated amylase value in the aspirate fluid may also be an indication for laparotomy if it is associated with abnormal physical findings.

In some centers, CT has replaced peritoneal lavage for diagnosis of occult intraabdominal bleeding after blunt abdominal trauma. To reiterate, if the patient's condition is unstable, he must be brought expeditiously to the operating room. If, however, the blood pressure and pulse are sustained after initial resuscitation, CT can make the diagnosis of blood in the peritoneal cavity and can demonstrate a ruptured spleen or lacerated liver. It can frequently demonstrate retroperitoneal hematomas. CT is especially helpful in trauma centers that have a radiologist and technician available 24 hours. In Case 13–1, the patient's condition was stable enough to make possible transport to the CT suite and to allow CT of the head. This ruled out a surgically correctable intracranial injury, and CT of the abdomen demonstrated the intraabdominal injuries.

At this point, the patient had received enough crystalloid to fill the vascular compartment and cause hemodilution, and his hematocrit value fell. At surgery, the liver laceration was left undisturbed and a closed drainage system was placed near it because it had stopped bleeding. Sometimes major débridement or formal resection of a lobe of liver is necessary to stop the hemorrhage (Fig. 13–3). Pringle's maneuver is finger compression of the hepatic artery and portal vein at the portal triad followed by application of a vascular clamp. This usually arrests the bleeding until definitive hemostasis can be achieved. If it does not stop the bleeding, the surgeon must consider the possibility that the bleeding is coming from one of the hepatic veins or its tributaries.

Splenectomy no longer is routinely performed for minor splenic injuries. It has become apparent that the spleen plays an important role in the immune response by virtue of its reticuloendothelial function, its ability to produce antibodies, and its defensive function against encapsulated bacteria. Splenectomized children have an increased incidence of

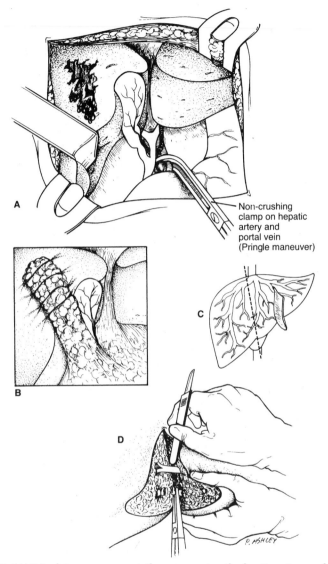

Non-crushing
clamp on hepatic
artery and
portal vein
(Pringle maneuver)

Figure 13–3. *(A)* Pringle's maneuver entails compressing the heptic artery and portal vein at the porta hepatis, temporarily curtailing massive hemorrhage in the wake of major liver trauma. Crushed tissue can often be débrided with specific ligation of grossly apparent vessels and bile ducts. *(B)* A flap of omentum on a vascular pedicle can be used to pack the defect. The area should be drained. *(C)* A major lobar resection may occasionally be required when damage is extensive. Depicted here is a right hepatic lobectomy. A line drawn from the inferior vena cava to the gallbladder fossa marks the division between the right and left lobes. The middle hepatic vein is preserved. *(D)* Blunt dissection of the liver parenchyma with the scalpel handle or finger (finger-fracture technique) allows accurate ligation of visible vessels and ducts, obviating anatomic resection of a lobe in most cases. Lobectomy is an operation of significant magnitude.

overwhelming sepsis due to encapsulated organisms such as pneumo-cocci *(Streptococcus pneumoniae), Haemophilus influenzae,* and *Neisseria meningitidis.* This observation, along with new techniques of salvage such as partial splenectomy, suture with pledgets, and application of topical hemostatic agents, has resulted in salvage of many spleens (Fig. 13–4). These techniques, however, take longer than splenectomy and do not guarantee that secondary hemorrhage will not occur. Accordingly, in patients whose condition is unstable or who have multiple injuries or extensive spleen damage, splenectomy may still be the prudent course of action.

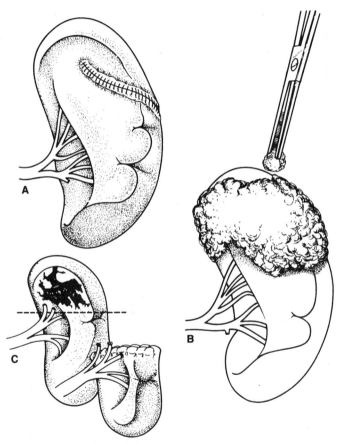

Figure 13–4. Splenic repair (splenorrhaphy) may be performed when the patient's condition has stabilized, if no other life-threatening injuries are present, and if the splenic damage is not too extensive. The spleen must first be mobilized completely. *(A)* A laceration that does not involve the pedicle can be repaired by suture. Pledgets may help to avoid tearing. *(B)* Avulsion of a segment of capsule may be prevented from bleeding if it is packed with topical hemostatic agents. *(C)* It has been recognized that the arterial supply to the spleen is segmental, and partial splenectomy can be performed between segments.

When preoperative CT or intravenous pyelography has shown good renal function, one tries to avoid opening Gerota's fascia in the case of a flank hematoma, as this could release the tamponade and necessitate nephrectomy. Laparotomy may, however, be unavoidable with serious renal injury. Pelvic hematomas likewise are not opened routinely, as hemostasis may be quite hard to achieve once the tamponade is released. If the hematoma is expanding, however, exploration may be necessary to rule out injury to a major vessel. Both hemidiaphragms must be inspected carefully to rule out traumatic rupture, as this could escape detection during hospitalization and present later as an incarcerated diaphragmatic hernia.

Postoperative Course

The patient in Case 13–1 had multiple conditions that cause right-to-left intrapulmonary shunt with arterial oxygen desaturation. The initial blunt trauma may be responsible for a lung contusion, which may cause ventilation-perfusion mismatch. In addition, shock itself liberates substances that interfere with surfactant, causing microatelectasis and perfusion of underventilated alveoli. The particulate matter in banked blood can also be responsible for lung injury after massive transfusion. This patient had an elevated amylase level, representative of either pancreatitis from the trauma itself or pancreatitis from the operative trauma of splenectomy. In pancreatitis, mediators that injure the lung and cause ARDS are liberated. This can cause microatelectasis, decreased compliance, and right-to-left shunting.

Adult respiratory distress syndrome (ARDS) is a constellation of entities whose common denominator seems to be collapse of the alveoli with ventilation-perfusion mismatch, right-to-left shunting, arterial hypoxemia, and bilateral diffuse fluffy infiltrates on chest x-ray. Supplemental oxygen and positive-pressure ventilation usually are required to support respiratory function. *Positive end-expiratory pressure* (PEEP) seems to be therapeutic for this condition by preventing collapse of the alveoli. The most important measure in treating ARDS is finding and eliminating the underlying cause, when possible. Fat emboli from long-bone fractures can cause mental confusion in addition to hypoxemia; early open reduction and internal fixation of the fracture may reduce the incidence of this complication.

Patients with major trauma have a fast metabolic rate and can require as many 45 kCal/kg of body weight, as opposed to the 25 to 35 kCal/kg required by normal healthy persons. This patient was therefore given total parenteral nutrition until normal gastrointestinal function returned. Nutritional support may be complicated because of glucose intolerance secondary to release of catabolic substances such as epinephrine and norepinephrine in the stress state. Thirty percent of nonprotein calories may be given as fat. Enteral feeding may provide substrate to the enterocytes in the small bowel, to give them enough energy so that they can prevent bacterial translocation from the gut lumen to the bloodstream.

SUMMARY

Prompt resuscitation, with attention to airway, breathing, and circulation, followed by definitive diagnosis and surgical intervention can salvage many young trauma patients. Meticulous attention to postoperative care is necessary. Prevention may ultimately be the most important measure in minimizing death from trauma.

Recommended Reading

1. Maull KI, Rodriguez A, Wiles CE III (eds): *Complications in Trauma and Critical Care.* Philadelphia: W.B. Saunders, 1996.
2. Jurkovich GJ, Carrico CJ: Trauma: Management of the acutely injured patient. In Sabiston DC Jr., Lyerly HK (eds): *Textbook of Surgery: The Biological Basis of Modern Surgical Practice,* ed 15. Philadelphia: W.B. Saunders, 1997.
3. Feliciano DV, Moore EE, Mattox KL (eds): *Trauma,* ed 3. Stamford, Conn: Appleton & Lange, 1996.
4. Ivatury RR, Cauten CG (eds): *The Textbook of Penetrating Trauma.* Baltimore: Williams & Wilkins, 1996.

14

Hernia

A hernia is a protrusion of one structure through a defect in another. Groin hernias include inguinal and femoral hernias; abdominal wall hernias consist of umbilical, epigastric, incisional, and spigelian hernias. As illustrated in Chapter 8 on intestinal obstruction, repair of hernias is usually recommended to prevent incarceration and possible strangulation or to relieve symptoms such as pain, which straining can induce.

CASE 14–1

Elective Repair of Indirect Inguinal Hernia

A 54-year-old man employed at a shipyard was referred for elective herniorrhaphy.

For the last 3 years, the patient had had a bulge in his left groin. His family doctor had prescribed a truss, but the hernia became increasingly uncomfortable and interfered with the patient's work. His fellow employees suggested that the patient have his hernia repaired. The patient was at all times able to push the bulge in, and he had never had any bouts of abdominal pain, nausea, or vomiting. There was no history of change in bowel habits or straining at stool, nor of nocturia, frequency, or hesitancy.

Past medical history was negative for heart disease, diabetes, and other serious medical illnesses. The patient had stopped smoking 15 years ago.

Physical examination of the heart and lungs was normal. Abdominal examination revealed no masses or organomegaly. The patient had a bulge in the left groin that was easily reducible. Rectal examination revealed no masses, and the prostate was not enlarged.

Laboratory examination was done on an outpatient basis to satisfy the requirements for anesthesia should supplementation of the local anesthesia by intravenous sedation prove necessary. The complete blood count, electrolytes, BUN, glucose, urinalysis, chest x-ray, and ECG were unremarkable.

In the ambulatory surgery suite the patient underwent repair of his indirect inguinal hernia under long-acting local anesthesia with Marcaine. The anesthesiologist supplemented this with intravenous sedation. The repair was performed by the method of Bassini.

The patient was allowed to go home with his wife that night, after being carefully counseled to notify his surgeon if there were any bleeding, difficulty in voiding, or fever. He remained comfortable, however, and his sutures were removed in the office a week later. At his follow-up appointment 1 year later, the repair was found to be sound.

DISCUSSION OF CASE 14–1

Diagnosis

Symptoms. An inguinal hernia may present with mild pain or discomfort in the groin, and the patient may experience a bulge. If the hernia is reducible, the patient is usually able to push the bulge back into the abdomen himself. Nausea, vomiting, and cramping abdominal pain suggesting small bowel obstruction occur only when the hernia becomes incarcerated.

Signs. The most obvious sign is a bulge in the groin. It may be necessary to ask the patient to cough or to perform the Valsalva maneuver to demonstrate the hernia. Examining the patient while he is in the standing position often makes the hernia apparent. It is sometimes helpful to insert the examining finger through the external inguinal ring into the inguinal canal to demonstrate an impulse with coughing or Valsalva. The mere presence of a dilated external inguinal ring is not indicative of a hernia. A tender, red mass in the groin suggests strangulation of intestine within the hernia sac. In infants, it may not be possible to demonstrate an inguinal hernia in the surgeon's office; one can rely on information the mother provides and perform herniorrhaphy on that basis.

Laboratory Examination. The diagnosis of an inguinal hernia is usually a clinical one that requires no laboratory examination. If the patient is to require supplementation of local anesthesia with intravenous sedation or other anesthetic agents, laboratory tests such as CBC and serum potassium are usually required to satisfy hospital protocol for patients undergoing anesthesia or with "anesthesia standby," and chest x-ray and ECG may be required by hospital policy if the patient is over 40 years old and may be indicated when associated medical problems are known or suspected.

Treatment

Once the diagnosis of an inguinal hernia is made, herniorrhaphy is usually indicated as prophylaxis against later incarceration and possible strangulation. If the hernia is incarcerated (i.e., cannot be reduced), herniorrhaphy should be performed expeditiously to prevent strangulation (gangrene of the bowel due to ischemia).

There are obviously circumstances in which the patient has a limited life expectancy or has serious medical illnesses that preclude surgery. In the usual situation, elective herniorrhaphy is recommended, since the morbidity and mortality are much greater when incarceration and strangulation supervene. In some patients of advanced age, the potential benefits and risks of surgery may approximate each other, and herniorrhaphy may be avoided if the hernia is not incarcerated and symptoms are not severe. Prescription of a truss (a belt to compress the hernia to keep it reduced) is of questionable efficacy.

The surgical technique of inguinal hernia repair has evolved over the years, with many great surgeons contributing to its development. Accordingly, there are eponyms (surnames) attached to the different types of hernia repair, and memorizing all of these is probably unnecessary for students. However, as one develops as a surgeon, the study of the history of hernia repair not only proves fascinating but affords insights into the anatomy of this area and the principles of sound repair. The Bassini and McVay repairs are discussed here, to provide a basic understanding of the principles involved.

Hesselbach's triangle (Fig. 14–1) is formed by the inferior epigastric artery (its lateral border), the inguinal ligament (its inferior border), and the lateral edge of the rectus sheath (its medial border). An *indirect inguinal hernia* (Fig. 14–2) protrudes through the deep inguinal ring, which is just lateral to the inferior epigastric artery; thus, this is outside of Hesselbach's triangle and is called *indirect*. A *direct inguinal hernia* (Fig. 14–3) is a weakness in the medial wall of the inguinal canal, medial to the inferior epigastric artery. A direct inguinal hernia is a protrusion through Hesselbach's triangle.

Technique or Repair

Because the skin incision for repair of both direct and indirect inguinal hernias is the same, it is no longer considered important to distinguish between them preoperatively. An incision is made in the skin crease two fingerbreadths above an imaginary line between the anterior superior iliac spine and the pubic tubercle. After incision of Camper's and Scarpa's fasciae, which are filmy, the aponeurosis of the external oblique is incised in the direction of its fibers and the superficial inguinal ring is transected (Fig. 14–4). The ilioinguinal nerve is preserved, because transecting it causes numbness of the scrotum and medial aspect of the thigh. The medial and lateral leaves of the aponeurosis of the external oblique are developed (Fig. 14–5); the cremasteric veil is incised (Fig. 14–6); and the spermatic cord is circumscribed with a Penrose drain (Fig. 14–7).

If an indirect inguinal hernia is present, the sac is skeletonized; that is, it is dissected free from the spermatic cord and from the lipoma of the cord (Fig. 14–8). The latter structure is really a projection of properitoneal fat; thus *lipoma* is a misnomer. High ligation of the sac (Fig. 14–9) is one of the most important principles of repair of an indirect inguinal hernia. A direct inguinal hernia is medial to the epigastric vessels and so is not found within the cremasteric veil. Its base is usually wide, and it may have bladder within it. It is thus usually imbricated, rather than ligated and excised, to avoid injury to the bladder (Fig. 14–10).

Text continued on page 198

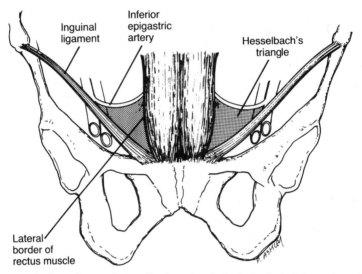

Figure 14–1. The boundaries of Hesselbach's triangle include the inferior epigastric artery, the lateral border of the rectus sheath, and the inguinal ligament.

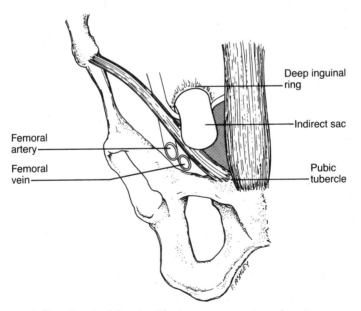

Figure 14–2. Indirect inguinal hernia. The sac, an extension of peritoneum, protrudes through the deep inguinal ring lateral to the inferior epigastric vessels. It does not, therefore, pass through Hesselbach's triangle.

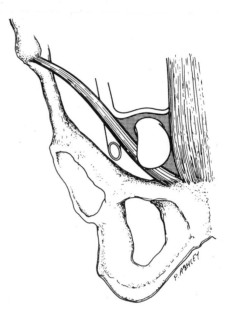

Figure 14–3. Direct inguinal hernia. The sac protrudes through Hesselbach's triangle medial to the epigastric vessels.

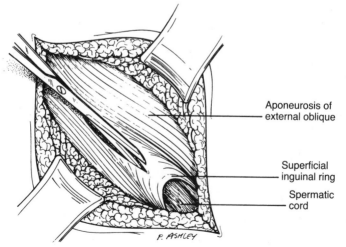

Aponeurosis of
external oblique

Superficial
inguinal ring

Spermatic
cord

Figure 14–4. In repair of groin hernias, the aponeurosis of the external oblique is incised in the direction of its fibers and the superficial inguinal ring is transected.

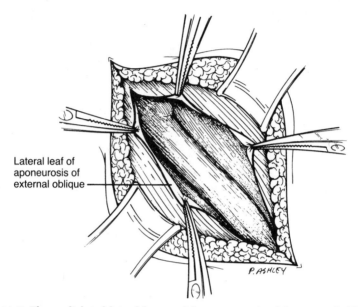

Figure 14–5. The medial and lateral leaves of the aponeurosis of the external oblique are developed.

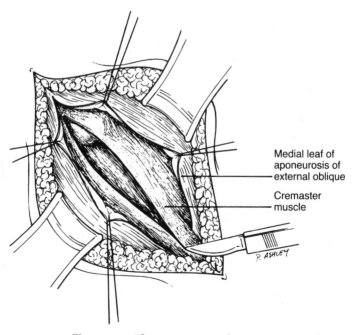

Figure 14–6. The cremasteric veil is incised.

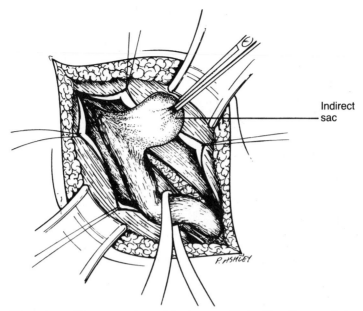

Figure 14–7. The spermatic cord is circumscribed with a Penrose drain.

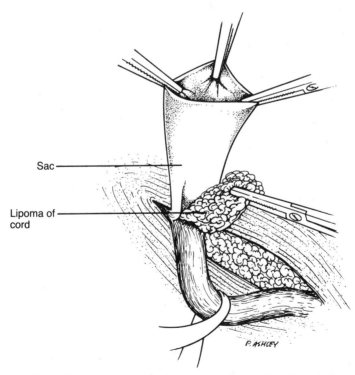

Figure 14–8. The indirect hernia sac is skeletonized; that is, it is dissected free from the spermatic cord and from the "lipoma" of the cord. These three structures, which are encountered after the cremasteric fascia is incised, can be remembered if one considers that Julius Caesar divided Gaul into three parts.

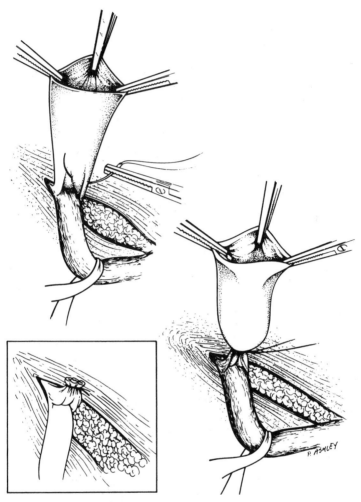

Figure 14–9. High ligation of the sac, as emphasized by Halsted, is an important principle of repair of an indirect inguinal hernia.

The floor of the inguinal canal must then be reconstructed. In the *Bassini repair* (Fig. 14–11), the medial leaf of the transversalis fascia and the conjoined tendon are approximated to the lateral leaf of the transversalis fascia and to the shelving edge of Poupart's ligament (inguinal ligament). In the *McVay repair* (Fig. 14–12), the medial leaf of the transversalis fascia and the conjoined tendon are approximated to Cooper's ligament. A transition stitch is required in the Cooper's ligament repair when the femoral sheath is reached.

The aponeurosis of the external oblique is then reapproximated (Fig. 14–13), although this layer adds no strength to the repair, and the skin

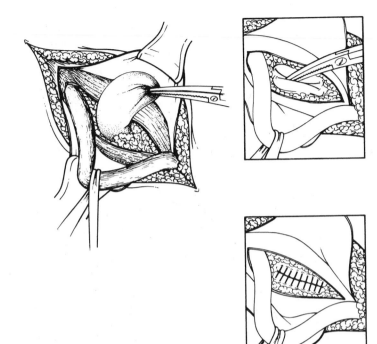

Figure 14–10. In a direct inguinal hernia, the sac is imbricated. Injury to the bladder must be avoided.

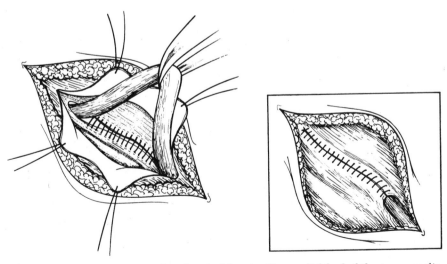

Figure 14–11. Bassini's repair of an inguinal hernia. The medial leaf of the transversalis fascia and the conjoined tendon are approximated to the lateral leaf of the transversalis fascia and the shelving edge of Poupart's ligament.

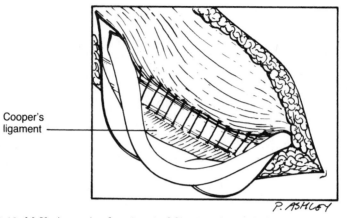

Figure 14–12. McVay's repair of an inguinal hernia. The medial leaf of the transversalis fascia and the conjoined tendon are approximated to Cooper's ligament.

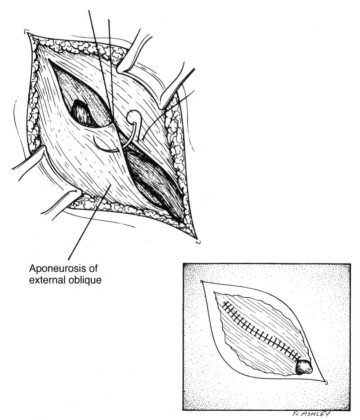

Figure 14–13. The aponeurosis of the external oblique is approximated, reconstructing the external inguinal ring.

is closed with sutures or staples. A normal diet is resumed the same day, and the patient should be out of bed walking the evening of the repair. Unless the patient is very elderly or frail or there are serious intercurrent medical problems, the repair is usually performed as an outpatient procedure.

CASE 14–2
Incisional Hernia

A 43-year-old woman was admitted for elective repair of an incisional hernia.

Six months before admission, the patient underwent total abdominal hysterectomy and bilateral salpingo-oophorectomy for a large leiomyoma of the uterus (fibroid uterus). A postoperative wound infection necessitated drainage of the lower part of the wound; this ultimately healed by secondary intention. She later developed a bulge in the lower end of her midline incision and was referred by the gynecologist to the surgeon for repair of this incisional hernia.

Past medical history included diabetes mellitus controlled by diet and a 40–pack-year history of cigarette smoking.

Physical examination revealed an obese female with a well-defined hernia defect at the lower end of the incision. The remainder of the physical examination was unremarkable.

Laboratory examination was negative except for a blood sugar of 180 mg/dL.

The patient underwent repair of her incisional hernia. She resumed eating on the first postoperative day and was discharged the same day.

DISCUSSION OF CASE 14–2

Diagnosis

History. It is significant that this patient had a postoperative wound infection; this is an important factor that frequently predisposes to incisional hernia. Other factors include chronic cough such as a heavy smoker might have, obesity, diabetes, malnutrition, cancer, use of steroids or chemotherapeutic agents, intestinal distention at the time of wound closure, and a drain or a stoma brought through the wound. However, no predisposing factors may be present; technical factors such as placing the sutures too loosely or too tightly (causing necrosis of the fascia) or taking too small bites of fascia may play a role.

Physical Examination. The fact that a well-defined hernia ring could be palpated suggests that there is good, strong tissue with which to close the defect. When healthy fascia is not available, synthetic material is sometimes required. A small defect is more likely to cause incarceration and strangulation of intraabdominal viscera than is a large defect.

Laboratory Examination. Although preoperative room air arterial blood gases were not drawn in this patient, they are indicated in patients with a history suggestive of significant pulmonary disease. An abdominal incision can compromise pulmonary function by discouraging coughing and deep breathing and can promote atelectasis and retained secretions. Moreover, with large incisional hernias, the intraabdominal contents may be lying within the hernia and may have lost their "right of domain" in the peritoneal cavity. Abrupt repositioning can increase intraabdominal pressure and interfere with diaphragmatic excursions and cause respiratory embarrassment. Having a baseline preoperative arterial blood gas value or pulmonary function tests can facilitate pulmonary management postoperatively.

Treatment

The goal of incisional herniorrhaphy is to close the defect by sewing good tissue to good tissue (Fig. 14–14). These hernias are repaired to

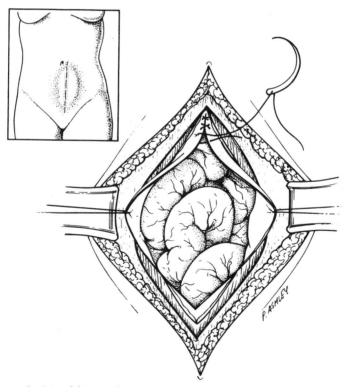

Figure 14–14. Incisional herniorrhaphy. The fascial defect is closed either longitudinally or transversely, depending on which approach causes the least tension. Nonabsorbable suture material is used, and generous bites of fascia are taken, at least 1 cm back from the edge.

prevent incarceration and strangulation. Moreover, they can become large, causing the patient vague abdominal distress, and they can become a cosmetic problem. When very large, they can become excoriated and even ulcerate. Nonabsorbable suture material should be employed in the repair. When the patient's own fascia cannot be approximated without tension, synthetic patches such as Marlex or Gore-Tex must be used to repair the defect (Fig. 14–15). In rare cases, progressive pneumoperitoneum can be employed. This technique consists of injecting more air into the peritoneal cavity each day, so that it "stretches out." When larger, it will accommodate the viscera being placed back into it without undue increase in intraabdominal pressure and its attendant respiratory embarrassment.

OTHER VENTRAL (ABDOMINAL WALL) HERNIAS

Umbilical hernias are congenital defects. They usually close spontaneously. If they have not done so by age four, repair is often recommended at that time. Incarceration and strangulation are not common in childhood, but they are more common in adults, so repair is usually recommended in the latter age group. The traditional repair has been the "vest

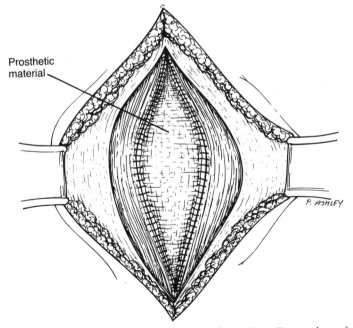

Prosthetic material

Figure 14–15. Prosthetic material such as Marlex mesh or a Gore-Tex patch can be used to repair large incisional hernias for which autogenous material is inadequate.

over pants" repair of Mayo (Fig. 14–16), although simple closure, sewing good fascia to good fascia, is now believed to be the best treatment.

An *epigastric hernia* is a defect in the linea alba above the umbilicus. Symptoms may be caused by incarceration of a piece of omentum or properitoneal fat in the hernia. These hernias are repaired via an incision in the midline. Since they tend to be multiple, the surgeon's finger should explore the midline from its peritoneal surface to seek additional hernias.

VARIETIES OF GROIN HERNIA

In addition to inguinal hernias, femoral and obturator hernias can be seen. In *femoral hernia* the sac protrudes medial to the femoral sheath, inferior to the inguinal ligament, lateral to the lacunar ligament, and superior to Cooper's ligament (Fig. 14–17). This hernia can be approached through the usual groin incision and repaired by the method

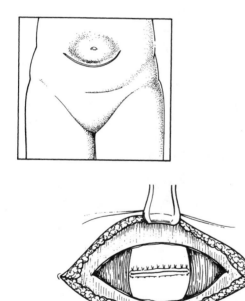

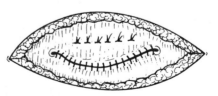

Figure 14–16. "Vest over pants" repair of an umbilical hernia, as advocated by Mayo.

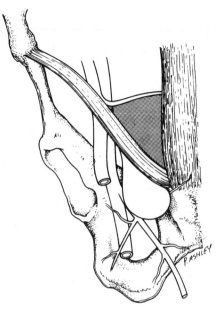

Figure 14–17. Anatomy of a femoral hernia. The sac protrudes medial to the femoral sheath, superior to the pubic bone, inferior to the inguinal ligament, and lateral to the lacunar ligament.

of McVay, as described for inguinal hernia. An obturator hernia occurs when the sac protrudes through the obturator canal (Fig. 14–18). This diagnosis can be difficult to make but should be suspected when there is evidence of intestinal obstruction and pain in the thigh.

A *sliding hernia* is a form of inguinal hernia in which a hollow viscus forms part of the sac. Care must be taken to avoid damage to the viscus and its blood supply. High ligation of the sac is not an option in a sliding hernia. The sac is inverted into the peritoneal cavity, and the inguinal floor is repaired. *Richter's hernia* (Fig. 14–19) is one in which a knuckle of the antimesenteric portion of small intestine becomes incarcerated. This is treacherous because gangrene of this knuckle can occur without producing the clinical picture of intestinal obstruction.

There are so many variations to the theme of hernia that, to paraphrase Dr. Mark Ravitch, if the practice of general surgery were limited to the repair of hernias, it would still be an interesting pursuit.

Some surgeons have advocated the use of synthetic mesh or synthetic plugs to avoid tension on the repair. It is true that tension on the suture line is a main cause of recurrence and of postoperative discomfort, but enthusiasm for this approach must be tempered by the fact that a foreign body can predispose to infection, which could necessitate removal of the mesh (although actual infection of the mesh itself is said to be uncommon).

Recently, laparoscopic herniorrhaphy has gained advocates because it allows patients to return to normal activity sooner than the traditional approach and it substitutes small stab wounds for a formal incision. It

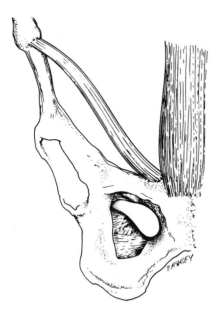

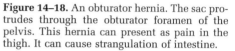

Figure 14–18. An obturator hernia. The sac protrudes through the obturator foramen of the pelvis. This hernia can present as pain in the thigh. It can cause strangulation of intestine.

also avoids damage to the inguinal canal, to the blood supply of the testicle, and to the ilioinguinal nerve. Detractors argue that the conventional approach is "surface surgery" that requires only local anesthesia and has proved safe and effective. Why, then, should one use the laparoscopic technique, which requires violation of the peritoneal cavity (although there are variants of the technique that do not) and carries the

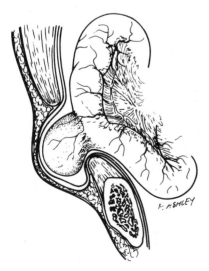

Figure 14–19. Richter's hernia. A knuckle of antimesenteric border of the intestines becomes incarcerated in the hernia ring. This knuckle may become gangrenous without obstructing the bowel lumen, and the gangrenous portion of bowel will cause sepsis.

potential for adhesions or visceral injury? Moreover, this latter approach generally is performed under general anesthesia, and synthetic mesh is usually employed. It remains to be seen whether laparoscopic herniorrhaphy will become the standard technique, but it seems likely that patients will request it because it seems to be associated with less postoperative discomfort and disability. Long-term outcome studies may further elucidate the issue.

Recommended Reading

1. Eubanks S: Hernias. In Sabiston DC (ed): *Textbook of Surgery: The Biological Basis of Modern Surgical Practice,* ed 15. Philadelphia: W.B. Saunders, 1997, pp 1215–1233.
2. Abrahamson J: Hernias. In Zinner MJ, Schwartz SI, Ellis H (ed): *Maingot's Abdominal Operations,* vol I. Stamford, Conn: Appleton & Lange, 1997, pp 479–580.
3. Zuidema GD, Nyhus LM (ed): *Shackelford's Surgery of the Alimentary Tract,* ed 4th, vol 5. Philadelphia: W.B. Saunders, 1996, pp 93–226.
4. Munson JL: Repair of inguinal hernia; Ventral herniorrhaphy with marlex mesh: and Repair of umbilical hernia. In Braasch JW, Sedgwick CE, Veidenheimer MC, Ellis FH Jr. (eds): *Atlas of Abdominal Surgery.* Philadelphia: W.B. Saunders, 1991, pp 421–434.

15

Surgery of the Breast

The incidence of breast cancer in the female population is high: it affects one in eight or nine women sometime in their lives. Early detection affords the best chance of cure. It thus behooves all physicians to watch vigilantly for this condition and to provide screening for their patients. Women with risk factors should be followed especially carefully, although it must be emphasized that many women with breast cancer have no known risk factors. A baseline mammogram should be performed at age 35 to 37 in asymptomatic women and then approximately every 2 years until age 50. Yearly mammography is indicated in women over 50 years of age, as it has been shown to help lower mortality from breast cancer.

One must keep pace with the literature in this rapidly changing field. The surgeon should use new treatment modalities that have been proven effective but should not abandon traditional methods for newer ones until the latter have been demonstrated to ensure equal or better life expectancy and quality of life over the long term.

The diagnosis of any disease state must be based on the history, a physical examination, simple laboratory tests, imaging, and possibly invasive procedures. With diseases of the breast the diagnosis may also be suggested by the patient's age and the presence or absence of other risk factors such as family history. The following hypothetical case studies illustrate the fundamentals of diagnosis and management of common breast conditions.

CASE 15–1

Breast Cancer

Six weeks before admission the patient, a 64-year-old woman, noticed a lump beneath the areola of her right breast while taking a shower. When the lump did not disappear she visited her family physician, who ordered a mammogram and referred her to a surgeon.

The patient's sister died of breast cancer at age 40, and her maternal aunt also died of breast cancer. The onset of menarche occurred when the patient was 12 years old. She was gravida I, para I; her daughter was born when the patient was 30. Menopause occurred at age 45. The patient had taken no hormones.

The medical history was negative for heart disease, diabetes mellitus, and other serious illnesses. There had been no previous surgery. The review of systems yielded no positive findings.

The physical examination revealed a nontender, hard mass measuring 3 cm in diameter subjacent to the nipple of the right breast. The mass did not appear to be fixed to the skin or chest wall, and there was no dimpling of the skin or *peau d'orange.* The breasts were symmetrical and small. Several lymph nodes were palpable in the right axilla, but they did not appear to be fixed to each other or to underlying structures. No supraclavicular nodes could be palpated. There was no hepatomegaly.

The alkaline phosphatase level was normal, and findings on chest x-ray examination were normal. The mammogram showed in the right breast a stellate density with a cluster of more than six microcalcifications, and there were diffuse microcalcifications throughout the involved breast. No mammographic abnormalities were noted in the other breast.

Permanent sections from a Tru-Cut needle biopsy done in the office revealed an infiltrating ductal carcinoma. When the patient returned with her daughter for counseling 3 days later she was informed of the diagnosis, given sympathetic support, and told about the various treatment options and their potential benefits and risks. The surgeon, the patient, and the daughter decided upon modified radical mastectomy, which was scheduled for 3 days later. She was admitted on the morning of surgery.

The surgical procedure was uneventful. No transfusions were required, and the patient was out of bed and tolerated food on the first postoperative night. The Hemovac drain was removed on the third postoperative day and the incision healed per primum. The pathology report of invasive ductal carcinoma noted that five of 25 axillary lymph nodes contained evidence of metastatic carcinoma.

The patient was seen in consultation by a medical oncologist, who arranged outpatient follow-up to consider chemotherapy and hormonal manipulation.

DISCUSSION OF CASE 15–1

Diagnosis

History. As in Case 15–1, many cases of breast cancer are discovered by the patient herself. When properly instructed by her physician in breast self-examination, the patient can become so familiar with her own breasts that she can discover a nodule early, when the possibility of cure is excellent.

Self-examination consists of looking at the breasts in the mirror, assuming different poses, and looking for nipple retraction, puckering of the skin, asymmetry of the breasts, and other skin changes such as skin edema (*peau d'orange*). The woman then feels each quadrant sequentially, using the pads of the fingers of the contralateral hand. It is important not to use a pinching motion, as this creates the sensation of a lump where none exists.

Risk factors are an important part of the history in evaluating a breast lump. Some women who possess one or more of the risk factors are at even greater risk. However, even patients with none of the risk factors can develop breast cancer and thus must be screened.

Advanced age is the most important risk factor. A family history of breast cancer increases a woman's risk of developing it especially if one or more relatives has developed premenopausal or bilateral breast cancer or, even worse, both. A paternal or maternal history of breast cancer increases the risk. Prolongation of the potential childbearing years (early menarche or late menopause, or both) increases the risk of breast cancer, as does having the first child at an older age. Ingestion of estrogen for whatever purpose may be a risk factor, although as of this writing this is not clear. Some types of cystic hyperplasia of the breast (fibrocystic disease) may prove to be risk factors. The proliferative type of cystic hyperplasia increases the risk, which is increased even further when there is atypia. A history of radiation of the chest is a risk factor. Much dietary fat can enhance the risk of breast cancer, and prolonged breast feeding may decrease the risk. Patients may increasingly come to the surgeon with a history of increased susceptibility to breast cancer by virtue of inheriting the genes BRCA1 or BRCA2, and the surgeon will need to learn how to address this problem.

The patient in Case 15–1 was coaxed by her family to seek medical attention; a patient's anxiety frequently prevents her from obtaining an early examination and so contributes to delay in diagnosis. In this case study the mammographic data were included in the history because mammography was recommended by the general practitioner before the patient was referred to the surgical service. The presence of a mass on physical examination demands biopsy (unless it is proven on ultrasound to be a pure cyst) because mammography detects only 85% to 90% of breast cancers. The absence of mammographic evidence of carcinoma does not relieve the surgeon of the obligation to biopsy the lump so that it can be examined histologically. One benefit of the mammogram when there is a palpable lump is that it may reveal an occult (impalpable) carcinoma in the other breast or elsewhere in the same breast so that it, too, can be extirpated. A dominant mass is a common mammographic finding in breast cancer, and these malignant lesions are likely to be spiculated or stellate. Clusters of more than five microcalcifications on mammography also suggest the presence of breast cancer, as do skin thickening, nipple retraction, and architectural distortion.

As always it is important to obtain an accurate medical history and a review of systems to detect other conditions that might influence the therapeutic plan. In this patient none were found.

Physical Examination. In addition to the complete physical examination for any patient for whom hospital admission is contemplated, one must pay special attention to the factors that will allow clinical staging of the breast cancer. One should characterize any nodules (lumps smaller than 2 cm diameter) or masses (lumps greater than 2 cm) by size, mobility, tenderness, regularity, and consistency. Nipple retraction and skin dimpling can be caused by tethering by Cooper's ligaments secondary to fibrotic reaction from even a relatively small cancer. Palpable axillary lymph nodes render the prognosis worse. Fixed or matted lymph nodes, arm edema, ulceration, satellite nodules, skin edema (*peau d'orange*), and tumor fixed to the skin or chest wall all imply locally advanced disease. Supraclavicular adenopathy indicates disseminated disease. Clinical staging not only helps in the formulation of a rational therapeutic plan but also facilitates gathering of data for clinical research.

To make possible the compilation of data for the largest possible number of patients, a uniform method of staging is needed. The system espoused by the American Joint Committee on Cancer (AJCC) and the TNM Committee of the International Union Against Cancer (UICC) is used commonly. The *T* value describes the size and nature of the primary tumor; *N* refers to the nodal status; and M to the presence or absence of distant metastases. Clinical diagnostic staging is done before surgery and is not revised after pathologic study. Pathologic staging of the surgical specimens is done by the pathologist. There is probably a 30% to 40% chance of error in clinical staging as compared with pathologic staging.

The TNM staging symbols, and their meanings, follow:

T0: No demonstrable tumor
T1: Tumor smaller than 2 cm in diameter
T2: Tumor larger than 2 cm but not more than 5 cm in diameter
T3: Tumor larger than 5 cm in diameter
T4: Tumor of any size with direct extension to the skin or chest wall (including inflammatory carcinoma)
N0: Ipsilateral axillary nodes thought not to contain tumor
N1: Ipsilateral axillary nodes thought to contain tumor but not fixed to one another or to the chest wall
N2: Ipsilateral axillary nodes thought to contain tumor and fixed to one another or to other structures
N3: Ipsilateral internal mammary nodes containing tumor
M0: No distant metastasis
M1: Distant metastasis (includes ipsilateral supraclavicular nodes)

Stage I: T1 N0 M0
Stage II: T0 N1 M0, *or* T1 N1 M0, *or* T2 N0 M0, or T2 N1 M0, *or* T3 N0 M0
Stage III: T0 N2 M0, *or* T1 N2 M0, *or* T2 N2 M0, or T3 N2 M0, or T3 N1 M0, or any T N3 M0 *or* T4 ANY N, M0
Stage IV: Any T, any N, M1

The lesion in Case 15–1 was classified as clinical and pathologic stage II. As will be seen when we discuss therapy, this information helped the physicians make appropriate decisions on therapy. Staging also allows information on the outcome of this patient's treatment to be combined with data from other cases, perhaps helping to improve methods of treatment for this disease.

Laboratory Examination and Imaging. Before mastectomy is done, a chest x-ray examination is performed to search for pulmonary metastases. CT and MRI have replaced liver scan in the diagnosis of liver metastasis in patients with breast cancer, but the indication for these studies remains controversial because their yield is low in patients without palpable axillary lymph nodes and elevated liver enzymes. Similarly, the indications for preoperative bone scan remain vague; the yield is low for stage I and II disease, and false-positive findings are not uncommon. Bone pain, abnormal skeletal x-rays, palpable axillary lymph nodes, or a tumor larger than 3 cm might be an indication for bone scanning, and some clinicians perform this test routinely. Again, the mammogram may suggest the presence of carcinoma, but biopsy is still required. The mammogram is helpful in evaluating the contralateral breast and other areas in the same breast.

Biopsy and Histologic Examination. The patient in Case 15–1 underwent a Tru-Cut needle biopsy in the physicians office. With this instrument a core of tissue is removed from which the pathologist can make a histologic diagnosis with permanent sections. The results are usually available within 2 or 3 days, and the patient and family can be brought back to the office for counseling and for help in making treatment decisions. This procedure is useful only for relatively large tumors, when the surgeon is relatively sure that the lesion is cancer and merely needs histologic confirmation. Needle biopsy examination without stereotactic guidance is of little use if it yields no evidence of malignant disease, as there is no guarantee that the core of tissue taken was representative of the lesion. An excisional or incisional biopsy is then required. When needle biopsy results are positive, the surgeon can counsel the family, obtain additional studies or additional consultations, and arrange for definitive surgery. Stereotactic needle biopsy under mammographic guidance is being performed more frequently, in preparation for definitive surgery (lumpectomy plus axillary dissection plus radiation therapy or modified radical mastectomy) if the biopsy should be positive for cancer. It may be useful in impalpable lesions or lesions so small that a needle biopsy is hard to obtain without stereotactic techniques. Stereotactic biopsy is discussed later in this chapter in the section on minimally invasive breast surgery.

In some centers needle aspiration is performed with a relatively fine-gauge needle, which collects cells rather than tissue. The specimen is submitted for cytologic, rather than histologic, examination. Surgeons in many centers are unwilling to proceed with mastectomy on the basis of cytologic examination alone.

If the diagnosis has not been established by needle biopsy, excisional biopsy is usually performed on an outpatient basis. It can be performed under general or local anesthesia. Margins of resection must be free of tumor, so that the excisional biopsy, along with axillary dissection and postoperative radiation therapy, can be employed as definitive therapy if the tumor proves malignant and the patient and surgeon so elect. Determination by the pathologist of whether or not the margins of resection are free of tumor can be facilitated if the surgeon orients the specimen and does not cut into it, so that the pathologist can paint the outside with ink. He can then determine under the microscope whether the neoplasm extends to the ink stain. If the lumpectomy margins are positive (tumor extends to the inked border of the specimen), the tumor bed can be re-excised at the time of the axillary dissection or encompassed in the specimen if modified radical mastectomy is elected. It is not clear whether radiation therapy can substitute for re-excision in "favorable" breast cancers with positive (involved with tumor) or narrow (less than 1 mm) margins. The time-honored procedure of breast biopsy, frozen section, and modified radical mastectomy at the same operation when biopsy findings are positive is now practiced infrequently.

Definitive Surgery

The patient in Case 15–1 underwent modified radical mastectomy because the tumor was so close to the nipple-areola complex that removal of the cancer would probably necessitate sacrifice of this complex, rendering conservation surgery (lumpectomy plus axillary dissection) irrelevant. Also, the relatively large tumor, in relation to the size of the breast, would have made lumpectomy (partial mastectomy) less cosmetically satisfactory. Moreover, this patient had an inordinate and irrational fear of radiation therapy, which would have been required after lumpectomy but was not after modified radical mastectomy. Another argument against conservation surgery for this patient was the diffuse microcalcifications on mammography that raised the specter of multifocal lesions. It should be noted, however, that the combination of local excision, axillary dissection, and postoperative radiation therapy is widely accepted as the treatment of choice for most stage I and II breast cancers because conservation surgery seems to achieve survival rates similar to those of modified radical mastectomy.

Some of the procedures performed for mammary carcinoma are depicted in Figures 15–1 through 15–6. The original operation described by William Halsted at Johns Hopkins University was the *radical mastectomy* (Fig. 15–1). This entailed resecting the involved breast en bloc along with the pectoralis major and minor muscles and the axillary contents. This procedure is now considered too deforming, as it leaves a concavity in the chest wall. However, it must be remembered that Dr. Halsted was seeing patients with large, neglected tumors, and removal of the pectoralis major probably offered the best chance of survival. This procedure may still be indicated for tumors impinging on the pectoralis fascia.

The *extended radical mastectomy,* an operation of considerable extent or magnitude, includes excision of the internal mammary lymph nodes (Fig. 15–2). The rationale for this operation is that, with lesions in the inner quadrants of the breast or under the areola there is a significant incidence of metastasis to this lymph node chain. This is especially true of large tumors. This more extensive operation is, however, likely to lead to more morbidity. Radiation of the internal mammary chain or chemotherapy may be helpful in such a situation, obviating extended radical mastectomy.

The *modified radical mastectomy* requires removal of the entire breast and pectoralis fascia en bloc with the axillary contents. In Patey's version the pectoralis minor muscle is removed (Fig. 15–3), whereas in Madden's version the muscle is lifted out of the way but not excised (Fig. 15–4). *Total mastectomy* (formerly called *simple mastectomy*) entails

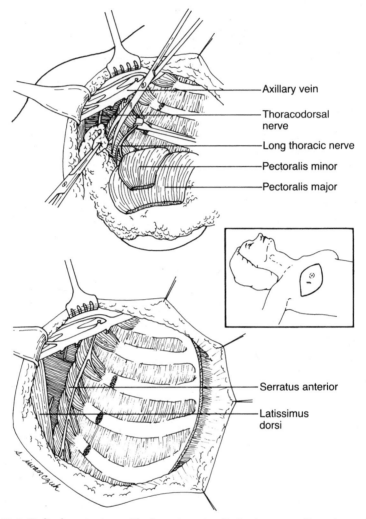

Axillary vein

Thoracodorsal
nerve

Long thoracic nerve

Pectoralis minor

Pectoralis major

Serratus anterior

Latissimus
dorsi

Figure 15–1. Radical mastectomy. The breast, pectoralis fascia, pectoralis major and minor muscles, and axillary contents are excised en bloc. The ribs and intercostal muscles lie beneath. This procedure is rarely done today, because it leaves the chest wall concave and function controlled by the large muscles is impaired.

removing the entire breast but preserves the pectoralis major and minor muscles and omits the axillary dissection (Fig. 15–5). It is most appropriate for palliation of locally advanced breast cancer (ulcerated, fungating tumors) or for cystosarcoma phylloides, in which case spread to axillary nodes is uncommon.

In most cases, *local excision with axillary dissection* (Fig. 15–6) and postoperative radiation therapy has become the treatment of choice for

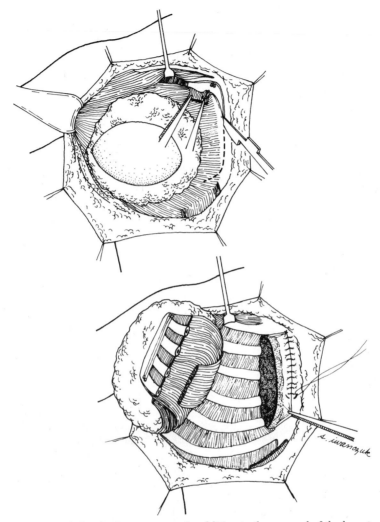

Figure 15–2. Extended radical mastectomy. In addition to the removal of the breast, axillary contents, and pectoralis major and minor muscles, the second through fifth ribs and ipsilateral half of the sternum are transected, to remove the internal mammary lymph node chain. This operation can be done for subareolar or medial breast cancers, which both are likely to metastasize to the internal mammary chain, but, it is extensive and associated with substantial morbidity. As an alternative, the internal mammary chain can be irradiated or treated with chemotherapy instead of being excised. This operation is not often done.

stage I and stage II breast cancers, as it achieves long-term survival rates equal to those for modified radical mastectomy. Best cosmetic results are usually obtained when no ellipse of skin is removed, when the incision is made directly over the lump in Langer's lines (the normal skin lines), and when the axillary dissection is performed through a separate inci-

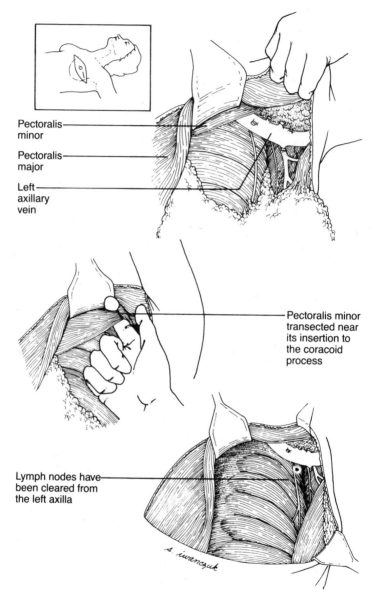

Pectoralis
minor

Pectoralis
major

Left
axillary
vein

Pectoralis minor
transected near
its insertion to
the coracoid
process

Lymph nodes have
been cleared from
the left axilla

Figure 15–3. Patey's modified radical mastectomy, which preserves the pectoralis major muscle, causing less cosmetic and functional deformity than radical mastectomy. The pectoralis minor muscle is removed en bloc with the breast, pectoralis fascia, and axillary contents. The long thoracic nerve innervates the serratus anterior and is preserved to prevent winging of the scapula. The thoracodorsal nerve innervates the latissimus dorsi and is also preserved. Rotter's nodes, found between the pectoralis major and minor muscles, are removed with the specimen.

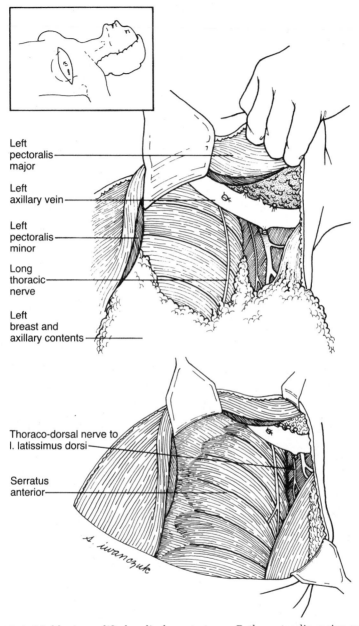

Figure 15–4. Madden's modified radical mastectomy. Both pectoralis major and minor muscles are preserved. The latter muscle can be elevated with a retractor, affording excellent exposure for the axillary dissection. The breast, pectoralis fascia, and axillary lymph nodes are resected en bloc.

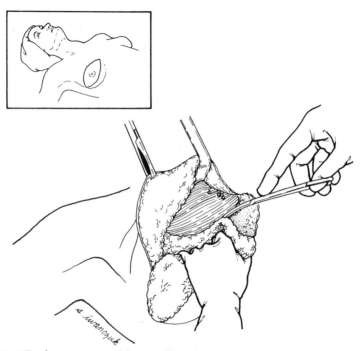

Figure 15–5. Total mastectomy without axillary dissection. The breast and pectoralis fascia are removed. This operation can be performed rapidly in poor-risk patients, although, when it is, the prognostic information that might be gained from examining the axillary lymph nodes histologically is not available. This procedure might be appropriate palliation for an elderly, poor-risk patient with a fungating, ulcerated, foul-smelling breast cancer (sometimes called a *toilet mastectomy*).

sion. One should obtain histologic confirmation of clean margins when local excision is employed. The axillary dissection provides useful prognostic information that is used to determine whether chemotherapy is indicated. At present, postoperative radiation therapy is mandatory after local excision of breast cancer, as this neoplasm is believed to be multicentric. There may be some limited exceptions in very early, less aggressive cancers.

Good cosmetic results may be impossible to obtain by local excision and axillary dissection when the tumor is large and the breast small or when the lesion is close to the nipple-areola complex, and modified radical mastectomy may be necessary in these cases. Breast reconstruction may yield satisfactory cosmetic results after this latter procedure. Reconstruction can be immediate or delayed. The simplest and quickest method is to place a saline implant under the pectoralis major muscle (Fig.15–7). Alternatively, a transverse rectus abdominis (TRAM) flap may be used to allow contouring while avoiding the introduction of foreign material. This involves swinging a flap of tissue that includes abdominal

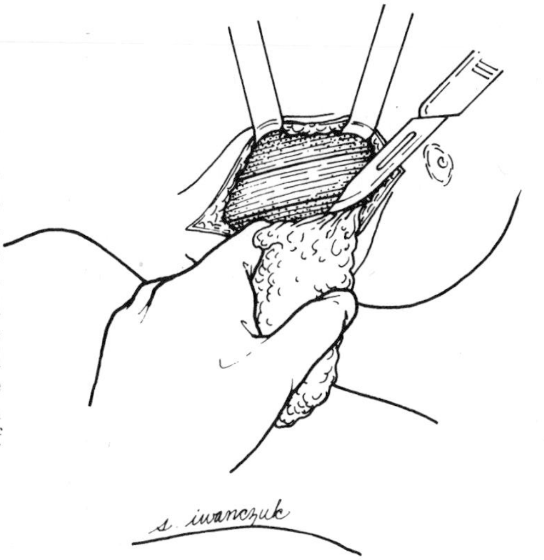

Figure 15–6. Local excision (also known as tyelectomy or partial mastectomy) plus axillary dissection. It is no longer recommended that an ellipse of skin be removed, as this measure does not improve survival and can interfere with the cosmetic result. Similarly, the skin incision should be made along the natural lines of the skin (Langer's lines), and the axillary dissection should be performed through a separate incision to achieve the best cosmetic result. The surgeon should obtain histologic confirmation of clear margins.

fat, rectus muscle, and skin based on the inferior epigastric artery to create a new breast mound.

Postoperative Management

Mastectomy does not require entrance into a major body cavity and thus should not produce the pulmonary complications to the same extent encountered after laparotomy and thoracotomy. There is no interference with gastrointestinal function, and generally the patient's normal diet can be resumed on the first postoperative night.

There can be significant blood loss. Transfusion usually can be avoided, and mild anemia can be treated with iron supplements. Usually one or two closed suction drains are left beneath the flaps, to prevent hematoma or seroma formation and to keep the flaps approximated to the chest wall by reason of the vacuum created. Because this facilitates wound healing, the drains are left in place until the drainage is less than 15 cc in 24 hours. A drain, after all, is a foreign body and also provides a portal of entry for microorganisms. They should be removed as soon as the drainage tapers off.

Prognostic Factors

Large tumors, involved lymph nodes, and greater numbers of involved nodes correlate with a poorer chance of survival. Most tumors are invasive ductal carcinomas with fibrosis. Uncommon special types represent only 20% to 30% of invasive cancers of the breast but have a more favorable prognosis than the more common tumors, which are classified as invasive ductal with fibrosis (or "no special type"). Examples of these

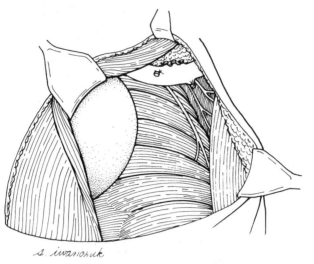

Figure 15–7. Breast reconstruction. For some women quality of life can be improved by breast reconstruction. This can be done at the time of mastectomy or later. The mound is recreated by placing a prosthesis under the pectoralis major muscle. Alternatively, the breast can be reconstructed with a musculocutaneous flap. The nipple-areola complex can be created by sharing tissue from the contralateral nipple, by using pigmented tissue from other parts of the body, or by tattooing.

more favorable invasive carcinomas include medullary, tubular, and mucinous.

High histologic grade, aneuploidy, or high S-phase values on flow cytometry, comedohistology, HER-2/neu overexpression, estrogen and progesterone receptor negativity, mutant p53 suppressor gene, among other factors, all seem to be associated with more aggressive breast cancers. However, since many of these factors correlate with each other, all do not have independent significance.

Breast Carcinomas In Situ

Ductal carcinoma in situ (DCIS) may be an intermediate point in the progression from proliferation with atypia to invasive cancer, and patients with DCIS are likely later to develop invasive ductal cancer in the same breast. Interestingly, patients with lobular carcinoma in situ (LCIS) may develop invasive ductal *or* invasive lobular carcinoma in the ipsilateral or contralateral breast.

Adjuvant Chemotherapy

Adjuvant chemotherapy is drug treatment given after potentially curative surgery, to improve survival. Lymph node–positive premenopausal women—and possibly node-positive postmenopausal women (especially those who are medically fit, who are estrogen receptor negative, or whose tumors have other characteristics suggesting they are aggressive)—should be treated with a standard chemotherapeutic regimen such as cytoxan, methotrexate, and 5-fluorouracil (CMF). Tamoxifen is sometimes added, especially for estrogen receptor–positive women. Lymph node–positive, postmenopausal, estrogen receptor–positive women are sometimes treated postoperatively with the antiestrogen agent tamoxifen alone, especially when they seem fragile or are so medically compromised that they may not tolerate chemotherapy. Estrogen receptor–positive patients are more likely to respond to hormonal manipulation. A postmenopausal, node-positive, estrogen receptor–positive woman who is in good health may be treated with both chemotherapy and tamoxifen. Chemotherapy is sometimes recommended even for node-negative women if they have features (listed above) that suggest that their tumors are more biologically aggressive. A simplified way of looking at this is that adjuvent chemotherapy is indicated for node-positive patients who are medically fit enough to tolerate it and for node-negative patients with poor prognostic indicators. If estrogen receptor status is positive, the tumor is more likely to be responsive to tamoxifen, and this might make the clinician more willing to accept hormonal manipulation alone for a postmenopausal patient who is borderline fit.

There is some indication that neoadjuvant chemotherapy (that given preoperatively, rather than postoperatively as *adjuvant* chemotherapy) for locally advanced disease (stage III) may shrink the primary tumor and facilitate breast conservation surgery (local excision plus axillary dissection plus radiation therapy). Neoadjuvant chemotherapy can also improve survival in locally advanced disease regardless of whether mastectomy or conservation surgery is chosen.

Radiation Therapy

Following breast conservation surgery, radiation therapy is used to decrease the chances of local recurrence and to destroy other foci of invasive cancers or cancers in situ that might be present in the same breast. Also, it is probably helpful to irradiate the internal mammary chain of lymph nodes when the primary lesion is medial or subareolar and axillary lymph nodes are found to be positive for tumor or if a medial or subareolar tumor is large, as it is highly likely in such cases that the internal mammary nodes are involved. Modified radical or radical mastectomy does not include extirpation of internal mammary nodes. Radiation therapy may be used in a neoadjuvent fashion for locally advanced (stage III) breast cancer.

Complications of radiation therapy are uncommon, but arm edema, inflammation of the lung, rib fractures, pericarditis, wound breakdown, and injury to the brachial plexus can, rarely, occur. Some patients refuse radiation therapy because of misconceptions they may have or because daily trips to the radiation therapy site are inconvenient or impossible.

Such a decision by the patient would argue for modified radical mastectomy over local excision, which requires radiation therapy to be effective.

Postoperative Support and Follow-Up

Reach for Recovery, a branch of the American Cancer Society, is a support group of women volunteers who themselves have undergone mastectomy. Most surgeons thoroughly and sympathetically discuss with their mastectomy patients such important matters as their feelings about change in body image, what to wear after mastectomy, available lingerie, and how to deal with a husband or lover who may be anxious about the mastectomy. The Reach for Recovery volunteer is often able to supplement this counseling.

Follow-up examination should be conducted at regular intervals and should consist primarily of the taking of a history and a physical examination. The scar must be examined for recurrence in the case of mastectomy, and new lumps must be sought in the same breast after lumpectomy. Supraclavicular and axillary regions must be examined for adenopathy. The liver should be examined for enlargement. Special attention should be devoted to the contralateral breast, as, discovered early, a primary tumor there might be cured. The surgeon should also look for a second primary cancer—of endometrium, ovary, or colon—as early discovery of these neoplasms can also improve life expectancy, and there may be an association between them and breast cancer. Chest x-ray can be done annually to look for distant metastasis. Bone scan and CT of the liver are less important unless symptoms supervene, because the discovery of distant metastases is not likely to result in cure and these studies often present a significant financial burden for the patient.

CASE 15–2

Early Breast Cancer Detected in a Screening Program

A 40-year-old woman was admitted for needle localization and biopsy of a suspicious area in the left breast detected by mammography. The mammogram had revealed suspicious microcalcifications in the upper outer quadrant of the left breast, but neither the nurse practitioner nor the consulting surgeon could feel a lump or any axillary lymph nodes.

The patient arrived at the hospital, bringing with her an envelope containing the history, the results of the physical examination performed by her doctor and of laboratory tests done 2 days earlier. In the x-ray department the suspicious lesion was localized with a hooked needle under mammographic control. The patient was brought to the operating room. Because the lesion was deep and close to the chest wall, general anesthesia was administered, an incision was made in the breast, and a wedge of tissue containing the tip of the needle was excised and sent to the mammographic suite and then to the pathology laboratory. An x-ray view of the specimen revealed the microcalcifications within. The patient was discharged the same afternoon with an appointment to see her surgeon 3 days later.

At the postoperative visit she was told that the pathology report revealed an invasive carcinoma of the breast 0.8 cm in diameter with good margins on all sides. The surgeon discussed the treatment options with her. Two weeks later the patient underwent axillary lymph node dissection with subsequent radiation therapy. No axillary lymph nodes were found to be involved, and no adjuvant chemotherapy was recommended.

DISCUSSION OF CASE 15–2

When a patient such as the one described in Case 15–2 with an impalpable breast cancer discovered by mammography undergoes local excision and axillary dissection and the nodes are found to be negative (which is usually the case), the prognosis is excellent and radical surgery usually is not required. Adjuvant radiation therapy is important, however, to achieve local control and to destroy other possible small foci of cancer in situ or invasive cancer in the same breast. Some oncologists are prescribing adjuvant chemotherapy even for selected stage I premenopausal patients.

CASE 15–3

Locally Advanced Breast Cancer

A 76-year-old woman was brought to her doctor by her daughter. Examination revealed a mass 5 cm in diameter in the lower outer quadrant of the right breast with ulceration of the overlying skin. There were two palpable lymph nodes in the right axilla. There was no supraclavicular adenopathy and no edema of the arm, nor was there evidence of distant metastasis.

The patient was referred to a surgeon, who carried out a Tru-Cut needle biopsy in his office, revealing invasive ductal carcinoma of the breast with productive fibrosis. The lesion was thought to be a stage III (T4 N1 M0) carcinoma and was initially treated with cyclophosphamide, methotrexate, and 5-fluorouracil. The ulceration resolved, and the lesion measured only 4 cm in diameter after the course of chemotherapy. It was, therefore, believed that modified radical mastectomy could be carried out with an acceptable risk of local recurrence in the chest wall. Postoperatively the patient was treated with radiation therapy of the chest wall and axilla. Since the estrogen and progesterone receptor determinations were positive, she received tamoxifen as well. Chemotherapy was continued postoperatively. Eighteen months later, there was no evidence of local or systemic recurrence.

DISCUSSION OF CASE 15–3

Locally advanced breast cancer is encountered in several settings. As in case 15–3, it can develop in patients who did not previously know they had breast cancer. It may also be encountered in patients who experience recurrence after radical or modified radical mastectomy and as a recurrence after conservation surgery such as partial mastectomy (also known as *lumpectomy, local excision,* or *tylectomy*), with or without axillary dissection.

The patient in this case had a stage III lesion (T4, N1, M0) (rated T4 because of skin ulceration). With such locally advanced breast cancer, the probability of distant metastasis (often occult) is high and the long-term prognosis is poor. Interpreting treatment trials for locally advanced breast cancer is difficult, because the studies usually are not randomized and are thus open to selection bias; however, total mastectomy with axillary sampling or with axillary dissection (the latter is the same as modified radical mastectomy) is an expeditious method of obtaining local control, and adding chemotherapy and radiation therapy may be of benefit. Neoadjuvant chemotherapy or radiation therapy may "downstage" the tumor, making it amenable to either mastectomy or conservation surgery. Neoadjuvant and adjuvant chemotherapy or radiation therapy may improve survival with locally advanced breast cancer.

Inflammatory carcinoma is an uncommon condition in which at least one third of the breast is edematous, enlarged, red, and often warm and tender, with or without an associated discrete mass. The term is a misnomer because no inflammatory cells are present. Rather, infiltration and obstruction of the dermal lymphatics by tumor cells causes the findings. This is a T4 lesion, rendering the cancer stage III unless, as is often the case, distant metastases are present, in which case, it is stage IV. Patients with inflammatory carcinoma are likely to have involved axillary lymph nodes and a poor prognosis. The preferred treatment combines mastectomy, radiation, and chemotherapy for local control and to improve survival.

CASE 15–4

Cystic Hyperplasia of the Breast

A 37-year-old woman was referred to the surgeon by her gynecologist after she discovered a lump 2 cm in diameter in her left breast that had not been palpable at her annual gynecologic examination 3 months earlier. There was no family history of breast cancer. The patient had been 22 years old at the time of her first pregnancy. She had never taken oral contraceptives. Her breasts tended to become painful and engorged at the time of menses.

The physical examination revealed a mobile, nontender, well-circumscribed lesion, 2 cm in diameter, at the 3:00 o'clock position in the left breast, 2 cm from the areola. There were no other discrete nodules or masses, but there was some thickening in the upper outer quadrants of both breasts. There were no palpable axillary or supraclavicular lymph nodes.

In the surgeon's office a 21-gauge needle inserted into the lesion yielded green fluid. The cyst was not palpable immediately after aspiration. The fluid was submitted for cytologic examination, which showed no evidence of malignant cells. One week after aspiration, the cyst was not palpable. A mammogram was unremarkable. The patient was told that no biopsy was necessary. She was instructed in and given a booklet on breast self-examination, and a follow-up appointment was scheduled 3 months later.

DISCUSSION: CYSTIC HYPERPLASIA OF THE BREAST AND OTHER BENIGN CONDITIONS

It is notable that this patient discovered the lump herself. Many women with breast lumps do so, and this is why instruction in breast self-examination is important. Some have questioned the utility of breast self-examination, but it can prove useful and there is very little, if any, risk to it. If the physician himself instructs the patient, she is more likely to perform monthly self-examinations than if a nurse or some other person provides the instruction. Again, it is important to note the presence or absence of risk factors, although even women without risk factors develop breast cancer.

Gross breast cysts, also called *blue-domed cysts,* like the one described in the hypothetical patient in Case 15–4, are often categorized as a form of fibrocystic disease of the breast. Other patients with fibrocystic disease may present with generalized, ill-defined "lumpiness" and tenderness. The terms *nonproliferative lesions of the breast, proliferative breast disorders without atypia,* and *atypical proliferative lesions* are useful because patients with these diagnoses have no increased risk, slightly increased risk, and substantially increased risk of malignancy, respectively. The term *fibrocystic disease* (also called *cystic hyperplasia* or *cystic mastitis*) is less useful for assessing a patient's risk for developing breast cancer, because it lumps together multiple disparate pathologic entities. Gross cysts are nonproliferative lesions. When green fluid is obtained on aspiration and the lump completely disappears, and if the fluid is not bloody and the lump does not return by examination 6 weeks later, no further treatment is indicated. Sending the fluid for cytologic examination is probably unnecessary unless it is bloody. Mammography is still performed in older patients, to look for suspicious lesions, both near the cyst and elsewhere, too small to be palpated. Avoidance of methylxanthine in the diet (coffee, tea, chocolate, and colas), although often recommended, probably cannot reduce the nodularity from these entities or decrease discomfort (mastalgia) associated with the physiologic breast engorgement often associated with menses. Ultrasonography is very useful for demonstrating that a lesion found on physical examination or mammography is a pure cyst or, alternatively, is solid. Sonography can also guide cyst aspiration.

A *fibroadenoma* is a benign breast tumor that usually occurs in adolescents and young women but is also found in postmenopausal breasts. These tumors are usually mobile and well-circumscribed and can be diagnosed preoperatively with a fair degree of certainty. Excisional biopsy is usually indicated, however, because of their tendency to enlarge and because malignant tissue must be completely ruled out. A variant called cystosarcoma phylloides tends to recur locally and may require total mastectomy if the tumor is large. When cystosarcoma phylloides is malignant, it tends to metastasize hematogenously rather than to regional lymph nodes.

An intraductal papilloma usually presents with bloody nipple discharge. It is treated by excision. Intraductal carcinoma must be ruled out as the cause of the bloody discharge.

Minimally Invasive Breast Surgery

Consistent with developments in other areas of surgery, techniques are evolving in breast surgery that are aimed at minimizing tissue trauma, effecting improved cosmesis, causing less discomfort or disability, and minimizing cost. Minimally invasive techniques that have been applied to palpable lesions for some time consist of attempts to establish a diagnosis by performing core biopsy or needle aspiration for cytology in the office, primarily to collect information to help the surgeon and patient decide upon which type of definitive procedure they wish to embark. The possibility that the retrieved tissue is not representative of the entire lesion must be considered, and subsequent incisional or excisional biopsy must be contemplated in the case of a negative result.

In the treatment of impalpable, mammographically detected breast lesions (a density or cluster of microcalcifications), several minimally invasive techniques have evolved in the hope of replacing the standard procedure, which is needle localization under mammographic guidance followed by moving the patient from the mammographic suite to the operating room, where the area about the needle is surgically excised for histologic examination. One such new, minimally invasive method is the automated, sterotactic, mammographically guided, large-core biopsy. Multiple passes can be made, and the lesion can essentially be obliterated. Because one can confirm mammographically that the core needle is encompassing part or all of the lesion, sampling error is minimized, though not eliminated. This has been recommended especially for impalpable lesions that on mammography the radiologist feels have low but not zero probability of malignancy, as in this setting the technique has a very small chance of missing a cancer, even when sampling errors occur. Advanced minimally invasive breast biopsy instruments can encompass and remove a core of tissue up to 2 cm in diameter under mammographic stereotactic guidance. The instrumentation may be able to demonstrate mammographically that the lesion is within the core and does not remain in the breast, eliminating sampling error. That is, the whole lesion may be removed in the one large core. In the future we may find out that even carcinomas, if they are very small, can be removed by this technique with an adequate margin. The technology is promising.

Recommended Reading

1. Farndon J: Breast and Endocrine Surgery. In Carter DC (ed): *A Companion to Specialist Surgical Practice.* Philadelphia: W.B. Saunders, 1997.
2. Iglehart IG: The breast. In Sabiston DC, Lyerly HK: *Textbook of Surgery: The Biological Basis of Modern Surgical Practice,* ed 15. Philadelphia: W.B. Saunders, 1997, pp 555–598.
3. Leitch M: Breast carcinoma. In McClelland RN, Weigelt JA (eds): *Selected Readings in General Surgery* vol 22, no 10–12; vol 23, no 1. Dallas: The University of Texas Southwestern Medical Center, Oct–Dec 1995, Jan 1996.

16

Vascular Surgery

The field of vascular surgery traditionally encompasses four areas: (1) surgery for stenosis, occlusion, or trauma of the arteries of the lower and upper extremities and for aneurysms of these vessels (peripheral arterial disease); (2) treatment of deep vein thrombosis (DVT); (3) treatment of cerebrovascular disease due to lesions in the carotid arteries; and (4) treatment of stenosis or occlusion of the visceral vessels such as the renal arteries or arteries to the gut. Coronary artery bypass for coronary artery disease is not usually considered peripheral vascular surgery, as bypass grafting is performed by cardiothoracic surgeons, whereas peripheral vascular surgery is performed by general vascular surgeons. Atherosclerosis is by far the most common cause of disease in these blood vessels. Appropriate decision making requires knowledge of the effects of atherosclerosis on arteries in all anatomic sites.

CASE 16–1

Combined Aortoiliac and Femoropopliteal Occlusive Disease

A 64-year-old retired mail carrier complained of a 2-week history of severe pain in the left foot that kept him awake at night.

For the past 6 months the patient had experienced pain in his left buttock and thigh after walking about a block and a half. He was forced to stop and rest each time before walking on. Upon questioning, he stated that he had been unable to attain an erection for the last year. Two weeks before admission, he had begun to experience severe pain in the left foot, which prevented him from sleeping. He was forced to sleep with his left foot over the side of the bed to minimize the pain, and he frequently arose to walk around the room, which afforded slight relief.

Past medical history was negative for heart disease or diabetes. He had a 40–pack-year history of cigarette smoking. Review of systems uncovered no history of angina pectoris, dyspnea on exertion, or paroxysmal nocturnal dyspnea, nor of transient ischemic attacks.

Physical examination revealed the blood pressure to be 160/90 mm Hg in each arm. Examination of the heart and lungs was unremarkable. The patient had 2 + carotid and radial pulses bilaterally. There were 1+ femoral pulses bilaterally, and no pulses were palpable below that. Shiny skin and absence of hair was noted on both feet, and the left foot was cool and exhibited pallor on elevation and dependent rubor. No carotid bruits could be heard, and no abdominal aortic aneurysm could be palpated.

Segmental pressures taken in the noninvasive vascular laboratory revealed these findings:

	Right (mm Hg)	Left (mm Hg)
Thigh	74	82
Calf	70	50
Ankle	69	30

The distal aortogram with runoff revealed bilateral aortoiliac stenosis and total occlusion of the left superficial femoral artery at its takeoff. There was reconstitution of the popliteal artery below the knee with the anterior tibial artery patent to the foot. The posterior tibial and peroneal arteries were occluded.

The patient underwent an intravenous dipyridamole-thallium stress test that showed no evidence of ischemic heart disease. Duplex scan showed no evidence of hemodynamically significant stenosis of either carotid artery. Preoperative pulmonary function tests revealed moderate obstructive pulmonary disease. Room air arterial blood gases were obtained as a baseline. The patient subsequently underwent aortobifemoral bypass without complications. He received aggressive pulmonary toilet postoperatively, including early ambulation and incentive spirometry, and was encouraged to cough and breath deep. He was discharged to home on the seventh postoperative day.

At the time of discharge, he was free of ischemic rest pain, but with increasing ambulation he began to experience one-block intermittent claudication in the left calf. This was quite limiting. Accordingly, he was readmitted and underwent left femoropopliteal bypass graft below the knee with a reversed autogenous saphenous vein. He was discharged to home on the sixth postoperative day and was without exercise limitation. He remained free of symptoms until he died of a massive myocardial infarction 4 years later.

DISCUSSION OF CASE 16–1

Diagnosis

Peripheral arterial occlusive disease is almost always caused by atherosclerosis; fibrous dysplasia runs a distant second. It involves the lower extremities much more often than the upper ones. Risk factors include smoking, various forms of hyperlipidemia, hypertension, diabetes mellitus, and, possibly, sedentary lifestyle.

Symptoms. Symptoms of peripheral arterial occlusive disease include, in order of increasing severity, intermittent claudication, ischemic rest pain, ulceration, and gangrene.

Intermittent claudication is pain in the thigh and buttock in the case of aortoiliac disease, or pain in the calf or foot in femoropopliteal disease. It is precipitated by walking a certain distance and is relieved by rest that allows the patient to resume walking, only to be forced to stop again after covering about the same distance. The natural history of intermittent claudication is that it improves over time (especially if the patient can stop smoking) as collateral channels develop. A certain number of patients progress to ischemic rest pain, ulceration, or gangrene.

Ischemic rest pain is pain in the foot caused by inadequate arterial circulation. It is often worse when the patient lies in bed at night, owing to the attendant decrease in cardiac output, and may be partially mitigated when the patient places the extremity in a dependent position. Gravity increases perfusion of the distal limb; thus, the classic description in which the patient with ischemic rest pain sleeps with the involved leg hanging over the side of the bed. Ischemic rest pain is a more ominous symptom than intermittent claudication, as its natural history is progression to gangrene and limb loss. Surgery for ischemic rest pain can be said to be for *limb salvage.*

Ulceration due to arterial disease can be precipitated by pressure over bony prominences, such as hallux valgus (bunions) or trauma from ill-fitting shoes to a foot that is relatively insensate from the peripheral neuropathy of diabetes mellitus. It is difficult to heal foot ulcers in patients with poor arterial circulation, especially when there is the "small vessel disease" typical of diabetes mellitus. Major amputation such as a below- or above-knee amputation may be necessary in this instance.

Gangrene of one or several toes or of the entire foot occurs when the arterial inflow is inadequate to support the metabolic needs of the tissues. This is often accompanied by black discoloration (mummification, dry gangrene). If superinfection can be prevented, a digit may become black and simply fall off (autoamputate); however, the dead tissue is devoid of defense mechanisms and bacterial infection with suppuration (wet gangrene) frequently occurs, which requires expeditious amputation to prevent generalized sepsis and death.

Chronic critical leg ischemia is said to be present when there is persistent ischemic rest pain or ulceration or gangrene of the foot or toes with low segmental pressures as measured by the vascular laboratory.

In summary, when taking a history from a patient with peripheral arterial occlusive disease, one must note whether claudication, rest pain, ulceration, or gangrene is present, as each of these symptoms has different implications for the potential benefits and risks of reconstructive arterial surgery. The surgeon must attempt to determine whether there are symptoms of ischemic heart disease or cerebrovascular disease. These entities make peripheral arterial surgery more risky. Coronary artery bypass grafting or carotid endarterectomy sometimes needs to be considered in preparation for major peripheral arterial surgery. Finally, one must determine whether the patient has had a cardiac arrhythmia such as atrial fibrillation or whether there has been a recent myocardial infarction that could have caused a mural thrombus in the heart. Such a thrombus can cause peripheral embolization to the arteries of the extremities. In this situation, acute arterial insufficiency might not be due to atherosclerotic narrowing at all but rather to blockage of the artery by a clot that originated in the heart and embolized distally.

Signs. Chronic peripheral arterial insufficiency is usually caused by atherosclerosis, and its signs are several. Loss of peripheral pulses is common. Absent or diminished femoral pulse suggests aortoiliac disease, whereas a strong, palpable femoral pulse with a diminished or absent popliteal pulse is suggestive of superficial femoral artery stenosis or occlusion. The student should be familiar with the term *Leriche's syndrome,* which denotes aortoiliac disease manifested by intermittent claudication, impotence, and absence of femoral pulses. A cool, pale extremity indicates arterial insufficiency. Absence of hair on the feet suggests established arterial disease. Pallor on elevation and dependent rubor indicate severe ischemia. Obviously, blackened gangrenous areas along with areas of ulceration must be noted. Auscultation over the groin and abdomen may suggest areas of narrowing, as manifested by an overlying bruit. A bruit is caused by turbulent blood flow through areas of atherosclerotic arterial narrowing.

Acute arterial insufficiency can be caused by trauma to a major artery, by sudden thrombosis of a previous area of atherosclerotic narrowing, or by embolization of a clot originating in the heart. In any event, acute arterial insufficiency is manifested by the five *P*s: *p*allor, *p*ulselessness, *p*aralysis, *p*aresthesias, and *p*ain. A sixth *p* has often been cited, *p*oikilothermia (body temperature follows environmental temperature—in this setting, coolness). These ominous signs suggest that surgical intervention must be done promptly, preferably within a few hours, if the chances of limb salvage are to be good. Occasionally, salvage is possible in an extremity where acute occlusion occurred several days earlier.

Noninvasive Vascular Laboratory. After the symptoms and signs are elicited by a thorough history and physical examination, the noninvasive vascular laboratory should be utilized to gather more information. It is in the vascular laboratory that one is able to quantitate the magnitude of peripheral arterial disease. Segmental pressures are one of the most useful noninvasive tests.

A basic understanding of how the *Doppler probe* functions is helpful. Ultrasound waves emitted by the Doppler probe hit the blood moving in a vessel and the frequency of the reflected wave is changed in proportion to the velocity of the blood in the conduit. The difference in frequency between the emitted signal and the reflected signal is detected by the Doppler probe and converted to an audible signal. The presence of an audible signal over a vessel simply means that some blood is moving within it. Segmental pressures are simply systolic blood pressures recorded in the brachial artery and at the thigh, calf, ankle, and sometimes the transmetatarsal level. This is usually done by placing a series of pressure cuffs at these levels and sequentially inflating each until the Doppler signal no longer can be detected in the distal vessels. What is thus determined is the pressure *under each* cuff, not the pressure at the level of the Doppler probe. A 20-mm Hg gradient is generally held to suggest a hemodynamically significant stenosis between the two sites. For example, when the brachial systolic pressure is 20 mm Hg greater than that in the thigh, aortoiliac occlusive disease or a very proximal femoral artery stenosis is likely. If there is a 20-mm Hg gradient between the thigh and the calf cuffs, a hemodynamically significant superficial femoral artery or popliteal artery stenosis would be suggested. Since blood flow in arteries is laminar (i.e., not turbulent, in layers, parallel to the vessel wall, and mostly through the center of the artery), the diameter must be reduced by 50% (representing a 70% diminution in cross-sectional area) before the atherosclerotic narrowing becomes hemodynamically significant.

Duplex ultrasonography with real-time color Doppler imaging, an important addition to many vascular laboratories, allows the clinician to map the vascular tree. The vessel is imaged and the velocity of blood in it is measured. The velocity at a stenosis is increased in the same way at an area of narrowing in a river produces rapids. Distal to a stenosis, spectral widening caused by many velocities translated into many Doppler frequencies, indicates turbulence.

Imaging. Angiography is the most definitive test for defining the pathologic anatomy in peripheral arterial occlusive disease, although the noninvasive laboratory may give more information about function (blood flow). A *distal aortogram with runoff* is usually performed by inserting a needle into a femoral artery, passing a guidewire through the needle into the aorta, and then threading a catheter over the guidewire (Seldinger's technique). Dye is then injected and radiographs are taken over the entire arterial tree, from above the renal vessels down to the feet. Delayed exposures are required to allow adequate visualization of the distal vessels in patients with significant occlusive disease.

Digital subtraction angiography is a modality whereby the image is digitalized and background noise is subtracted. It can be used in conjunction with an arterial injection, to decrease the amount of contrast medium required to get a high-resolution image.

Magnetic resonance angiography is a technique that may allow accurate visualization of the arterial tree without the use of dye.

Treatment

The procedure of choice for hemodynamically significant aortoiliac disease is usually *aortobifemoral bypass* (Fig. 16–1). This has a high 5-year patency rate (approximately 90%); however, because it involves entering a major body cavity (the abdomen), it can have a significant mortality rate in poor-risk patients with conditions such as coronary artery disease, chronic obstructive pulmonary disease, and cerebrovascular disease. Accordingly, in medically compromised patients an "extraanatomic" bypass such as the *axillobifemoral* (Fig. 16–2) or *femoro-femoral* (Fig. 16–3) is often performed. They have perhaps lower 5-year patency rates but also lower mortality for patients with serious associated medical problems.

The operation usually performed for femoropopliteal stenosis or occlusion is *femoropopliteal bypass graft* (Fig. 16–4). The preferred conduit for this is the patient's own greater saphenous vein, because of its low thrombogenicity and the advantage it provides of avoiding a foreign body. The vein, of course, must be reversed to avoid obstruction of flow

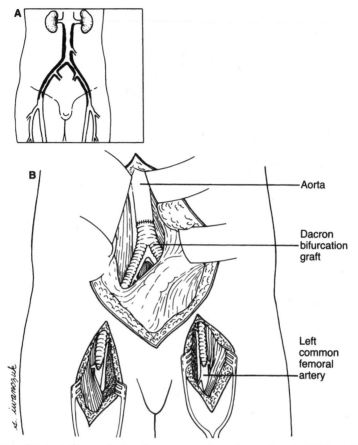

Figure 16–1. *(A)* Aortoiliac occlusive disease caused by atherosclerosis. *(B)* Aortobifemoral bypass graft performed with a bifurcated Dacron graft for arterial reconstruction for aortoiliac occlusive disease. The procedure is performed through a midline abdominal incision and a longitudinal incision in each groin.

by the valves. If the vein is too narrow or too short, or if there is a desire to save it for future coronary artery bypass grafting, expanded polytetrafluoroethylene (Gore-Tex) can be used as a conduit, especially above the knee. For grafting to the popliteal artery below the knee or to the anterior or posterior tibial or peroneal arteries, the autogenous saphenous vein offers a patency rate far superior to those of artificial conduits. Bypasses "in situ," in which the greater saphenous vein is left in position and anastomosed to the common femoral artery proximally and the popliteal artery or its branches distally is a good alternative. The valves must be destroyed intraoperatively to allow caudad flow. Tributaries of the saphenous vein must be ligated to prevent arteriovenous fistulas. Bypass in situ has the advantage of requiring less dissection, and perhaps

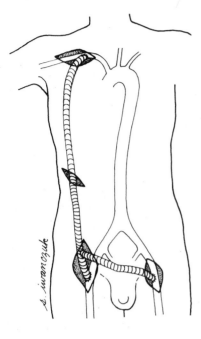

Figure 16–2. Axillobifemoral bypass graft performed by anastomosing a synthetic conduit to the axillary artery and passing it through a subcutaneous tunnel to the right femoral artery. Also, there is an extension from the graft to the left femoral artery. This extension may be prefabricated or may be sutured in place. This "extra-anatomic bypass" obviates entering a major body cavity and thus may have a lower mortality rate in patients with severe concomitant cardiorespiratory problems. It is also indicated as a bypass for patients with aortoiliac disease who also have a septic intraabdominal focus (e.g., after removal of an infected aortic graft). This long bypass graft has a lower 5-year patency rate than an aortobifemoral bypass.

less intimal damage to the vein. It allows a better match, size-wise, by anastomosing the larger proximal saphenous vein to the larger proximal artery and the small distal saphenous vein to the smaller distal artery. In spite of this, the results of bypass in situ have not been proven superior to those achieved with the reversed autogenous saphenous vein. Traditionally, the common femoral artery has been chosen as the site of proximal anastomosis (that is, the site where inflow is obtained). If however, the vein is not long enough to extend from the common femoral artery to the appropriate site of distal anastomosis, the superficial femoral artery or popliteal artery can be chosen as the site of proximal anastomosis, so long as there is no stenosis farther cephalad.

Some areas of arterial stenosis can be opened up by percutaneous transluminal balloon catheter angioplasty. In this procedure, a puncture is made in the groin and a guidewire is passed across the stenosis (Seldinger's technique). In some centers, when occlusion is complete, the laser is used to make a small passage for the guidewire. A balloon is passed over the guidewire and across the stenosis, and is then inflated, dilating the narrowed area. Recurrent stenosis is a concern with transluminal angioplasty, especially when the original stenosis was long. Transluminal angioplasty rivals bypass when the stenosis is short, disease is not diffuse, or the patient is a poor anesthesia risk. Stents have been used in the hope of preventing recurrence of stenosis or occlusion.

In a patient with acute arterial insufficiency manifested by pallor, paresthesias, paralysis of the extremity, pulselessness, pain, and poikilo-

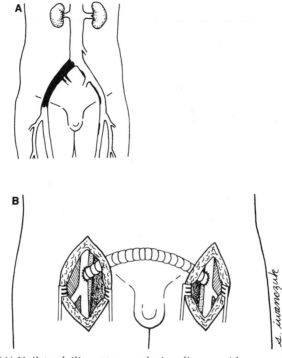

Figure 16–3. *(A)* Unilateral iliac artery occlusive disease with a nonstenotic aorta and widely patent contralateral iliac artery is a good indication for femorofemoral bypass. *(B)* Femorofemoral bypass can be performed under local anesthesia and does not require entering a major body cavity. Thus, it is good for medically compromised patients. A Dacron or Gore-Tex graft is placed through a subcutaneous suprapubic tunnel from one common femoral artery to the other. Because the graft is short and in a high-flow environment, its 5-year patency rate is good. This is an effective operation for unilateral iliac artery disease.

thermia, it is necessary to distinguish between embolization and thrombosis of a preexisting stenosis that has been caused by atherosclerosis. In the former case, embolectomy with a Fogarty catheter (Fig. 16–5) may be very successful and salvage the extremity. In the latter case, merely removing the clot with a catheter is unlikely to be successful, because thrombosis will recur owing to low flow in the stenotic segment. In this case, formal arterial reconstruction, such as an aortobifemoral bypass or a femoropopliteal bypass (depending, of course, on which segment is narrowed) is necessary if revascularization is to be achieved. In the latter case, an alternative is to lyse the clot with thrombolytic agents such as urokinase and then to dilate the stenosis with balloon catheter angioplasty in the hope of preventing recurrent thrombosis. When blood flow is restored to a very ischemic limb, the muscle swells. The compartments in the leg cannot expand because of the tight fascial envelope, and the elevated pressure can injure the muscle and nerves therein, causing

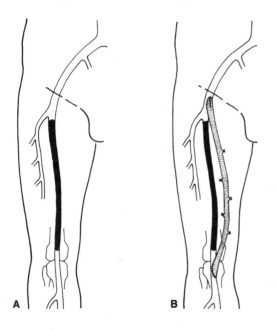

Figure 16–4. *(A)* Femoropopliteal occlusive disease. In this example, the superficial femoral artery is occluded at its takeoff from the common femoral artery. The occlusion could also occur at the adductor hiatus. *(B)* The stenosis or occlusion of the superficial femoral artery can be bypassed with a reversed saphenous vein graft as a conduit and anastomosis of this conduit to the common femoral artery cephalad and the popliteal artery either above or below the knee, caudad.

compartment syndrome. Fasciotomy (incising the enveloping fascia) may be required to sustain the gain achieved by restoration of flow in the arterial system.

While patients with diabetes mellitus are at increased risk for large-vessel occlusive disease such as aortoiliac or femoropopliteal disease, they are also at risk for severe atherosclerotic narrowing of the small arteries of the extremities. Since these small arteries cannot be bypassed, many diabetes patients develop refractory (nonhealing) foot ulcers and diabetic foot infections that cannot be helped by arterial reconstruction. That many diabetics suffer from peripheral neuropathy compounds the issue, because they may suffer trauma to the feet from ill-fitting shoes or walking barefoot without feeling the pain that would warn a normally innervated person. Proper control of the blood sugar may enhance wound healing. Diabetics, as well as their nondiabetic counterparts with peripheral arterial occlusive disease, must be encouraged to stop smoking.

Surgeons often regard *amputation* as an admission of a failure in patients with peripheral vascular disease. Amputations certainly represent a liability to the patient because of the attendant loss of function and the interference with body image. However, for some patients with severe atherosclerotic peripheral arterial occlusive disease, major amputation is unavoidable, and a properly conducted amputation with expert rehabilitation can often restore excellent function. Many patients ambulate well on a below-knee or above-knee prosthesis. Transmetatarsal amputation of a toe or of the foot may be successful (Fig. 16–6), especially when perfusion of the extremity can be improved with an arterial recon-

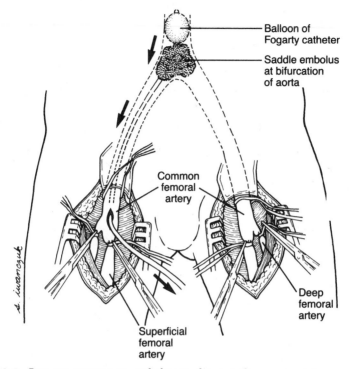

Figure 16–5. One can remove an embolus to the aortoiliac segment by exposing the common femoral artery in the groin, obtaining proximal and distal control with umbilical tapes, and passing a Fogarty balloon catheter through an arteriotomy past the embolus with the balloon deflated. Once the tip is past the embolus, the balloon is inflated and the catheter withdrawn, bringing the embolus with it. One must make sure that no clot has been broken off to lodge in the contralateral iliac or femoral artery.

struction. Frequently, however, below-knee (Fig. 16–7) or above-knee amputation (Fig. 16–8) is necessary. The below-knee amputation is preferred in most instances, because it improves the chances of rehabilitation of geriatric patients. Above-knee amputation has a somewhat greater chance of healing, however, and may be indicated for patients with no chance of rehabilitation or those with infection up to the site of transection for a below-knee amputation.

CASE 16–2

Ruptured Abdominal Aortic Aneurysm

A 70-year-old man was brought to the emergency department with severe back pain, diaphoresis, and hypotension. He was known to have a "small" abdominal aortic aneurysm, but his physician had discouraged elective resection because of his moderately severe coronary artery disease and heavy smoking history.

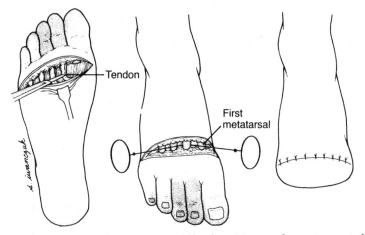

Figure 16–6. Transmetatarsal amputation of the foot. Metatarsals are transected with a Gigli saw.

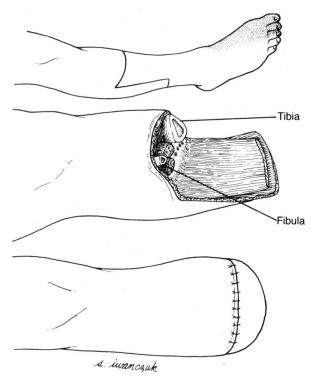

Figure 16–7. Below-knee amputation. A long posterior skin flap is fashioned. The tibia is transected approximately one third of the way down the leg, and the fibula is transected several centimeters above the tibia. The skin is sutured in the most atraumatic fashion possible, to maximize healing.

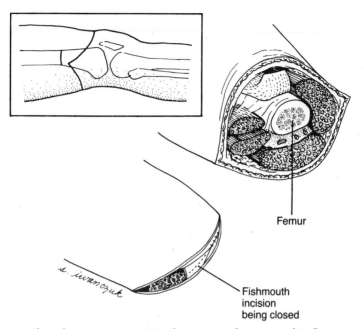

Femur

Fishmouth
incision
being closed

Figure 16–8. Above-knee amputation. Equal anterior and posterior skin flaps are made in a "fish-mouth" fashion. The femur is transected at the midthigh. Again, it is important to suture the skin atraumatically.

Past medical history included a myocardial infarction 2 years before admission. The patient was taking digoxin, 0.25 mg daily, and furosemide (Lasix), 40 mg PO daily, for congestive heart failure.

Physical examination on admission revealed a pale, diaphoretic, elderly man in moderate distress. The blood pressure was 70 palpable and the pulse was 130 and thready. The patient was confused and agitated. There was no neck vein distention. Abdominal examination revealed a tender, pulsatile mass in the epigastrium. Femoral pulses were 1+ palpable bilaterally, and no pulses were palpable below. Both legs were cold and mottled.

An intravenous line was inserted, blood sent for typing and cross-matching, and the patient was brought immediately to the operating room. Proximal and distal control of the aorta was achieved, and the aneurysm was incised. The clot was evacuated, and a woven Dacron tube graft was placed from within the aneurysm. A Foley catheter, Swan-Ganz catheter, and arterial line were inserted intraoperatively.

The patient initially required inotropic agents postoperatively and had a transient bout of oliguric renal failure that resolved spontaneously. He required prolonged intubation because of the known chronic obstructive pulmonary disease from cigarette smoking. He was ultimately weaned from the ventilator and was discharged home on the 20th postoperative day.

DISCUSSION OF CASE 16–2

An *abdominal aortic aneurysm* is a ballooning out of the abdominal aorta (Fig. 16–9), that puts the patient at great risk because of the likelihood of rupture. Some students call it a *dissecting aneurysm,* but this is incorrect. Dissection can occur in the thoracic aorta as a result of cystic medial necrosis, whereby blood dissects between the layers of media, causing a false and a true channel. Rupture is the untoward event that typically is associated with abdominal aortic aneurysm. Smoking, hypertension, and genetic factors can predispose to abdominal aortic aneurysm. Traditionally aneurysms were considered to reflect atherosclerosis, but there is some evidence that they may be related to excess degradation of collagen by collagenase and of elastin by elastase in relation to their rates of synthesis.

Diagnosis

Symptoms. Abdominal aortic aneurysms can be asymptomatic, and the first clinical manifestation can be fatal rupture. When they become symptomatic they may present as *back pain.* This is taken to indicate that they are expanding and that rupture is imminent, and may precipitate surgery even in a poor-risk patient who was being followed nonoperatively. Patients with abdominal aortic aneurysms surprisingly often do not have peripheral arterial occlusive disease and may have no claudication or rest pain.

Signs. An abdominal aortic aneurysm may be discovered as a *pulsatile epigastric mass* on routine physical examination. When this

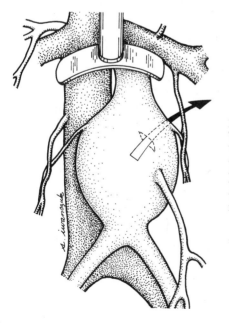

Figure 16–9. Abdominal aortic aneurysm. The aneurysm is usually below the renal arteries, and the inferior mesenteric artery arises from the aneurysmal aorta. When the aneurysm ruptures, it often does so retroperitoneally, and the bleeding may be controlled temporarily by tamponade from the surrounding tissue.

pulsatile mass is tender, it suggests rupture or impending rupture. The most important thing the surgeon can do for a patient with a ruptured abdominal aortic aneurysm is immediate operation. Time should not be wasted with diagnostic tests of *any* sort, although blood should certainly be prepared for transfusion. The most important step is to bring the patient immediately to the operating room.

Imaging. An abdominal aortic aneurysm may be apparent on plain film of the abdomen as a shell-like rim of calcification outlining the aneurysmal aorta, and this may be more obvious on cross-table lateral or oblique films of the abdomen. An aneurysm may likewise become apparent on *intravenous pyelography* (IVP) performed for complaints of severe flank pain (a not uncommon presentation of abdominal aortic aneurysm). IVP may demonstrate displacement of the ureter by the aneurysm. It is not unheard of for a patient with back or flank pain to suffer rupture of an abdominal aortic aneurysm in the x-ray department while awaiting IVP, that was ordered on the mistaken assumption that the patient was suffering from urolithiasis.

The abdominal aortic aneurysm can be imaged by ultrasonography, CT, or magnetic resonance angiography, and these modalities can accurately determine the size of the lesion. An arteriogram is not good for diagnosing an aneurysm, because thrombus can exist within the aneurysm so that the actual channel does not differ much in size from the rest of the aorta (Fig. 16–10). In a patient known to have an unruptured abdominal aortic aneurysm, however, arteriography may be useful for demonstrating (1) the runoff vessels, such as the iliac and femoral arteries, (2) anomalies of the renal and mesenteric vessels that would have a bearing on the operative approach, and (3) horseshoe kidney, which would complicate the operative approach some-

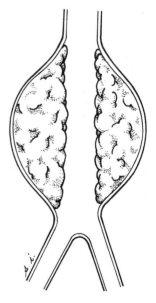

Figure 16–10. Clot within an abdominal aortic aneurysm. At the time of arteriography, the channel through the clot may be the same size as the remainder of the aorta, and the size of the aneurysm may not be appreciated. Thus, ultrasonography or CT is better for assessing the size of the aneurysm.

what. More than 90% of abdominal aortic aneurysms originate below the renal arteries.

Natural History and Treatment

Although aneurysms larger than 5 cm have a much higher incidence of rupture than smaller ones, the small ones can rupture; in any event, they tend to enlarge at the rate of about 0.4 cm per year. For abdominal aortic aneurysms larger than 5 cm, the annual rate of rupture begins at 5% and increases to 20% per year for very large ones. The mortality rate for resection of unruptured aneurysms is 3% to 4%, whereas for ruptured aneurysms treated surgically it is approximately 50%. Accordingly, for most patients resection of an abdominal aortic aneurysm is in their best interest. It is true that many of these patients are medically compromised by atherosclerotic cardiovascular disease, and perhaps cerebrovascular disease. Thus, the benefits and risks of surgery must be weighed extremely carefully by the surgeon and explained fully to the patient.

The patient undergoing elective resection of an abdominal aortic aneurysm should be tested preoperatively for pulmonary function and room air blood gases. Preoperative duplex scans of the carotid arteries and a cardiac stress test may be indicated. A Swan-Ganz catheter and arterial line can be inserted, to allow extra fluid to be given to patients who are dehydrated (as manifested by a low pulmonary capillary wedge pressure, low cardiac output, and high total peripheral resistance). Patients with low cardiac output and high wedge pressure may benefit from infusion of an inotropic agent. Monitoring the physiologic profile with the Swan-Ganz catheter may help the surgeon and the anesthesiologist address the hemodynamic derangements encountered intraoperatively attendant with administration of anesthetic agents, blood loss, and clamping and unclamping of the aorta. Urine output must be monitored and is usually a good reflection of the patient's volume status. Real-time transesophageal echocardiography (TEE) may facilitate monitoring of the function of the left side of the heart. The autotransfusion device may minimize the need for transfusion of homologous blood, with its risk of blood-borne infection. This maximization of the patient's hemodynamic status can reduce the incidence of postoperative complications such as renal failure. The operative technique for resection of an abdominal aortic aneurysm is depicted in Figure 16–11.

As mentioned earlier, patients with a ruptured abdominal aortic aneurysm are brought immediately to surgery. Anesthesia is induced with the team scrubbed and the patient prepped and draped. Once proximal and distal control of the aorta is achieved, the patient can be given heparin ("heparinized") to prevent thrombosis of the distal arterial tree, and the procedure can be conducted in a manner similar to that shown in Figure 16–11.

When an abdominal aortic aneurysm ruptures, it often bleeds into the retroperitoneum, and the bleeding can be temporarily controlled by

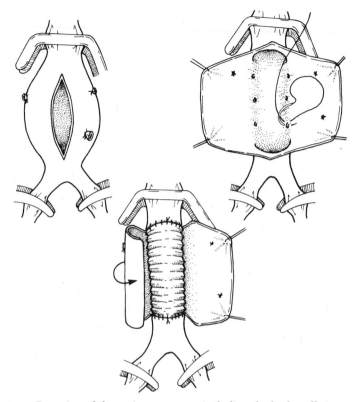

Figure 16–11. Resection of the entire aneurysm, including the back wall, is unnecessary and carries too much risk for blood loss. Accordingly, the surgeon incises the aneurysm and opens it up like a book. The lumbar arteries and inferior mesenteric artery can be oversewn from within the aneurysm, and a Dacron graft can be anastomosed to the proximal and distal aorta from within the aneurysm. The wall of the aneurysm can then be closed over the graft, to separate it from the duodenum and thus help to prevent future development of an aortoduodenal fistula.

tamponade by the surrounding tissue, affording a little extra time. In the group of patients with ruptured aneurysms who preoperatively had a stable blood pressure and good urine output, the operative mortality is less than the 50% cited earlier for ruptured aneurysm, whereas patients presenting with shock and anuria have an operative mortality rate substantially higher than 50%.

CASE 16–3

Deep Vein Thrombosis

A 41-year-old, obese woman developed pain and swelling in her left lower extremity 4 days after total abdominal hysterectomy.

Past medical history included three cesarean sections and chole-cystectomy. She had hypertension treated by diet. There was no history of heart disease or diabetes, no known allergies, and no history of bleeding disorders.

Physical examination at the time of surgical consultation for the swollen left leg revealed no abnormalities of the cardiorespiratory system. The abdomen was soft and not tender, with a healing lower midline hysterectomy incision. Rectal examination was normal. There were good pedal pulses bilaterally, and both feet were warm and well-perfused. The left lower extremity was swollen from the foot to the lower thigh, with edema of the foot and pretibial region. The calf was tender, and Homans' sign was positive. No cords involving the greater or lesser saphenous veins were palpable. The patient had brown pigmentation and dry, scaly skin of both lower legs.

Impedance plethysmography was performed and revealed the patient to have deep vein thrombosis above the knee. After the initial prothrombin time and partial thromboplastin time were confirmed to be normal, the patient was given a bolus of heparin, 10,000 units IV push, and a continuous infusion of heparin at 1000 units per hour was instituted. The partial thromboplastin time was repeated 4 hours after the bolus, and the continuous heparin infusion was titrated to keep the partial thromboplastin time 1.5 to 2 times the control value. The patient was initially kept on bed rest with feet elevated above the heart. After she had received heparin for 4 days, Coumadin was begun by mouth. Four days later, the International Normalized Ratio (INR) for the prothrombin time was found to be 2.5, and heparin was discontinued the next day. The swelling and pain in the left lower extremity resolved, and the patient was allowed out of bed for progressively longer periods. Coumadin was continued indefinitely as the patient's brown pigmentation and dry scaly skin (postphlebitic syndrome) suggested that this was not this patient's first bout of deep vein thrombosis. The patient was fitted for compression stockings and instructed to keep the foot of the bed elevated at night and to avoid prolonged sitting and standing still.

DISCUSSION OF CASE 16–3

Venous disorders are frequently treated nonoperatively, but the care of patients with venous disease is, in any event, traditionally rendered by general and vascular surgeons. This section deals with deep vein thrombosis of the lower extremities, and the possible sequelae of pulmonary embolus and postphlebitic syndrome, and briefly with varicose veins.

The anatomy of the venous drainage of the lower extremities is such that blood returning to the heart drains from the superficial system to the deep veins (Fig. 16–12) via perforating veins that course through the fascial layer, and a system of valves prevents the blood from refluxing caudad.

Factors that contribute to venous return include (1) the pumping action of the muscles through which the veins course, such as the gastrocnemius and soleus muscles (the *muscle pump*); (2) the changes

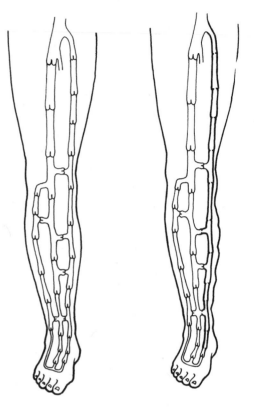

Figure 16–12. The superficial venous system empties into the deep venous system via perforating veins. Valves help to prevent reflux. Deep vein thrombosis may destroy the valves, even though the vein ultimately recanalizes.

in intrathoracic and intraabdominal pressure that occur with respirations; and (3) the head of pressure generated by arterial inflow. Factors that predispose to deep vein thrombosis include stasis, hypercoagulability of the blood, and damage to the intimal surface of the veins. This is called *Virchow's triad.* Stasis may occur during anesthesia, when muscle relaxants paralyze the muscle pump and the patient is lying supine on the operating table. Alternatively, stasis can occur in a patient who sits for a long time. Hypercoagulability can occur in cancer patients, those with polycythemia, and those undergoing surgery (when tissue thromboplastin is released into the circulation by the operative trauma). Inherited deficiencies of substances such as antithrombin III, protein C, or protein S can cause hypercoagulability. Intimal damage may be caused by invasive procedures in which the vein is cannulated, by direct trauma, or by a previous episode of deep vein thrombosis.

Diagnosis

Symptoms. Symptoms of deep vein thrombosis of the lower extremities include *pain* in the calf, the popliteal fossa, or the thigh, though deep vein thrombosis can be asymptomatic ("silent"). One should also question the patient about pleuritic chest pain, dyspnea, or hemoptysis, which would suggest that a pulmonary embolus has developed as a result of the deep vein thrombosis.

Signs. Signs of deep vein thrombosis include swelling, tenderness, pallor of the limb, fever, and tachycardia. Homans' sign is said to be positive when pain in the calf is elicited by dorsiflexion of the foot. It is now recognized that Homans' sign is *not* pathognomonic for deep vein thrombosis and is likely to be positive whenever a significant pathologic lesion is present in the calf, such as a tear of the plantar tendon. In fact, the clinical diagnosis of deep vein thrombosis is inexact even in experienced hands, and the noninvasive vascular laboratory has come to play a major role in the diagnosis of deep vein thrombosis. There are times, however, when the findings are not subtle. An ileofemoral vein thrombosis, by completely halting venous return from the lower extremity, can produce a markedly swollen, painful, blue leg, a condition called *phlegmasia cerulea dolens,* which can progress rapidly to venous gangrene and limb loss.

Noninvasive Vascular Laboratory Studies. Although the venogram is considered the prototype for the diagnosis of deep vein thrombosis, it is invasive and one should be reluctant to order it if the index of suspicion is low. The ramifications of missing a case of deep vein thrombosis are so serious, however, that one is obliged to initiate workup when there is any suspicion at all.

Noninvasive tests such as duplex ultrasonography and *impedance plethysmography* (IPG) correlate so well with venography findings that they have largely replaced it in many centers. To make the diagnosis of deep vein thrombosis duplex ultrasound scanning relies on the presence of (1) a filling defect in the venous lumen, (2) inability to compress the vein, or (3) decreased flow. The technique can be brought to the bedside, is quite reliable in experienced hands, and is in wide use. IPG requires that an occluding cuff be placed around the thigh and a circular electrode around the calf. The electrode around the calf measures impedance or resistance that, because blood conducts electricity well, decreases as the calf fills with blood and increases as blood drains from the leg. When the occluding cuff is inflated above venous pressure but below arterial pressure, the amount of blood in the leg (*venous capacitance*) increases and impedance decreases; that is, conductance increases. When the occluding cuff is deflated, blood rapidly drains from the leg (*venous outflow*) and conductance decreases. If a clot is occluding the deep venous system above the knee, venous outflow is diminished. The patient's values are compared against a series of normal values (Fig. 16–13). IPG is a selective and specific test for deep vein thrombosis, and therapeutic decisions are often based on the results.

Treatment

Anticoagulation provides an important facet of the treatment of deep vein thrombosis. After the diagnosis of deep vein thrombosis has been made, the patient is usually given 100 to 150 IU/kg of heparin, IV push,

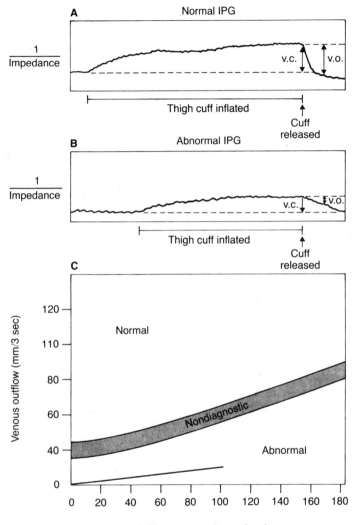

Figure 16–13. *(A)* Impedance plethysmography in the diagnosis of deep vein thrombosis. Conductance falls rapidly (impedance increases) when the occluding cuff is deflated and blood flows rapidly out through the veins of a normal lower extremity. *(B)* Conductance falls more slowly after release of the occluding cuff if the major veins draining the extremity are occluded with thrombus. *(C)* The patient's venous capacitance (VC) and venous outflow (VO) are compared against a table of normal values to determine whether the test patient has deep vein thrombosis.

and then continuous drip with an infusion pump is instituted. The PTT is monitored, and the continuous heparin infusion is titrated to keep the PTT at 1.5 to 2 times control. After a day or two, oral Coumadin is begun, and when the INR reaches 2.0 to 3.0 (this usually takes about 3 days), the heparin is discontinued. There is a suggestion that keeping the anticoagulation at the minimum therapeutic level may reduce the likelihood of hemorrhagic complications. Accordingly, heparin can be infused to keep the partial thromboplastin time 15 to 25 seconds beyond the initial baseline value and, if a baseline value has not been obtained, 15 to 25 seconds beyond the middle of the hospital's normal range. The Coumadin should be continued for at least 3 months, keeping the INR between 2.0 and 3.0, and may be necessary indefinitely for patients with recurrent deep vein thrombosis or pulmonary embolus or those with malignant disease or another hypercoagulable state. Sometimes, deep vein thrombosis is treated with thrombolysis. Thrombolytics such as urokinase, streptokinase, and recombinant tissue plasminogen activator can decrease the risk of post-phlebitic syndrome.

The treatment of deep vein thrombosis is geared toward prevention of *pulmonary embolus,* a life-threatening lesion, and toward prevention of *postphlebitic syndrome,* which can have long-term morbidity. The symptoms of pulmonary embolus include pleuritic chest pain, shortness of breath, and hemoptysis. Signs include tachycardia, hypotension, a loud pulmonic component of the second heart sound (P_2), a pleural friction rub if pulmonary infarction has occurred, and sometimes an irregular rhythm, as atrial fibrillation can result from pulmonary embolus. Arterial blood gases may show arterial oxygen desaturation (a decreased PaO_2) and decreased $PaCO_2$ due to hyperventilation. The chest x-ray may show a wedge-shaped infiltrate at the periphery when a pulmonary infarct has supervened. An area that is well-ventilated but not perfused on a ventilation-perfusion scan (lung scan) suggests a pulmonary embolus, and this can be confirmed by pulmonary arteriograpy, if necessary.

Pulmonary embolus can be treated with a regimen of anticoagulation, as outlined earlier. Rarely, in severe cases, the clot in the pulmonary artery can be dissolved with either streptokinase or urokinase. Attempts have been made in desperate cases to perform pulmonary embolectomy, either operatively or with a specially designed catheter inserted via the femoral or jugular vein through the right side of the heart into the pulmonary circulation.

The best treatment of deep vein thrombosis and resultant pulmonary embolus is prevention. It has been shown in a large series of general surgical patients that prophylactic low-dose (also called *minidose*) heparin, 5000 units administered subcutaneously 2 hours preoperatively and continued every 12 hours postoperatively, can lower the risk of fatal pulmonary embolus in general surgical patients. This is especially so for patients older than 40 years, obese patients, those with cancer, those undergoing prolonged surgery or pelvic operations, and patients with a past history of phlebitis, MI, congestive heart failure, paralytic stroke, prolonged bed rest, pregnancy, or oral contraceptive use. The patient in Case 3 was over 40, was obese, and had stasis pigmentation and stasis dermatitis, suggesting that she had had a "silent" episode of deep vein thrombosis, probably at the time of one of the cesarean sections or at cholecystectomy. These factors all placed her in a moderate to high-risk group, and she would have been better served had subcutaneous heparin or a sequential compression device been started preoperatively. External intermittent compression devices placed around the calves have also proved effective prophylaxis against deep vein thrombosis. They are believed to work by decreasing stasis and by increasing activity of the body's thrombolytic system.

Patients with documented deep vein thrombosis are anticoagulated in an attempt to prevent pulmonary embolus. Patients on adequate anticoagulation who develop a recurrent pulmonary embolus, and patients with pulmonary emboli and an absolute contraindication to anticoagulation such as a berry aneurysm, a brain tumor, or active GI hemorrhage, have an indication for venous interruption.

One method of doing this is to operatively place a clip around the vena cava (Fig. 16–14) in an attempt to prevent emboli from the deep veins in the legs from reaching the pulmonary circulation. Another method of accomplishing the same thing is to cut down on the internal jugular vein and fluoroscopically insert a vena cava filter through the internal jugular vein, superior vena cava, and right atrium, into the inferior vena cava until it sits in the inferior vena cava just below the renal veins, preventing pulmonary embolus (Fig. 16–15). This now can also be done percutaneously by either the jugular or the femoral route.

Postphlebitic syndrome is a consequence of deep vein thrombosis that, in contradistinction to pulmonary embolus, is not ordinarily life threatening. It can result, however, in long-term morbidity and should be avoided or minimized when possible. The syndrome consists of ulceration of the skin, frequently that overlying the medial malleolus (*stasis ulcer*), scaly, erythematous skin (*stasis dermatitis*), pedal edema, and brown discoloration of the skin (*stasis pigmentation*) from deposition of pigments released from the breakdown of hemoglobin.

Although the deep veins usually recanalize after a bout of deep vein thrombosis, postphlebitic syndrome occurs because the competence of the valves has usually been destroyed. This allows the full hydrostatic force of the column of blood from the heart to the distal limb to be conducted retrograde through incompetent valves in the deep venous system and in the perforating veins, which course through the fascia. This is responsible for the breakdown of overlying skin, deposition of pigment, and swelling.

Medical management of this entity consists of elevating the foot of the bed at night, avoiding prolonged sitting and standing still, and wearing specially fitted stockings that provide a pressure gradient from caudad to cephalad. Weekly wrapping of the extremity from the foot to just below the knee with a zinc-impregnated wrap (an *Unna boot*) is successful in treating postphlebitic ulcers. The main disadvantage of this

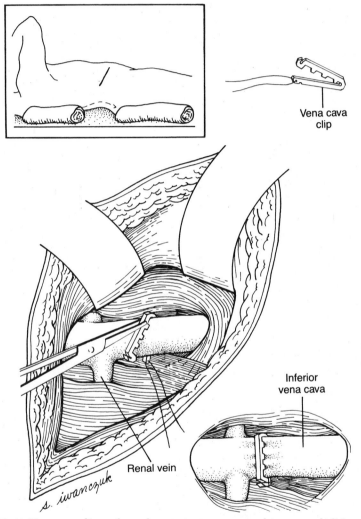

Figure 16–14. Vena cava clip performed to prevent recurrent pulmonary emboli in a patient with deep vein thrombosis of a lower extremity who has already had a pulmonary embolus while taking adequate anticoagulants or has had a pulmonary embolus and has a contraindication to anticoagulation. An incision is made in the right flank, and the peritoneum with its contents is pushed anteromedially. The vena cava is circumscribed and a serrated clip is placed around it. This clip "compartmentalizes" the vena cava, so that a large clot cannot reach the pulmonary circulation.

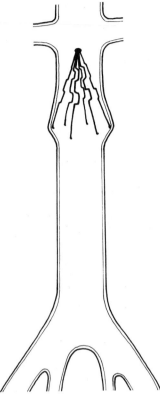

Figure 16–15. A Kimray-Greenfield filter can be passed on a catheter through a cutdown on the internal jugular vein or by percutaneous Seldinger's technique and passed through the superior vena cava, through the right atrium, and into the inferior vena cava. The filter should be disengaged in the inferior vena cava just inferior to the renal veins. Access can also be obtained via a puncture in the femoral vein.

method is that the ulcer can take many months to heal. The boot must be changed once a week, and it is hot and sometimes malodorous in summer, not to mention unsightly. In spite of this, it can often be employed successfully.

Stripping of the greater saphenous vein and ligation and avulsion of tributaries may play a role in the treatment of selected cases of stasis ulcers, as reflux back into the greater saphenous vein from an incompetent saphenofemoral junction can exacerbate the usual underlying pathophysiology, which is incompetent valves in the deep venous system and perforators. Mere skin grafting of the ulcers is unlikely to produce long-term success, as the underlying lesion remains unchanged. Subfascial ligation of perforators, or Linton's procedure (Fig. 16–16), does deal with the underlying pathophysiology and is likely to produce mild to moderate success. The limiting factor in subfascial ligation of perforators has been the high incidence of wound complications related to the necessity of making the incision through diseased skin. Accordingly, new techniques of minimally invasive surgery have been applied to this problem. Subfascial endoscopic perforator surgery (SEPS) allows use of a small

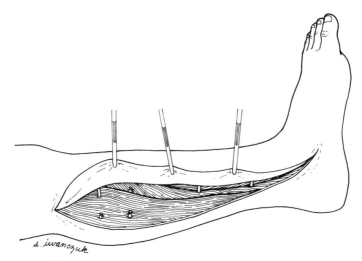

Figure 16–16. Subfascial ligation of perforators (Linton's procedure) performed to treat venous stasis ulcer overlying the perforators at the medial malleolus. The perforators are ligated in a plane just below the fascia.

incision that can be made through healthy skin remote from the ulcer and areas of stasis dermititis. This is thought to minimize wound infection and breakdown.

Some preliminary work has been conducted with the autotransplantation of valves from expendable venous segments such as the greater saphenous vein. Venous bypasses have been attempted in the small percentage of people who have no recanalization of the deep venous system after deep vein thrombosis. The low flow in the venous system, as compared with the arterial side, tends to decrease the patency rate of venous bypass, as stasis leads to thrombosis.

Varicose Veins

Many patients complain of varicose veins along the course of the greater saphenous vein (which drains into the femoral vein in the groin) or along the course of the lesser saphenous vein. The lesser vein empties into the popliteal vein posteriorly. Although many patients complain of aching legs at the end of a long day, it is often difficult to be sure that the symptoms are caused by varicose veins and that the patient will derive symptomatic improvement from stripping and ligation. Many patients are more concerned about the unsightly appearance of the varicose veins.

Some patients have recurrent episodes of superficial phlebitis in the greater saphenous vein, presenting as a tender, red cord along the course of the vein. In contradistinction to deep vein thrombosis, superficial phlebitis is not treated with anticoagulation but usually on an "ambulatory basis," with warm packs and nonsteroidal antiinflammatory drugs (NSAIDs). Recurrent attacks of superficial phlebitis are a reasonable indication for *stripping and ligation,* the procedure illustrated in Figure 16–17. Another indisputable indication for vein stripping is recurrent marked bleeding from erosion of a superficial varix at the ankle, which affects only a small group of patients.

CASE 16–4

Carotid Endarterectomy for Transient Ischemic Attacks

A 64-year-old man was admitted to the hospital with an episode of slurred speech and weakness of the right arm and leg. The episode had resolved completely 8 hours later.

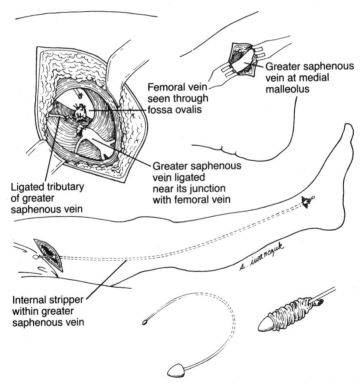

Figure 16–17. Stripping and ligation of the greater saphenous vein. The tributaries of the greater saphenous vein are doubly ligated and transected near the saphenofemoral junction. The vein is transected in the groin and is dissected free through a small incision at the medial malleolus. Proximal and distal control are obtained, an internal stripper is passed from the ankle to the groin, and the vein is stripped.

Past medical history included a myocardial infarction 4 years before admission and a 40–pack-year history of cigarette smoking.

Physical examination at the time that the surgical consultation was called revealed only a left carotid bruit. There were no focal neurologic deficits. Although no pulses were palpable below the femoral pulses bilaterally, the lower extremities were warm and well-perfused.

A duplex scan revealed an ulcerated plaque at the bifurcation of the left common carotid artery extending into the internal carotid artery, and this was confirmed by arteriography, which included views of the major vessels as they came off the aortic arch.

The patient was taken to the operating room, where an arterial line was inserted to monitor blood pressure and left carotid endarterectomy was performed. The patient had an unremarkable postoperative course. On the first postoperative day, a regular diet was resumed and the peripheral IV and the arterial line were removed. The patient was ambulating independently with no neurologic deficit, and he was discharged on the 2nd postoperative day.

DISCUSSION OF CASE 16–4

Surgeons become involved in the treatment of cerebrovascular disease because many strokes are due to atherosclerotic plaques in the common and internal carotid arteries. By reason of their accessible location in the neck, they can be corrected by the surgeon before the catastrophe of stroke occurs.

Diagnosis

Symptoms and Signs. A transient ischemic attack (TIA) is an instance of neurologic defect lasting less than 24 hours that results from decreased blood flow to an area of the brain. A patient might have aphasia and right hemiparesis that last less than 24 hours. The patient might have *amaurosis fugax* (transient loss of vision in one eye) secondary to embolization of the ophthalmic artery, which is a branch of the internal carotid artery inside the cranial vault. The importance of transient ischemic attacks is that they often provide a warning that, if no treatment is given, the patient will later suffer a stroke. A *stroke* (cerebrovascular accident, CVA) not only has a significant mortality rate but produces profound morbidity in those who survive. Many of these patients are incapable of functioning independently, in spite of prolonged attempts at rehabilitation, and they may even need to be confined to a skilled nursing facility. Accordingly, it is exceedingly important to prevent the development of stroke in these patients, whose TIAs serve as a warning.

Some transient ischemic attacks resulting from extracranial cerebrovascular disease are caused by hemodynamically significant stenosis (greater than 50% of vessel diameter) of the carotid and vertebral arteries which produce decreased cerebral blood flow. Others are caused by embolization to the end arteries of the brain by platelet emboli or atherosclerotic debris that originates in an ulcerated plaque in the carotid artery. Such plaques can occupy less than 50% of the diameter of the vessel and still be the source of platelet emboli to the brain, causing TIAs or CVAs without impeding blood flow in the carotid arteries. Other physical findings in addition to the neurologic defects caused by cerebrovascular disease may include diminished or absent carotid pulses or a carotid bruit. A carotid bruit is caused by turbulence of blood flow around a carotid plaque (obstructing or nonobstructing). When an artery is completely obstructed, blood flow ceases entirely and the bruit disappears.

Noninvasive Vascular Laboratory Studies. Oculoplethysmography by the method of Gee is a noninvasive technique for detecting a hemodynamically significant plaque in the carotid arteries. This test uses eye cups to measure the pressure in both globes, which reflects the pressure in the ipsilateral ophthalmic artery and, thus, the pressure in the ipsilateral internal carotid artery. When the pressure on one side is 5 mm Hg less than that on the other side or when it is less than approximately 70% of brachial systolic pressure, significant (greater than 50%) stenosis of the carotid artery is likely. The limitation of this technique is that it does not pick up ulcerated, nonobstructing plaques, which can be sources of stroke-producing emboli. Because this patient had rather unequivocal symptoms of TIAs, oculoplethysmography could have been foregone because arteriography was required in any event. Duplex ultrasonography, often with color images, is now often done in the vascular laboratory or the radiology department. Correspondingly, oculoplethysmography is done less frequently. Duplex scanning can be used to evaluate asymptomatic carotid bruits, to screen the carotid arteries of candidates for cardiac or peripheral vascular surgery or patients with symptomatic cerebrovascular disease. The latter indication is less clear cut, as arteriography will be required for symptomatic patients, especially when the symptoms are hemispheric (in the distribution of the middle cerebral artery). Duplex scanning detects a hemodynamically significant stenosis (greater than 50% of the luminal diameter) because of increased velocity of blood through the narrowing and because of turbulent flow at stenoses causing spectral widening. However, even a stenosis that is not "hemodynamically significant" can be the source of microemboli that cause transient ischemic attacks and strokes. Thus, arteriography may be required even when duplex scanning is negative.

Imaging. Arteriography—demonstrating the aortic arch; the great vessels including the innominate artery, both common, internal, and external carotid arteries; the vertebral arteries; and the intracranial vessels—is critical to diagnosis. It is usually required to decide whether surgical correction of a carotid artery lesion is indicated. MRI or CT is sometimes helpful because both can identify areas of infarction in the brain. *Magnetic resonance angiography* can provide excellent images of the carotid arteries without injection of contrast medium. Its role is evolving.

Treatment

The best treatment for carotid artery plaques is determined by the patient's history and by the morphology of the lesion. A high grade of stenosis, the presence of ulceration or soft plaque, and the presence of frequent transient ischemic attacks are all ominous signs. Patients who develop transient ischemic attacks in the distribution of a carotid artery with a hemodynamically significant stenosis (greater than 50% reduction in diameter, which translates to a 70% reduction in cross-sectional area), especially if the plaque is ulcerated or mixed consistency (which may be soft and prone to embolize), may benefit from carotid endarterectomy (Fig. 16–18). Patients with a 70% reduction in diameter should undergo carotid endarterectomy, even after one TIA.

Some patients with a history of stroke due to carotid artery disease

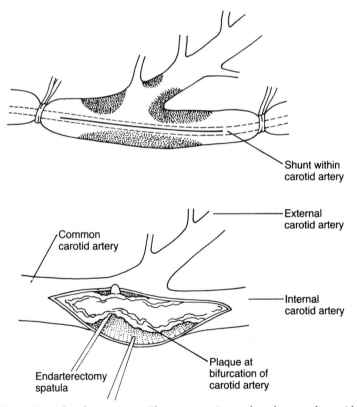

Figure 16–18. Carotid endarterectomy. The common, internal, and external carotid arteries are dissected free, care being taken that no atheromatous debris is dislodged to enter the cerebral circulation. Arteriotomy is performed, and an internal shunt can be placed if collateral circulation via the circle of Willis is judged to be inadequate for cerebral protection. The plaque is removed with a spatula, and the arteriotomy is closed with No. 6–0 Prolene.

who have good residual function may benefit from carotid endarterectomy to protect residual function of the cerebral hemisphere if an appropriate lesion (greater than 50% stenosis) is found by angiography or duplex scan. The surgery is often done after the patient's rehabilitation reaches a plateau. Patients with asymptomatic carotid bruits and more than 60% stenosis may benefit from carotid endarterectomy. Patients with coronary artery disease and high-grade stenosis in one or both carotid arteries may benefit from prophylactic carotid endarterectomy before coronary artery bypass grafting, whether or not they have symptoms of cerebrovascular disease. Global ischemic symptoms (such as the vague impression of decreased intellect), completed stroke, and stroke in evolution are much less acceptable indications for carotid endarterectomy.

OCCLUSIVE DISEASE OF THE VISCERAL VESSELS

Atherosclerotic narrowing of the visceral vessels may be amenable to surgical intervention. Stenosis of a renal artery may cause renovascular hypertension (Goldblatt's kidney) by stimulating release of renin, which converts angiotensin I to angiotensin II. The latter is a potent vasoconstrictor and can be responsible for marked hypertension. It also stimulates aldosterone secretion from the adrenal gland, causing sodium resorption in the renal tubules and adding to the hypertension. This can sometimes be corrected by bypassing the stenosis with a saphenous vein graft, removing the stimulus for renin release.

If two of the three major splanchnic vessels (celiac trunk, superior and inferior mesenteric arteries) are stenosed or occluded, the patient may develop intestinal angina. This presents as abdominal pain precipitated by eating and resulting from the increased demand for blood that eating produces. This is analogous to angina pectoris and can sometimes be corrected by a procedure that bypasses the areas of narrowing or occlusion, thus preventing the evolution of frank mesenteric infarction and relieving the symptom of pain upon eating. Mesenteric infarction necessitates resection of the involved segment of bowel and has a high mortality rate from resulting sepsis. Even if the patient survives, massive resection may result in short-bowel syndrome, making the patient an "intestinal cripple" who must rely on parenteral nutrition.

Atherosclerosis is a generalized, degenerative process. Someone making the decision to intervene surgically to combat its ravages in one anatomic location must take into consideration the complications likely to be caused by the presence of atherosclerotic occlusive disease in other sites plus the shorter life expectancy associated with generalized severe atherosclerosis. The ultimate goal is prevention, but, for the moment, we must exercise sound judgment and good surgical technique to preserve function, salvage limbs, and prolong good-quality life.

Recommended Reading

1. Moore WS (ed): *Vascular Surgery, A Comprehensive Review,* ed 5. Philadelphia: W.B. Saunders, 1998.
2. Valentine RJ (ed): Peripheral Arterial and Aortic Surgery. In McClelland RN (ed): *Selected Reading in General Surgery,* vol 24, no 9–11, 1997; vol 25, no 1, 1998. Dallas: The University of Texas Southwestern Medical Center.
3. Omert LA, Rich NM: Peripheral vascular complications. In Maull KI, Rodriguez A, Wiles CE III (eds): *Complications in Trauma and Critical Care.* Philadelphia: W.B. Saunders, 1996, pp 333–344.

17

Critical Care and the Surgeon

The modern critical care unit provides sophisticated intensive care to patients with life-threatening illnesses. As part of the typical surgical residency training program, the surgeon plays an integral role in the care of critically ill patients. A surgeon with a special interest in critical care is often the director of a critical care unit. In many institutions, there is a medical-surgical *intensive care unit* (ICU) where patients with illnesses classified as either medical or surgical can be managed. This type of unit is sometimes advantageous, as the boundary between the two disciplines is often fuzzy or nonexistent. Many institutions have a combination of other superspecialized units, an arrangement that can be desirable because it allows specialized training of nursing personnel and concentration of equipment unique to each unit.

A *cardiac care unit* is one where patients undergoing cardiac surgery are cared for. The cardiac care unit nurses can be specially trained in the use of special equipment such as the intraaortic balloon pump. Physiologic monitoring with the Swan-Ganz catheter and arterial line, along with cardiac pacemakers and multiple pressor agents, are also used routinely in the medical-surgical ICU. Care in a cardiac ICU may be under the direction of a cardiothoracic surgeon, an anesthesiologist, a cardiologist, or another intensivist, other specialists consulting as necessary.

A coronary care unit (CCU) is one in which patients whose principal problem is heart disease are treated under the care of a cardiologist. Emphasis is on early detection and treatment of complications of heart disease such as myocardial infarction, cardiogenic shock, and life-threatening arrhythmias. It must be remembered that no physiologic system operates in a vacuum. Other systems such as the respiratory, renal, and gastrointestinal can become involved in CCU patients, and the cardiovascular system is frequently involved in patients in the general medical-surgical ICU. Other specialized care units that exist in many institutions include the respiratory care unit, the neurosurgical ICU, the trauma unit, the burn unit, the pediatric ICU, and the neonatal ICU. A new specialty of critical care is evolving that encompasses care of patients in all of these areas.

The initial approach to a critically ill patient parallels the *ABC*s of *a*irway, *b*reathing, and *c*irculation that guide the resuscitation of any patient. This fundamental strategy must not be forgotten in the discussion of the more sophisticated techniques.

The first priority is to establish an airway. A trauma patient's neck must be immobilized until a cervical spine injury is ruled out by appropriate x-rays. The tongue is a common cause of airway obstruction in obtunded patients, and it can be dislodged by head tilt with the chin lift or jaw thrust. The chin lift can be performed without hyperextending the neck, an important consideration when cervical spine injury is suspected. Blood and secretions should be removed with a tonsil tip sucker unless a fracture of the cribriform plate is suspected. In such a case, great care must be used to avoid passing the instrument into the cranium. The airway can then be maintained by an oropharyngeal airway. If breathing is inadequate or the airway is still threatened, endotracheal intubation can be accomplished through the oral or nasal route. Care must be taken to avoid hyperextension of the neck if cervical spine films have not completely ruled out a cervical spine fracture. Nasotracheal intubation is contraindicated when fracture of the cribriform plate is suspected. Even in patients with severe fractures of the facial bones, orotracheal intubation can often be accomplished by a skilled clinician. If this cannot be accomplished, cricothyroidotomy or emergency tracheostomy can be performed; however, it should be noted that an emergency tracheostomy in the intensive care unit setting without proper lighting, assistance, and instruments can be a difficult procedure.

The surgeon can assess breathing for adequacy by watching the excursions of the chest, by listening for breath sounds, and by looking for cyanosis. If breathing is believed to be inadequate, the patient can be ventilated first with a face mask and an Ambu bag and then with intubation and positive-pressure ventilation.

One can rapidly assess the circulation by feeling for the strength of the peripheral pulse and by noting whether the extremities are warm, with good capillary filling. The circulation is initially supported by expansion of the intravascular volume with normal saline or Ringer's lactated solution, as this improves cardiac output in most patients, regardless of the underlying cause of hypoperfusion. If there is no effective heartbeat, closed chest massage must be instituted. If the heart is empty from severe hemorrhage, open heart message is sometimes indicated. After the ABCs of airway, breathing, and circulation are considered, definitive diagnosis and treatment are instituted.

In ICU patients, the ABCs are dealt with first when rapid resuscitation is required. Thereafter, each physiologic system is surveyed. The progress note in the critical care unit takes on much importance, because its proper organization provides a "database" from which the surgeon can comprehend the patient's problems and formulate a rational therapeutic plan. The physiologic systems that are usually considered in each note are:

1. Cardiovascular
2. Respiratory
3. Renal
4. Gastrointestinal/nutritional

5. Central nervous system
6. Endocrine
7. Hepatobiliary
8. Hematologic
9. Infectious disease (not really a physiologic system but listed as such)

Each system can be equated with a "problem" in the problem-oriented record (see Chapter 3), because it can be assumed that, if the critically ill patient does not already have at least one derangement in each physiologic system he might well develop one, and early detection and treatment will be facilitated by daily consideration of each system. The consideration of each system in the daily progress note may include *subjective* and *objective data,* an *assessment,* and a *plan* (the so-called SOAP format).

CASE 17–1

ICU Care of a Patient After Resection of a Ruptured Abdominal Aortic Aneurysm

A progress note written on the first postoperative day for a hypothetical patient who has undergone resection of a ruptured abdominal aortic aneurysm might read like this:

Postop day 1 for a 58 y/o M s/p resection of a ruptured AAA. Associated illnesses include a history of mild hypertension controlled by diet.

Problem 1: Cardiovascular

Subjective: Denies chest pain.
Objective: Heart rate 105, sinus tachycardia, BP 140/80. No JVD, no sacral or peripheral edema. Wedge pressure 12, cardiac output 5.6 L/min. ECG shows no change from preop. Strong dorsalis pedis and posterior tibial pulses bilaterally.
Assessment: Stable from a cardiovascular point of view.
Plan: Remove Swan-Ganz catheter and arterial line.

Problem 2: Respiratory

Subjective: Denies air hunger.
Objective: Tolerated mechanical ventilation well overnight in the assist/control mode. ABGs adequate on assist/control with a rate of 10 early this AM, now on CPAP of 5 cm H_2O with an FIO_2 of 40% with PO_2 of 120 mm Hg, PCO_2 of 35 mm Hg, and pH of 7.40. The forced inspiratory pressure (FIP) is -30, the tidal volume is 400 ml, and the vital capacity is 1100 ml. Lungs are clear to auscultation, and chest x-ray done this AM shows no infiltrate and no increased prominence of the vascular markings. The endotracheal tube and pulmonary artery catheter are in good position.

Assessment: Weaning from respirator progressing satisfactorily. Should be able to extubate.

Plan: Extubate. Place on 40% face mask. Repeat ABGs one half hour thereafter. Aggressive pulmonary toilet, including chest physiotherapy and incentive spirometry. Patient to be out of bed ambulating at least tid.

Problem 3: Renal

Subjective: Denies thirst.

Objective: Intake in the 16 hours since surgery, 2000 ml Ringer's lactated solution. Output 820 ml urine, 200 ml from NG tube. Serum electrolytes reveal Na of 140, K of 4.5, a Cl of 100, and a CO_2 of 30. BUN is 10.

Assessment: Renal status stable.

Plan: Maintenance IV fluid. Follow urine output. Check serum creatinine and daily weights.

Problem 4: GI/nutritional

Subjective: No nausea.

Objective: Abdomen soft, nondistended. Bowel sounds absent. Only 200 ml from NG tube. No flatus or BM.

Assessment: Should be able to reinstitute adequate nutritional intake via the enteral route in a few days.

Plan: D/C NG tube tomorrow.

Problem 5: Central nervous system

Subjective: Alert. Responds appropriately to commands.

Objective: Cranial nerves intact, no motor weakness, DTRs intact. No pathologic reflexes.

Assessment: No evidence of perioperative stroke.

Plan: Continue to monitor neurologic and psychologic status.

Problem 6: Endocrine

Subjective: [No entry]

Objective: No polyuria. Finger stick blood sugars all under 200.

Assessment: No evidence of glucose intolerance at present.

Plan: Continue to monitor blood sugars.

Problem 7: Hepatobiliary

Subjective: No pruritus. No RUQ abdominal pain.

Objective: Bilirubin, alkaline phosphatase, LDH, and SGOT all WNL.

Assessment: No evidence of hepatic dysfunction at present.

Plan: Monitor liver function tests.

Problem 8: Hematologic

Subjective: No entry

Objective: Has received 4 units packed red cells intraop and 2 units in recovery room. Has also received 2 units of fresh-frozen plasma. Hematocrit at 8 PM yesterday was 33. At 6 AM this morning hematocrit is 34, platelet count 80,000. Protime (INR) and partial thromboplastin time are WNL.

Assessment: No evidence of continuing blood loss, hemolysis, or coagulopathy. Platelet count adequate.
Plan: Continue to monitor. Keep hematocrit above 30.

Problem 9: Infectious

Subjective: No shaking chills.
Objective: Maximum temperature 100.4°F. WBC 11,000. On IV cephalothin.
Assessment: Nothing to suggest a septic complication at present.
Plan: Continue prophylactic antibiotics for a maximum of 48 hours. Monitor temperature curve and serial white counts.

DISCUSSION OF CASE 17–1

This progress note is similar to a note the ICU resident might write on the first postoperative day for a patient who underwent resection of a ruptured abdominal aortic aneurysm. It demonstrates many important points in the critical care of the surgical patient and serves as a point of departure for discussion of these concepts. Again, it should be recognized that the progress note provides not only a method of ensuring continuity of care but a template upon which one can conceptualize the patient's actual or potential problems and provide a plan for care.

Cardiovascular System

Subjective. Describing the subjective aspects of the cardiovascular system in this patient, the note states, "Denies chest pain." Other symptoms that might be elicited include, orthopnea, palpitations, and paroxysmal nocturnal dyspnea. Since the patient has an endotracheal tube in place, the subjective data base is necessarily abbreviated, yet the patient can often answer questions by nodding yes or no, providing important information. The patient also is comforted by communication with the physician. The subjective data base becomes more complete in subsequent notes after the patient has been extubated and is able to verbalize his complaints.

Objective. The objective portion of the cardiovascular data base indicates that the patient has mild sinus tachycardia. This is not a primary arrhythmia but is usually due to an underlying cause such as pain, fever, sepsis, atelectasis, hypovolemia, incipient congestive heart failure, anxiety, pulmonary embolus, myocardial infarction, or hypoxia. That is, sinus tachycardia is a nonspecific finding that can suggest any number of derangements, some more serious than others. Thus, sinus tachycardia is not usually treated with drugs to slow the heart rate, but attempts are made to correct the underlying cause. Sinus tachycardia of 105 is not unusual after an operation of this magnitude, and it will probably resolve after the patient is extubated and proper analgesia is provided.

Arrhythmias such as atrial fibrillation and frequent premature ventricular contractions can also have an underlying cause such as electrolyte disturbance, pulmonary embolus, hypoxia, or underlying coronary artery disease. Although the underlying cause should be sought and treated if found, the arrhythmia itself often requires treatment because of the hemodynamic derangements it can cause. Atrial fibrillation with a rapid ventricular response may result in decreased cardiac output and inadequate peripheral perfusion. This is often manifested by hypotension and oliguria, as the ventricle is prevented by the rapid rate of contraction from properly filling during diastole.

In atrial fibrillation, slowing the ventricular response by increasing the block across the AV node may improve cardiac output by slowing the rate at which the ventricle beats and allowing proper filling during diastole. Drugs that can do this include digoxin, propranolol (Inderal), and the calcium-channel blockers. Frequent premature ventricular contractions (PVCs) may require treatment to prevent evolution of ventricular fibrillation. The fact that this patient has good cardiac output with reasonable pulmonary capillary wedge pressure is noted in the data base. The wedge pressure is a reflection of left atrial pressure as ascertained by the flow-directed pulmonary artery catheter, (the Swan-Ganz catheter; Fig. 17–1). Cardiac output is determined by means of the thermodilution technique, which uses a thermistor at the end of the Swan-Ganz catheter (Fig. 17–2).

Assessment and Plan. Swan-Ganz catheters and arterial lines are often placed before elective resection of an abdominal aortic aneurysm. This may be done immediately before the surgery once the patient is asleep. When it is done the evening before surgery, examples of cardiac output can be obtained at several wedge pressures and a left ventricular function curve can be constructed (Fig. 17–3). The patient who is hypovolemic can have volume expansion with normal saline, Ringer's lactated solution, or 5% albumin. If left ventricular function is depressed, as manifested by a cardiac output that is low in the face of normal wedge pressure, an inotropic agent such as dopamine or dobutamine can be added. Present cost-saving trends dictate that even patients undergoing very major surgery be admitted the morning of the procedure; however, if preoperative testing of cardiac function suggests a derangement, such early admission and maximization of cardiac status may be justified.

Since this patient had a ruptured abdominal aortic aneurysm, the surgical team would not have had the luxury of inserting the Swan-Ganz catheter and arterial line preoperatively. These could have been inserted intraoperatively without interfering with the surgical field or immediately postoperatively to facilitate cardiorespiratory monitoring and fluid management. In this case, the pulmonary artery catheter and radial artery line are being removed on the first postoperative day because the patient's condition is hemodynamically stable and it is believed that the potential benefits are outweighed by the risks, such as line sepsis and pulmonary infarction.

It is often reasonable to leave the lines in place longer, for physiologic monitoring. Although it is recommended that a Swan-Ganz catheter not be left in situ longer than 48 to 72 hours, it can be changed over a guidewire if necessary. Postoperative ECG was performed because it is not uncommon to see a perioperative myocardial

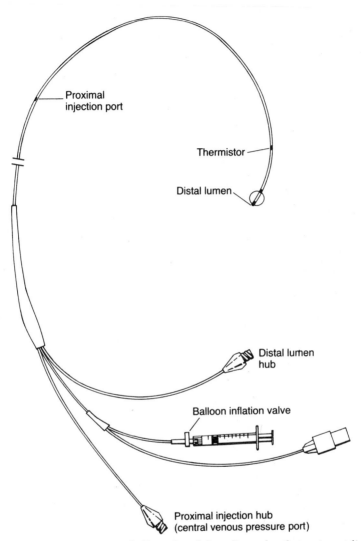

Figure 17–1. The Swan-Ganz is a balloon-tipped flow-directed catheter. A port lies in the right atrium to measure CVP. Moreover, iced saline can be injected through the CVP port to determine cardiac output by means of the thermodilution technique. When the balloon is inflated, the flow of blood in the right side of the heart pushes the catheter through the tricuspid valve, and then through the right ventricle and pulmonary artery into the right or left pulmonary artery. With the balloon inflated, the catheter wedges in a small vessel of the pulmonary circulation, and antegrade blood flow ceases. Thus, the pulmonary capillary wedge pressure is a reflection of left atrial pressure. In other words, the pressures in the left heart are estimated by performing right-sided heart catheterization, which obviates catheterizing the left side through the systemic arterial tree.

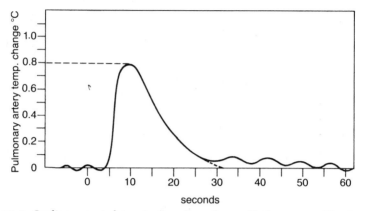

Figure 17-2. Cardiac output determination from thermodilution curve. The Swan-Ganz catheter has at its tip a thermistor that measures the temperature at the tip. This temperature decreases as the bolus of injected cold saline passes by the catheter tip. The computer takes the integral of the area under the curve and calculates cardiac output. When a pulmonary artery catheter with the ability to measure continuous mixed venous oxygen saturation is used, continuous cardiac outputs can be calculated and displayed if the arterial oxygen saturation is also measured with a pulse oximeter.

infarction in a patient who has suffered the hemodynamic insult of a ruptured abdominal aortic aneurysm. By stating that the pedal pulses were present, the resident has made a comment about the status of the peripheral vascular system in this patient, whose abdominal aorta has been replaced by a Dacron graft. It is often possible to achieve palpable peripheral pulses in patients with aneurysmal disease, because often they do not have associated significant peripheral arterial occlusive disease.

Respiratory System

Next, the respiratory system is dealt with in the daily ICU note. It is obvious that the cardiovascular and respiratory systems are inextricably interwoven. It will become apparent, shortly, that this is true of the other physiologic systems as well and that a derangement in one system can cause dysfunction of the others.

Subjective. Again, the fact that the patient is intubated forces a caregiver to be brief when eliciting subjective complaints, but the fact that the patient has no air hunger is significant. This patient has remained on the respirator since the first postoperative night because he has a large incision, and upper abdominal surgery can diminish respiratory function by approximately 70%. This occurs because incision pain prevents the patient from coughing and breathing deep, predisposing to atelectasis and retained secretions. In addition, the anesthetic agents and muscle relaxants decrease the force of respiration, again causing atelectasis and retained secretions.

Objective. There are various ways of ventilating a patient. *Assist/ control* is the mode in which the respirator delivers a preset tidal

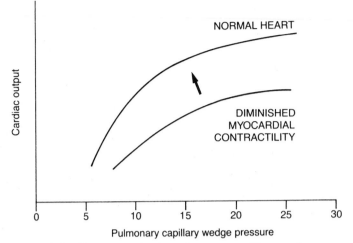

Figure 17–3. Frank-Starling curve. As the pulmonary capillary wedge pressure (which reflects left atrial pressure) increases, cardiac output increases. In a failing heart, the increment in cardiac output for each increment in wedge pressure is smaller. A positive inotropic agent may help to put the patient's heart on a more favorable curve.

Pulmonary capillary wedge pressure estimates left atrial pressure, which estimates left ventricular end-diastolic pressure, which roughly correlates with left ventricular end-diastolic volume. It is this latter measurement that most closely determines cardiac output. Left ventricular end-diastolic volume can be measured with transesophageal echocardiography.

volume to the patient at a preset minimum number of breaths per minute. In addition, every time the patient makes even a minimal respiratory effort, the machine "kicks in" and delivers the preset tidal volume. The minute ventilation is the product of the tidal volume and the respiratory rate. If the preset tidal volume and respiratory rate are large enough, the minute volume will be adequate to maintain P_{CO_2} in the physiologic range, even if the patient's own respiratory muscles are not strong enough to generate adequate tidal volume.

The ventilatory mode called *intermittent mandatory ventilation* (IMV) consists of delivering a preset tidal volume a minimum number of times per minute. The patient is allowed to take extra breaths, as determined by his respiratory drive, but the machine does not "kick in" for these extra breaths when it is in the IMV mode. Thus, when the number of breaths the machine delivers is decreased, the patient is forced to maintain adequate ventilation by generating an adequate tidal volume at an adequate number of times per minute. If he cannot do this, his P_{CO_2} rises because P_{CO_2} is a reflection of ventilation.

Possible advantages of IMV over assist/control ventilation are that IMV causes less barotrauma, it may be less deleterious to venous return to the right heart, it may cause less ventilation-perfusion mismatch, and it may cause less atrophy of the respiratory muscles. SIMV implies that the respirator *synchronizes* the breaths it delivers with those of the patient, to improve comfort. In pressure support ventilation, spontaneous inspiratory effort of the patient is supplemented by added gas flow to overcome the work of breathing caused by the ventilator and tubing. If the pressure support administered is greater than the work of breathing caused by the machine, one cannot predict that the patient will breathe adequately after discontinuation of the ventilator.

Assessment and Plan. An upper abdominal incision can compromise respiratory function by 70% because it hurts so much to cough and sigh that the patient is unable to mobilize secretions and keep the alveoli open. He may thus retain secretions and develop atelectasis with hypoxia and hypercapnia and require emergency reintubation. The signs of this are agitation, hypertension, and tachycardia (i.e., signs of increased catecholamine release due to an important and primitive reflex). In this example, the patient's arterial blood gases were adequate on assist/control ventilation, there was nothing in his past medical history (no chronic obstructive pulmonary disease, no restrictive lung disease) to suggest that the patient would be unable to breathe on his own on postoperative day 1, weaning parameters (see below) were adequate, and the patient was thus placed on CPAP 5 (continuous positive airway pressure of 5 cm H_2O). This is nothing more than a T piece through which the patient can breathe spontaneously (receiving no breaths from the machine), but with a valve that causes positive airway pressure to be present at all times, minimizing atelectasis. The patient does the work of ventilation; the CPAP keeps the alveoli open at end-expiration. If ventilation is adequate for a time on CPAP (i.e., the respiratory rate is not too rapid and the $Paco_2$ does not rise above physiologic limits), it suggests that the patient may be strong enough to tolerate extubation

Respiratory parameters (spontaneous tidal volume, vital capacity, and forced inspiratory pressure) can be obtained with a spirometer to help predict whether the patient will tolerate weaning from the respirator.

The *tidal volume* represents a normal inspiration followed by a normal expiration, and the patient should have a tidal volume of 5 ml/kg to have a reasonable expectation of being able to tolerate extubation.

The *vital capacity* represents maximal inspiration followed by a maximal expiration, and along with tidal volume it can be measured with a spirometer. The vital capacity should be 15 ml/kg before extubation is considered.

The *forced inspiratory pressure* (also known as *negative inspiratory force*) is the negative pressure that can be generated by forceful inspiration and the value should be less than -25 mm Hg to make weaning possible. Parameters in this range are required for the patient to generate a large enough cough and sigh to clear secretions and prevent atelectasis. In this case, the patient's parameters fall into a satisfactory range, and since the patient's arterial blood gases were satisfactory on CPAP of 5 cm H_2O, the plan is to remove the endotracheal tube, giving supplemental oxygen by face mask without positive-pressure ventilation. If the PCO_2 had risen on CPAP of 5, the patient would be hypoventilating and would therefore need to be placed back on positive-pressure ventilation.

During the weaning process, oxygen saturation can be monitored on a real-time basis by using pulse oximetry in which oxyhemoglobin saturation is determined by an apparatus placed on the finger. Pco_2 can be measured on a real-time basis by a mass spectrometer (a device that measures the end-tidal Pco_2, which correlates nicely with the arterial Pco_2). Thus, an increase in Pco_2 reflecting hypoventilation can be determined early.

Extubation in the face of inadequate parameters exposes the patient to possible emergency reintubation if respiratory insufficiency should result from retained secretions and atelectasis. Again, encouraging coughing and deep breathing and incentive spirometry help to prevent postoperative pneumonia and atelectasis. Early ambulation (on the first postoperative night or first postoperative day) not only helps to prevent atelectasis and pneumonia but probably reduces the possibility of developing deep vein thrombosis.

Renal System

Subjective. Next, attention is turned to the renal system. The complaint of thirst may be an important clue that the patient is dehydrated, as receptors in the hypothalamus respond to hypertonicity, causing the sensation of thirst. This is a homeostatic mechanism, as it prompts the dehydrated patient to drink if he is able. It may suggest to the clinician that supplemental intravenous fluids are necessary for a patient who is NPO and is thus unable to manage his own fluid status.

Objective. Patients are frequently placed on normal saline or Ringer's lactated solution the first day after aortic surgery, because they lose serum into the retroperitoneum secondary to the surgeon's dissection, and the volume can best be repleted with a solution, such as saline or Ringer's, whose salt content approaches that of serum. Thereafter, the daily fluid requirement is determined by adding up *maintenance requirements, initial deficit,* and *ongoing losses.*

The maintenance fluid requirement is the fluid the patient would require were he NPO with no abnormal losses such as nasogastric drainage and no preexisting deficits like those a patient would have who had been vomiting for a week before admission. The volume of the maintenance fluid requirement is the sum of urine output, fecal water loss, perspiration, and insensible losses and is related to body surface area. Since the ratio of body surface area to body weight is greatest in small children and small adults and does decrease with increasing weight, the maintenance fluid requirement does not increase linearly with weight. The formula for calculating maintenance fluid requirements over a 24-hour period is as follows:

100 ml/kg for the first 10 kg
50 ml/kg for the next 10 kg
20 ml/kg thereafter

In addition, maintenance fluid requirement over 24 hours is increased 7 ml/kg/°F above normal. Thus, when this patient reaches the point at which there are no ongoing losses (such as extravasation of serum into the retroperitoneum or loss of nasogastric tube drainage) and if he weighs 70 kg and his temperature averages 101°F, his maintenance requirement will be:

100 ml/kg × 10 kg = 1000 ml
50 ml/kg × 10 kg = 500 ml
20 ml/kg × 50 kg = 1000 ml
70 kg = 2500 ml   24-hour maintenance fluid requirement if the patient is afebrile

7 ml × 70 kg × 2 degrees F = 980 ml

Therefore, the maintenance fluid requirement in this patient who has undergone resection of an abdominal aortic aneurysm would be approximately 3500 ml in 24 hours when he reaches a point at which there are no abnormal fluid losses and his temperature averages 101°F.

Maintenance requirements for sodium and potassium are 30 mEq/L and 20 mEq/L, respectively. Since the sodium content of D5-¼ NS would approximate 30 mEq/L, this patient's maintenance requirement would be approximated by infusing D5-¼ NS + 20 mEq of KCl per liter at 150 ml per hour for 24 hours, which would provide 3600 ml in 24 hours. If the patient is afebrile, the intravenous rate could be set at 100 ml per hour, which would provide 2400 ml per 24 hours. If the patient is having significant nasogastric losses, they could be replaced volume for volume every 8-hour shift with D5-½ NS, a solution that approaches gastric juice in electrolyte content.

Once the intravenous fluids are ordered, one must continue to monitor the patient's fluid status closely and to adjust the fluids as necessary. Manifestations of hypovolemia include oliguria and tachycardia early and hypotension later, as the sympathetic response to hypovolemia causes an outpouring of catecholamines. These compounds increase the heart rate to improve cardiac output and cause constriction of the afferent arterioles in the kidney to conserve intravascular volume. Poor skin turgor, dry mucous membranes, and, in an infant, sunken fontaneles can suggest hypovolemia.

If a Swan-Ganz catheter is in place, low pulmonary capillary wedge pressure may suggest hypovolemia. Dyspnea may be a symptom of overhydration and congestive heart failure. Signs of overhydration include bibasilar rales, wheezes (so-called *cardiac asthma,* which can be an early manifestation of congestive heart failure), neck vein distention, hepatojugular reflux, a ventricular diastolic gallop (S3), and pedal or sacral edema. Steady weight gain over the course of several days may alert the astute doctor to the fact that the patient is in positive fluid balance and may allow correction of the situation before the patient develops frank pulmonary edema. Running totals of input and output (allowing for insensible losses) since admission may also be helpful. It must be noted, however, that the fluid administered often seeps into the interstitium or a "third space" such as the peritoneal cavity, requiring a positive fluid balance and increased weight to maintain a filling pressure (e.g., PCWP) that is high enough to allow adequate cardiac output and tissue perfusion.

A central venous pressure (CVP) reading may provide some information at the extremes. A patient with a CVP of 0 is unlikely to be overhydrated, and a patient with a CVP of 14 is unlikely to be underhydrated. One must remember, however, that the CVP does not accurately reflect action of the left side of the heart, and a patient may be in florid left ventricular failure with a normal central venous pressure. This is because there is great compliance on the right side of the heart, so that a massive amount of fluid can be accommodated in the venous system. Thus tremendous changes in volume may be met with only minor changes of pressure on the right side of the heart. Compliance on the left side of the circulation is much less, so changes in volume are manifested more quickly as changes in pressure, making the left atrial pressure as approximated by the pulmonary capillary wedge pressure a more accurate reflection of left heart action. The wedge pressure rises as intravascular volume increases. A rational plan of fluid management is formulated and ordered, as outlined, but one must constantly monitor the fluid balance in critically ill patients and alter the orders according to the values of the aforementioned parameters. The interrelationship between the cardiovascular, respiratory, and renal systems is obvious in the next example.

Gastrointestinal System

Strict attention must be given to the gastrointestinal system in critically ill patients, and this includes meticulous attention to the patient's nutritional status. As previously emphasized, each physiologic system is inextricably interwoven with the others, and a derangement in one can cause derangements in one or many of the others. For example, a low-flow state like that that might occur with cardiogenic shock can cause a nonocclusive mesenteric infarction, as blood is shunted away from the splanchnic circulation in this situation. This can cause gangrene of the entire midgut from the jejunum to the distal third of the transverse colon.

Another example of a derangement in one system's causing a derangement in another would be development of bleeding stress ulcers in a patient with respiratory failure. If surgery is required to stem the bleeding from stress ulceration, mortality and morbidity are increased. Conversely, if there is "GI failure," such as one might see with anastomotic disruption, the syndrome of multisystem failure can ensue, with the constellation of respiratory failure, heart failure, renal failure, and hepatic insufficiency. Moreover, it is the gut through which people obtain nutrition, and it is well-known that when a surgical patient is malnourished, sepsis is more likely to occur. Sepsis is also frequently the underlying cause in multisystem failure.

In a patient who has just undergone resection of an abdominal aortic aneurysm, it is likely that peristalsis will return in several days, allowing the patient to eat and thus to maintain his own nutritional status. However, some patients may develop prolonged ileus after aortic surgery, perhaps because of blood in the retroperitoneum, and the nutritional status of these patients may be problematic.

Subjective. The subjective data base is important in evaluating the gastrointestinal system. Abdominal pain, nausea, or vomiting can signal a problem arising in this system. Cramping abdominal pain can, however, signal the return of peristalsis. Hunger is a good sign.

Objective. The critically ill patient is examined frequently for abdominal tenderness, rebound, and involuntary guarding, any of which may signal that peritonitis has occurred. Abdominal distention may indicate ileus or the evolution of mechanical small bowel obstruction, whereas tympany in the left upper abdominal quadrant suggests acute gastric dilatation. After resection of an abdominal aortic aneurysm, bloody diarrhea should prompt suspicion of ischemic colitis. This can occur, albeit uncommonly, because of sacrifice of the inferior mesenteric artery at the time of aneurysmorrhaphy if the remainder of the visceral vessels are also narrowed. A dropping hematocrit or blood in the nasogastric tube can indicate upper gastrointestinal bleeding from stress ulceration.

Assessment and Plan. The surgeon must determine whether normal gastrointestinal function is likely to return soon. If not, total parenteral nutrition may be necessary to ensure that malnutrition, and its associated anergy, do not occur. If the gastrointestinal tract is functioning but the patient is unable to eat because of CNS depression or the presence of an endotracheal tube, enteral tube feedings are preferred over total parenteral nutrition because enteral feeding provides energy substrate to the gut mucosa. It may also be cheaper and have less complications; however, judgment is required because if GI function is marginal, vomiting with aspiration of GI contents causing aspiration pneumonia increases morbidity and mortality.

Central Nervous System

The progress note on the first postoperative day for this patient does not reflect any central nervous system abnormalities. However, it is important to consider this system in a critically ill patient so that any deviations from homeostasis can be quickly identified.

Subjective. The patient should be questioned for symptoms such as headache, dizziness, and diplopia. Visual hallucinations suggestive of delirium tremens from alcohol withdrawal are part of the subjective data base.

Objective. The patient's mental status as determined by the examiner is part of the objective data base. That this patient is "alert and responsive to commands" is useful information. It is important to describe the level of consciousness in terms of things the patient can do, instead of using vague terms such as *stuporous, comatose,* or *semicomatose,* which can have different meanings to different observers. To say that the patient knows his name, where he is, and the day of the month is specific and can be a useful parameter to follow. Clearly, a patient who can follow simple commands is functioning at a higher level of consciousness than a patient who responds, but only inappropriately, to noxious stimuli. The objective data base on this patient includes the fact that he moves all four extremities well, suggesting that there are no gross focal motor abnormalities. One might also check the deep tendon reflexes and attempt to elicit pathologic reflexes.

Assessment and Plan. The underlying cause of a central nervous system abnormality is sought in a systematic fashion. The patient in a critical care unit may develop "ICU psychosis," which may be caused at least in part by sensory deprivation, inability of the patient to follow his usual routine, anxiety over being very sick, and separation from family. In the modern ICU measures to minimize these pressures include providing music or television when possible, following a comprehensible schedule with lights on during the day and off at night, serving three meals on a regular schedule to patients who are able to eat, providing wall clocks and windows if possible, and having unlimited visiting hours. These elements of normalcy that encourage psychological recovery often take on added importance because the patient's defense mechanism can be weakened by toxic-metabolic derangements in one or several of the physiologic systems or by drugs that alter the sensorium.

Patients with inadequate cardiac output may exhibit confusion because of poor cerebral perfusion, and if there is superimposed carotid artery narrowing due to atherosclerosis, a cerebrovascular accident (frank stroke) may ensue. Hypoxia resulting from respiratory insufficiency can certainly cause confusion and agitation. Hyponatremia caused by inability of the kidney to regulate the amount of free water can result in mental obtundation, as can a hyperosmolar state like those associated with patients on total parenteral nutrition who develop hyperglycemic, hyperosmolar nonketotic coma. Hepatic insufficiency can result in hepatic encephalopathy, and sepsis can produce mental obtundation in and of itself. Hypoglycemia can cause unconsciousness along with permanent central nervous system damage. Again, the interdependence of the various physiologic systems becomes apparent. Analgesics and sedative-hypnotics required by these critically ill patients can also produce confusion, agitation, or somnolence, often requiring discontinuation or alteration in dose.

Endocrine System

One must consider the endocrine system when writing a daily progress note on a surgical patient in the ICU, as failure to do so may cause an important imbalance to be overlooked. The known diabetic who undergoes surgery may require an increase in insulin dose because of the stress of surgery with its attendant outpouring of catecholamines and glucocorticoids, and a diabetic whose disease was previously controlled by diet or oral hypoglycemics may require insulin for the first time. One must always remember, however, that hypoglycemia is much more dangerous than hyperglycemia as it can cause permanent brain damage, and thus, must be carefully guarded against. Intravenous hyperalimentation, with its increased glucose load, may necessitate use of exogenous insulin to facilitate entry of glucose into the cells, and failure to take this into account and to monitor blood sugar levels can lead to hyperglycemic, hyperosmolar nonketotic coma in a patient taking parenteral nutrition. The fact that a *glucose intolerance* of new onset can signal incipient *sepsis* should be noted.

Another endocrine abnormality for which one must be vigilant is *hypoadrenalism*. Many patients take exogenous glucocorticoids (e.g., prednisone) for conditions such as asthma or inflammatory bowel disease. If they have been taking these agents within the past year, they may have suppression of the hypothalamic-pituitary-adrenal axis and be unable to secrete the greater amounts of glucocorticoids necessary to compensate for increased stress. This can result in addisonian crisis, a potentially life-threatening problem characterized by fever, nausea, vomiting, abdominal pain, hypotension, and tachycardia. Accordingly, patients who have been taking steroids within the last year are routinely covered with a "steroid prep" of 300 mg of hydrocortisone per day in the perioperative period. Hypoadrenalism should be suspected and exogenous glucocorticoid administration considered when any patient develops circulatory collapse of indeterminate cause. The cause of the addisonian crisis could be unrecognized glucocorticoid ingestion during the past year or damage to the adrenal glands (e.g., by hemorrhage into them from sepsis, shock, or trauma).

Hyperthyroidism can result in atrial fibrillation of new onset and can be the cause of high-output heart failure. Conversely, hypothyroidism can cause mental deterioration or cardiorespiratory dysfunction. These diagnoses will be overlooked in critically ill surgical patients unless the physician maintains a reasonable index of suspicion.

Interpretation of thyroid function tests in critically ill patients may be difficult because of "euthyroid sick syndrome." In this entity, the abnormal thyroid function results may be an adaptive mechanism rather than an abnormality that requires treatment.

Hepatobiliary System. The hepatobiliary system should be carefully monitored and its status recorded in the daily progress note of the surgical patient in the ICU. Abnormalities of the hepatobiliary system may be prehepatic (from increased pigment load), hepatocellular, or posthepatic (from bile duct obstruction). Prehepatic jaundice may be caused by hemolysis of any cause (e.g., a hemolytic transfusion reaction) or resorption of an excess load of pigment from a resorbing intraabdominal or retroperitoneal hematoma. Hepatocellular disease can be preexisting, as in a patient with alcoholic cirrhosis, or it can be caused by the ongoing disease process or its treatment. Some of the inhalational anesthetic agents are believed to cause liver damage, if uncommonly. Hepatitis can certainly be transmitted via blood transfusion. It is now well-known that sepsis can cause hepatic insufficiency, probably because the endotoxins lower the liver's threshold for hypoxic damage, and this may be an important component of multisystem failure.

Postoperative obstructive jaundice can occur after iatrogenic injury to the common duct. This would be unlikely in association with aortic surgery and more likely after biliary tract or gastric surgery. *Acalculous cholecystitis* can occur in the postoperative period, probably because the gallbladder does not empty in the fasting state and so becomes distended. The increased tension can cause ischemia of the gallbladder wall with necrosis, especially when cardiac output is down as a result of dehydration. The exact cause of acalculous cholecystitis is a matter of speculation. Postoperative acalculous cholecystitis is particularly treacherous because it can be difficult to diagnose in postlaparotomy patients, as abdominal pain and tenderness are to be expected, and fever and ileus not unusual. The fact that the signs and symptoms of postoperative cholecystitis can be as vague as "failing to rebound from the initial surgery" compounds the difficulty of diagnosis, which may not be made until biliary sepsis intervenes. It is not clear how acute cholecystitis of any sort can cause jaundice, even in the absence of a common bile duct stone, but it can, perhaps because of the effects of sepsis on the liver or compression of the bile duct by the distended gallbladder. Acalculous cholecystitis can be treated by open or laparoscopic cholecystectomy, cholecystostomy (placing a tube in the gallbladder) under local anesthesia, or percutaneous drainage under ultrasound or CT guidance.

Hematologic System. Many aspects of the hematologic system must be followed in the surgical patient. The hemoglobin and hematocrit are important values that may drop with blood loss once the fluid compartments have time to equilibrate and interstitial fluid enters the vascular compartment. It is widely known that hemoglobin and hematocrit values can be normal early in acute blood loss, even if it is massive, since hemodilution has not yet had time to occur. Blood may be lost acutely into the abdomen, chest, or thigh after trauma or surgery. Blood lost into the chest is readily apparent on chest x-ray. It is not possible to lose enough blood into the cranial vault to cause hemodynamic instability or for the hematocrit to drop without first developing neurologic deterioration from increased intracranial pressure. Blood can be lost into the lumen of the gut over time, causing drops in hemoglobin and hematocrit. When the bleeding is slow, it may not be readily apparent that the blood is being lost into the GI tract. One can sometimes make the diagnosis of upper GI bleeding from, for example, stress ulceration or acute hemorrhagic gastritis by passing an NG tube in search of "coffee ground" aspirate. The hematocrit can also be low from hemolysis or bone marrow suppression. There is no conclusive evidence that there is such a thing as an optimal hematocrit value; however, it is common practice to keep the hematocrit about 30% and the hemoglobin about 10 g, on the assumption that this will help to ensure a adequate oxygen-carrying capacity.

Some advocate allowing the hemoglobin to fall even lower than 10 g, predicated on the concept that this will result in decreased viscosity with improved tissue perfusion and thus avoid subjecting the patient to the dangers of transfusion and preserve a precious resource, blood. It must be realized, however, that cardiac output, hemoglobin, oxygen saturation, and the oxyhemoglobin dissociation curve determine oxygen delivery to the tissues and the hemoglobin may be easier than the other factors to increase significantly. The relationship between oxygen demand at the cellular level and oxygen delivery is an important therapeutic end point.

The white blood count may be elevated over 10,000 when infection is present, and this may be associated with a leftward shift in the differential (more segs and bands and fewer lymphocytes). It is widely known, however, that overwhelming sepsis can actually cause leukopenia.

Platelet number can be decreased in *diffuse intravascular coagulation* (DIC). This is a consumptive coagulopathy in which clotting factors and platelets are consumed in an overvigorous process of thrombus formation and fibrinolysis, frequently triggered by sepsis and manifested by diffuse bleeding from surgical wounds and raw surfaces, venipuncture sites, and mucosal surfaces. The resultant intravascular thrombus formation can also result in ischemic damage to end organs. In addition to thrombocytopenia (decreased platelet number), there is usually prolongation of the prothrombin and partial thromboplastin times, a decrease in fibrinogen level, and an increase in fibrin degradation products and D-dimer (a product of the degradation of cross-linked fibrin). Some investigators have, paradoxically, tried to treat DIC with intravenous heparin or by administering clotting factors in the form of fresh-frozen plasma or cryoprecipitate, but the most important treatment is to eliminate the underlying cause, such as sepsis from an intraabdominal abscess.

Other causes of thrombocytopenia include hypersplenism from portal hypertension or leukemia, immune thrombocytopenic purpura, thrombotic thrombocytopenic purpura, dilution from massive transfusion, and bone marrow depression from cytotoxic drugs. Platelets may be accreted onto intravascular devices like a prosthetic graft or intraaortic balloon pump. Normally, undue bleeding does not occur until the platelet count goes below 50,000; platelet transfusions are not usually given until this level is reached. Patients with immune thrombocytopenic purpura may have immature platelets in the peripheral circulation. These are efficient, and even smaller numbers of the young platelets may be sufficient for clot formation. Qualitative platelet abnormalities such as those seen in renal failure, or ingestion of aspirin or NSAIDS may be corrected by administration of desmopressin (DDAVP). Hypothermia can cause a qualitative platelet abnormality and must be avoided by using a rapid infuser/warmer during resuscitation. IV fluids are at room temperature (25°C), and banked blood may be at 4°C while body temperature is 37.5°C, necessitating the use of the warmer during rapid infusion.

Patients taking broad-spectrum antibiotics may have decreased numbers of bacteria in the gut, bacteria that are responsible for vitamin K production. In addition, with extrahepatic biliary obstruction insufficient bile may be delivered to the intestines to emulsify fat, and the resultant inability to absorb fat may prevent absorption of fat-soluble vitamins such as vitamin K. Both of these phenomena can result in prolonged prothrombin and partial thromboplastin times because of the inability of the liver to make the vitamin K–dependent clotting factors II, VII, IX, and X. Both problems can be corrected by parenteral administration of vitamin K, whereas clotting abnormalities resulting from hepatocellular disease cannot be so corrected and may require administration of fresh-frozen plasma.

Infectious. Category 9 in the daily ICU progress note is *Infectious disease*. Although this is the only category that is not a physiologic system (the immune system, with which microorganisms interact *is* a system), it is an exceedingly important category because serious infection can cause septicemia and sequential failure of the other systems (multisystem organ failure). Even with our sophisticated techniques of supporting the various physiologic systems, the patient will have an inexorable downhill course if the underlying infection cannot be eradicated. In addition, derangements in many of the other physiologic systems can predispose to infection, also demonstrating the interdependence of the various systems.

The case of the second patient discussed in this chapter illustrates the process of multisystem failure. The patient is typical of those who are likely to have a protracted stay in the surgical ICU. He has uncontrolled sepsis and failure of several physiologic systems, each requiring sophisticated supportive measures. These supportive measures will avail nothing unless the underlying septic process can be eradicated. The progress note is an example of one that might be written for such a patient.

CASE 17–2

Multisystem Failure

This is the first ICU day for a 59-year-old man admitted from the surgical floor last night in respiratory distress, 6 days after resection of the sigmoid colon with primary anastomosis for carcinoma. Mild hypertension is the only associated preexisting problem.

Problem 1: Cardiovascular

Subjective: No chest pain.
Objective: No jugular venous distention or sacral edema. Pulse 124 and regular. BP, now 112/60. A Swan-Ganz catheter was placed last night on admission to the ICU. Wedge pressure at that time was 3 mm Hg with cardiac output of 7 L per minute and low total peripheral resistance. The patient's blood pressure and urine output are being maintained on dopamine at 300 μg per minute (5 μg/kg body weight per minute). There is ST-T wave depression in the lateral precordial leads.
Assessment: High cardiac output and low total peripheral resistance due to sepsis; low wedge pressure due to low total peripheral resistance in addition to intravascular volume depletion.
Plan: Maintain cardiac output by volume expansion and positive inotropic agents like dopamine. Try to identify and treat underlying cause of sepsis. Cardiac enzymes and serial ECGs to evaluate for an associated myocardial infarction, which may have been precipitated by the septic episode.

Problem 2: Respiratory

Subjective: No evidence of air hunger while on the ventilator.
Objective: Lungs clear to auscultation. No cyanosis. Arterial blood gases reveal PaO_2 of 74 mm Hg, $PaCO_2$ of 38 mm Hg, and pH of 7.25 on the ventilator with assist/control of 10, tidal volume of 720 ml, FIO_2 of 40%, and PEEP of 5 cm H_2O. Chest x-ray reveals bilateral fluffy infiltrates. Endotracheal tube is in good position above carina, and Swan-Ganz catheter is in the right pulmonary artery.
Assessment: Probable ARDS due to sepsis, with right-to-left shunt causing arterial oxygen desaturation.

Plan: Support respiration with supplemental oxygen, positive-pressure ventilation, and PEEP. Seek cause of ARDS (suspect sepsis) and attempt to eradicate.

Problem 3: Renal

Subjective: No entry.
Objective: Urine output 15 ml per hour for 2 hours; increased to 30 ml per hour after volume expansion and institution of inotropic agent (dopamine). BUN 44, creatinine 1.6.
Assessment: Prerenal azotemia due to inadequate renal perfusion.
Plan: Expand volume to maintain renal perfusion. Dopamine at this dosage should help by increasing cardiac output (and thus renal perfusion) without causing vasoconstriction.

Problem 4: GI/nutritional

Subjective: Complaining of nausea, vomiting, and left lower quadrant abdominal pain.
Objective: Moderate left lower quadrant abdominal tenderness. No involuntary guarding or generalized rebound. Mild distention. Bowel sounds hypoactive. CT shows intraabdominal abscess.
Assessment: Possible disruption of the anastomosis as the source of sepsis and resultant multisystem failure.
Plan: Follow temperature curve. Serial examinations and white counts. Needs broad-spectrum antibiotics and percutaneous drainage under CT guidance. NPO and NG tube to help decompress GI tract and prevent vomiting and aspiration. Institute total parenteral nutrition.

Problem 5: Central nervous system

Subjective: No entry.
Objective: Receiving IV morphine to help tolerate respirator. Responds appropriately to noxious stimuli.
Assessment: Level of consciousness depressed because of narcotics and systemic toxicity from sepsis.
Plan: Heel pads to prevent pressure sores. Turn from side to side every 2 hours to prevent sacral decubitus ulcers.

Problem 6: Endocrine

Subjective: No entry.
Objective: Blood sugar 150 mg/100 ml.
Assessment: No evidence of glucose intolerance at present.
Plan: Monitor blood sugars.

Problem 7: Hepatobiliary

Subjective: No entry.
Objective: Sclera appear icteric. Total bilirubin 3.4, with alkaline phosphatase of 130, LDH of 400, SGOT of 120.
Assessment: Probably hepatic dysfunction from sepsis.
Plan: Follow liver function tests. May need IV hyperalimentation solution rich in branched-chain amino acids and low in aromatic amino acids.

Problem 8: Hematologic

Subjective: No entry.
Objective: Hematocrit 33%, white blood cell count 3400 with 90% polys, 3% bands, and 7% lymphocytes.
Assessment: Hematocrit adequate. Low white count may be caused by overwhelming sepsis.
Plan: Serial CBCs.

Problem 9: Infectious disease

Subjective: Wife states patient is complaining of chills.
Objective: Has been spiking fevers to 101.5°F for past 2 nights. Blood cultures growing gram-negative rods. Rectal exam shows fluctuant mass in pelvis. CT suggests pericolic abscess.
Assessment: Probably has an intraabdominal septic focus without peritonitis.
Plan: Percutaneous drainage under CT guidance. Reoperate if percutaneous drainage unsuccessful or if peritonitis occurs. IV antibiotics, including gentamicin, ampicillin, and Flagyl.

*Signed*_____

DISCUSSION OF CASE 17–2

Complications of colon surgery can be responsible for significant morbidity and mortality and can be the cause of a protracted stay in the ICU. This patient has multiple system failure. If he is to survive, each system must be supported until the underlying cause can be eradicated.

Cardiovascular

Subjective. This patient had no subjective complaint of chest pain to signal myocardial infarction. A perioperative myocardial infarction can often be silent, however, and communication with an intubated patient may be difficult.

Objective. This patient's cardiovascular system is manifesting the typical changes of sepsis, with high cardiac output, low total peripheral resistance, and low wedge pressure. The high cardiac output partially compensates for the fact that extraction of oxygen by the tissues is decreased with sepsis, partly because of left-to-right shunts away from the nutrient vessels and partly because of a cellular derangement that interferes with oxygen consumption, resulting in a shift to anaerobic metabolism. This causes an increase in mixed venous Po_2 and promotes lactic acidosis. The low pulmonary capillary wedge pressure is caused partly by the low total peripheral resistance and partly by the fact that these patients are often dehydrated because of vomiting, fever, hypovolemia from inadequate PO or IV intake, or peritonitis with loss of fluid into the peritoneal cavity (third-space loss). The bacterial endotoxins are thought to release a myocardial depressant factor that has a negative inotropic effect. By the time cardiac output is low, rather than high, the patient is probably in irreversible septic shock. With sepsis the systemic blood pressure may initially be normal; however, peripheral vasodilatation with low total peripheral resistance, coupled with decreased cardiac output from hypovolemia or myocardial depressant factor, can ultimately cause hypotension. It must be emphasized that the high cardiac output seen in sepsis is a homeostatic mechanism, and in such patients it is worrisome when the cardiac output falls into the so-called normal range.

Assessment and Plan. The resident who wrote this progress note recognized that volume expansion and inotropic agents might help to support the cardiovascular system in this patient with sepsis, but that eradication of the underlying cause would ultimately be necessary for survival.

Respiratory System

Subjective. Since the patient is intubated, he may not be able to report that he has "air hunger." His hypoxia may be manifested by tachycardia, tachypnea, agitation, or hypertension.

Objective. Adult respiratory distress syndrome (ARDS) is caused by the response of the lungs to sepsis or other insults such as trauma, pancreatitis, inhaled toxins, aspiration of stomach contents, or massive transfusion. Presumably, with sepsis the endotoxins released by the bacteria interfere with surfactant, the surface-active agent that prevents the alveoli from collapsing under physiologic conditions. Interference with surfactant causes "stiff lungs" (decreased compliance) and microatelectasis with right-to-left shunting, producing arterial oxygen desaturation (venous admixture), a phenomenon that occurs when alveoli are perfused but not ventilated. Complement-mediated sequestration of white blood cells in the lung may play a role in the pulmonary insult of ARDS. There may be increased capillary leak with "wet lungs." An inciting insult, bilateral fluffy infiltrates on chest x-ray, arterial hypoxemia (e.g., PaO_2–FIO_2 ratio less than 200) and a PCWP that is not so elevated as to suggest left ventricular failure all suggest ARDS.

Assessment and Plan. The treatment of ARDS is usually institution of PEEP to prevent the alveoli from collapsing. A PaO_2 of 74 mm Hg on an FIO_2 of 40% is adequate for oxygen delivery, but it indicates a significant right-to-left shunt. The pH of 7.25 with a normal $PaCO_2$ indicates metabolic acidosis (not compensated by hyperventilation), presumably caused by lactic acid production from sepsis. Again, the resident writing this progress note recognized that the underlying theme is undrained sepsis, and although oxygenation can be temporarily supported with positive-pressure ventilation with increased concentration of oxygen in the inspired gases and PEEP, the septic focus must be eradicated if the patient is to survive.

Renal System

Subjective. Thirst, the subjective manifestation of hypovolemia, was not elicited in this intubated patient.

Objective. Hypovolemia or decreased cardiac output of any cause results in prerenal azotemia. The juxtaglomerular apparatus "sees" a contracted intravascular volume and stimulates the renin-angiotensin-aldosterone axis, causing resorption of salt and water. The rising BUN and creatinine values, and a BUN-creatinine ratio greater than 20:1 in this patient suggest prerenal azotemia.

Assessment and Plan. Hypovolemia and sepsis are more likely than hypovolemia alone (e.g., hemorrhagic shock) to result in acute renal failure. In this patient, oliguria necessitated volume expansion to improve renal perfusion. In some patients with myocardial depression from sepsis or with underlying coronary artery or valvular disease, volume expansion results in hydrostatic pulmonary edema with increased right-to-left shunt, resulting in hypoxia. A positive inotropic agent such as dopamine can selectively dilate the renal arterioles in small doses (2 µg/kg/min), and with larger doses (about 5 µg/kg/min) may have a positive inotropic effect, increasing cardiac output and improving renal perfusion. When dopamine is given in excess of above 5 to 10 µg/kg/min, it can have primarily an alpha effect, raising blood pressure by increasing systemic vascular resistance but actually having a deleterious effect on the kidneys and other organs and tissue beds secondary to vasoconstriction and ischemia. If acute tubular necrosis should occur, the patient can be supported with either hemodialysis or peritoneal dialysis; however, as more physiologic systems become involved, management becomes more complicated, and a patient with multisystem failure will not survive unless the underlying cause is eradicated.

Gastrointestinal System

Subjective. Nausea, vomiting, and abdominal pain are symptoms that can suggest a gastrointestinal derangement.

Objective. The GI tract is involved in this case, because it is the site of suspected sepsis, as anastomotic disruption could account for the previously outlined constellation of findings in this patient. The tenderness on rectal examination and the CT findings suggest a pericolic abscess that will require percutaneous or operative drainage if the patient is to be saved. The GI tract can be involved in multisystem failure, even in patients whose source of sepsis lies elsewhere. For instance, critically ill patients are prone to develop upper GI bleeding from stress ulcers, and this can be prevented by keeping the pH of the stomach above 5.0 with hourly doses of antacid or with H_2 blockers. Alternatively, sucralfate can be used to protect the mucosa of the stomach. Acalculous cholecystitis must be considered when the condition of a patient with a critical illness deteriorates inexplicably. The early signs and symptoms may be vague, leading to delay in diagnosis. These patients may have prolonged ileus after abdominal surgery, and many are catabolic; total parenteral nutrition needs to be considered in this setting.

When enterocytes are deprived of substrate (e.g., glutamine) in patients who are NPO or when they are deprived of oxygen in patients with a low cardiac output state, they may lose their barrier capability between bacteria in the lumen of the gut and the bloodstream. Translocation of such bacteria from the gut to the blood can be the engine for continued sepsis, multisystem organ failure, and death, even when the underlying cause of sepsis can be eradicated. That is, once the process of sepsis has reached a certain point—liberation of cytokines and other mediators—the process may be irreversible.

Assessment and Plan. The derangement in the gastrointestinal system, disruption of a colonic anastomosis, is believed to be the underlying cause of this patient's multisystem failure. An intraabdominal abscess can sometimes be treated with percutaneous drainage under CT control. If the sepsis cannot be eradicated with percutaneous drainage or if generalized peritonitis occurs, laparotomy with drainage plus proximal stoma for diversion will be necessary.

Central Nervous System

There are many causes of mental obtundation in critical illness. Morphine administered to relieve pain and to help the patient tolerate the respirator can cause mental abnormalities. Decreased cardiac output, hypoxia, uremia, hepatic insufficiency, and sepsis all can decrease the level of consciousness. ICU psychosis or delirium tremens must also be considered as possible causes of altered mental status.

Hepatobiliary System

Objective. The elevations in liver function tests (bilirubin, SGPT, LDH) seen here are probably due to bacterial endotoxins' lowering the threshold of the liver to hypoxic damage. The liver is an organ difficult to support, and the protein load must not be too great if hepatic encephalopathy is to be avoided in patients with very poor liver function. Parenteral nutrition high in branched-chain amino acids and low in aromatic ones may lessen the risk of hepatic encephalopathy. Other complications of hepatic failure include inability to biometabolize drugs and toxins, coagulopathy, cerebral edema, renal failure (hepatorenal syndrome), portal hypertension with hypersplenism or bleeding esophageal varices, and impairment of the ability to clear infection owing to derangements in the liver's reticuloendothelial system.

Assessment and Plan. Although the sequelae of hepatic insufficiency can be minimized with nutritional supplements rich in branched-chain amino acids and low in aromatic ones, progressive hepatic failure can be prevented only if the septic focus can be eradicated.

Infectious

Although leukocytosis with a leftward shift is very suggestive of infection, it is also true that overwhelming infection can cause leukopenia. The total lymphocyte count is calculated by multiplying the WBC count by the percentage of lymphocytes; when the product is less than 1000, it can indicate anergy, often caused by malnutrition.

Assessment and Plan. This patient clearly has an undrained septic focus and needs adequate drainage if he is to survive. A pelvic abscess could be drained extraserously through the rectum if fluctuance can be palpated on digital examination. Abscesses are also drained percutaneously with a catheter under CT control. If percutaneous drainage does not eliminate the septic focus or if peritonitis supervenes, surgical drainage with a proximal stoma will be necessary.

In summary, each physiologic system needs to be considered and supported. Good surgical principles, such as drainage of abscesses and débridement of devitalized tissue, need to be observed if critically ill patients are to recover.

Recommended Reading

1. Shoemaker WC, Ayres SM, Grenvik A, Holbrook PR (Eds): *Textbook of Critical Care,* ed 3. Philadelphia: W.B. Saunders, 1995.
2. Maull KI, Rodriguez A, Wiles CE III (Eds): *Complications in Trauma and Critical Care.* Philadelphia: W.B. Saunders, 1996.
3. Anderson RW, Vaslef SN: Shock, causes and management of circulatory collapse. In Sabiston DC Jr., Lyerly HK (Eds): *Textbook of Surgery: The Biological Basis of Modern Surgical Practice,* ed 15. Philadelphia: W.B. Saunders, 1997.

18

Milestones in Surgical Training

The development of a surgeon is a protracted process and, ideally, extends over a lifetime. There are, however, certain milestones along the way. In my experience, an understanding of these points helps nascent surgeons develop. Some students will branch out before becoming fully trained in general surgery, but it is to be hoped that the principles learned in the core curriculum of general surgery will help the doctor in whatever field he chooses.

Each third-year medical student is required to take a clerkship in surgery. This is indispensable. It is hard to imagine a medical discipline that can be practiced competently without a basic understanding of surgery. Most disease states are amenable to either medical or surgical intervention, depending on the stage of evolution, and the proper indications for surgery in a given disease state must be understood by internist and surgeon alike. Radiologists and pathologists must understand basic surgical principles if they expect to interact appropriately with the clinicians. Subspecialists such as urologists and orthopedists must be grounded in good surgical technique in order to practice their art.

A fourth-year surgical clerkship may take the form of an "acting internship," in which the student takes on more responsibility under supervision. This allows time for a greater understanding of surgical problems and participation in depth in preoperative, operative, and postoperative care. Many medical schools allow electives to be taken at other designated institutions. This not only allows students to gain a more diverse experience but lets them take electives at institutions where they might wish to do a surgical residency. Thus, the prospective resident can evaluate the program and the program director can evaluate the student. By rendering students somewhat less "unknown quantities," this experience can enhance their chances for selection into the given program. Not all program directors agree that an "audition elective" is useful. Some feel that it takes time away from other important electives in the medical subspecialities. Some feel that it doesn't really enhance an applicant's chance for acceptance into a program.

The process by which students are selected for surgical residency is administered by the National Interns and Residents Matching Program, which offers a computerized system that matches students with the most desired venue that will accept them. Individual surgical residency programs rank candidates on the basis of grades and class standing (when available), letters of recommendation, scores on the USMLE I and II (United States Medical Licensing Examination parts I and II), and interviews, as well as by the quality and reputation of the applicant's medical school. Students who desire a full 5 years' training in general surgery should apply to a categorical program. Residents in such a program who perform satisfactorily and are able to complete become eligible to practice general surgery or to enter further subspecialty training. Students who wish 1 or 2 years of general surgical training in preparation for residencies in ENT, orthopedics, urology, or neurosurgery should apply to a preliminary general surgical program.

There are definite goals that surgical residents must achieve to successfully complete their residency. The first postgraduate year (pgy-1) is spent becoming familiar with preoperative and postoperative care. Some skill is acquired in operative technique, but the former pursuits take precedence. With each succeeding year, more operative responsibility is given, under supervision, for more complex surgical procedures, and more opportunity available for the exercise of judgment in the surgical management of patients. The resident becomes facile with the performance of procedures such as insertion of Swan-Ganz catheters and arterial lines. The Association of Program Directors in Surgery (APDS) has developed a curriculum for general surgery residents, and the American College of Surgeons (ACS) has developed a *Guide for Medical Students and PGY-1 Surgical Residents,* outlining the knowledge and skills that students should acquire before and shortly after beginning a general surgical or surgical subspecialty training program.

The American Board of Surgery in-Training Examination is offered every year. Performance on the examination is often an important criterion for promotion, although certainly not the only one, since judgment, integrity, and operative skill are at least as important as test performance. The chief surgical resident, besides obtaining intensive operative and clinical decision-making experience, has administrative responsibilities and is required to do the work necessary to ensure smooth functioning of the service.

After completing a surgical residency, the physician is eligible to practice general surgery and to be granted general surgical privileges at a hospital. In common usage, he is called *board eligible,* although the American Board of Surgery does not use this term. To sit for the qualifying examination of the American Board of Surgery, the resident must have graduated from an approved medical school, completed an approved surgical training program, be licensed in a state, have submitted a satisfactory operative list, be approved by his Program Director, and be actively engaged in the practice of surgery or in further postgraduate surgical education. After successfully completing the written qualifying examination surgeons may the next year sit for the certifying examination, which is oral. If they pass the certifying examination, they become

Diplomates of the American Board of Surgery—that is, specialists in surgery. Certification must be renewed every 10 years by examination.

After 5 years' training in general surgery, the resident may go on to further postgraduate training. Training programs that lead to further board certification, such as cardiothoracic surgery or colon and rectal surgery, are called *residencies.* Programs such as critical care, vascular surgery, pediatric surgery, and hand surgery, which lead to certificates of added qualification or special qualification, are called either *residencies* or *fellowships.* The former has become the preferred term.

The next milestone in a surgeon's career is to become a Fellow of the American College of Surgeons (FACS). The College is dedicated to upholding high standards in surgery and to furthering surgical education among its practitioners. To be eligible to apply to the College, one must be a Diplomate of the American Board of Surgery and must have been in practice in one geographic location for 2 years. The applicant is interviewed, and a list of his operative cases is reviewed. A judgment is made about the applicant's ethical standards and professional qualifications, and if these are found acceptable he is admitted to fellowship. In addition to fellowship, the American College of Surgeons admits people into a candidate group when they are residents and to an associate group after they finish their residencies but before they become fellows.

In addition to these milestones, it is obvious that a surgeon's skill should continue to evolve during the course of his entire career and that he should acquire further knowledge and skills to serve his patients. In so doing, he will find surgery a most worthwhile pursuit. Proof of continued medical education is required in most locales, but for most surgeons this is "a given," since they are self-motivated to continue to learn and improve their skills. Meetings such as the Clinical Congress of the ACS provide continued medical education; there is also a wealth of excellent books and journals to keep surgeons and trainees up to date on the latest developments. Many of these sources are described in Chapter 19.

19

Educational Resources in Surgery

TEXTBOOKS

A widely used textbook of surgery is the 15th edition of the *Textbook of Surgery: The Biological Basis of Modern Surgical Practice,* edited by David C. Sabiston, Jr. and published by W. B. Saunders in 1997. It is more than 2000 pages in length. In my opinion, it or another such textbook should be read in its entirety before completing the first post-graduate year in surgery. *General Surgery*, by Ritchie, Steele, and Dean, and *Current Surgical Therapy*, by Cameron, are two additional important sources of information. In addition to reading one of these textbooks cover to cover, clerks and junior residents should read the appropriate section the evenings before the operations for which they are to scrub. Reading about the problems in the context of a real patient is assimilated more easily than information gathered in a vacuum.

ONGOING SERIES OF MAJOR IMPORTANCE

Selected Readings in General Surgery, edited by Robert N. McClelland, consists of important papers culled from the surgical literature. These papers are read by the surgical house staff at The University of Texas Southwestern Medical School Affiliated Hospitals in Dallas, Texas, as part of their curriculum. Each month, a series of papers representing the most important work on a general surgical topic are sent to subscribers, along with an overview. The reading program is set up so that one cycle lasts 5½ to 6 years, after which most of the major topics in general surgery have been covered. The cycle then begins again, outdated papers having been replaced by more current ones. Just as these readings are helpful to the residents at The University of Texas, they can be valuable to those in other programs and can form the basis for a journal club. Anyone who wishes to read the most important surgical papers over a 5- or 6-year period should take advantage of this resource.

The *Surgical Clinics of North America,* published bimonthly by

W. B. Saunders Company, consists of nicely bound monographs on surgical topics. The topics are timely and relevant, and each monograph can be read at a leisurely pace over the course of a week or two. This is a pleasant way to keep abreast of surgical knowledge.

JOURNALS

Journal of The American College of Surgeons (JACS), formerly called *Surgery, Gynecology, and Obstetrics* (SG&O), is the official scientific journal of The American College of Surgeons and so is a must for every surgical resident. Papers submitted to this publication are subjected to rigorous peer review before being accepted for publication, and authors usually employ sound scientific method. The journal is published monthly. An important section of JACS, "The Surgeon at Work," features surgical techniques that may prove useful to readers.

Annals of Surgery, published by J. B. Lippincott Company, contains original scientific work subjected to rigorous review before acceptance for publication. It is therefore an important source of information for surgical residents. *Current Surgery,* the official journal of the Association of Program Directors in Surgery, is published by Williams & Wilkins nine times a year. It presents overviews of surgical topics as well as abstracts with commentary and is an efficient way for students and residents to learn. Moreover, being the journal of the program directors, it emphasizes surgical education.

BOOKS ON SPECIFIC SUBJECTS

Basic Science Review for Surgeons, edited by Simmons and Steed and published by W. B. Saunders Company, reviews physiology as it relates to surgery and critical care. I recommend it enthusiastically for surgical residents and medical students. The *Physiologic Basis of Surgery* by O'Leary is another great source of surgical basic science. It has been developed as a project of The Association of Program Directors in Surgery and has a companion computerized tutorial and question bank.

Another book that is in my opinion indispensable to all surgical residents is John Madden's *Atlas of Technics in Surgery.* This work, published in two volumes by Appleton & Lange, describes common general and thoracic operations with line drawings. The drawings are so clear that the reader can almost immediately comprehend the essentials of a given operation. This atlas is excellent. Many other fine atlases are available, such as Sabiston's *Atlas of General Surgery* published by W. B. Saunders. Students and residents use these to review the steps of an operation before scrubbing.

Cope's Early Diagnosis of the Acute Abdomen, revised by William Silen, is a classic in surgery covering one of the most basic, yet most important, surgical topics. This is a must for every student and resident;

its readers will gain much in confidence and understanding. *Abdominal Operations*, by Rodney Maingot, will help residents to gain further insight into both surgical principles and surgical technique. *Surgery of the Colon, Rectum, and Anus*, edited by Mazier, Levien, Luchtefeld, and Senagore and published by W. B. Saunders Company, covers in depth the broad field of colorectal surgery.

Care of the Surgical Patient, published by *Scientific American* in collaboration with The American College of Surgeons, is updated periodically and is highly recommended as a source of information on preoperative and postoperative care. *The Management of Trauma*, 4th edition, by Zuidema, Rutherford, and Ballinger and published by W. B. Saunders Company, is an important work for those interested in trauma. *Trauma*, edited by Feliciano, Moore, and Mattox, is quite comprehensive. *Vascular Surgery*, edited by Robert B. Rutherford and published by W. B. Saunders Company, provides an extensive explication of the principles of vascular surgery.

Most medical libraries can provide a computer-aided search on any medical topic and on works by any author. The *Index Medicus* provides similar information.

With increasing frequency, students, residents, and attendings are learning to be proactive, doing their own searches with services such as *Ovid* and *Physician On Line*. This allows the individual more control, as the search can be continued if the appropriate information is not retrieved. Moreover, many of the references are stored in the data base in full text form, enhancing the utility of this modality for direct patient care. The day has already come when the practitioner uses a desktop computer to find relevant literature while the patient is in the office.

Index

Note: Page numbers in *italics* refer to illustrations; those followed by t refer to tables.